Clinical Cases in Paramedicine

Dedication

This text is being finalised for publication during the COVID-19 global pandemic. Many healthcare workers have lost their lives during this time while looking after those who contracted the SARS-CoV-2 virus. Therefore this text is dedicated to all those healthcare workers and paramedics who continue to look after the sick when faced with adversity and at risk to their own lives.

Also in memory of Brian Mfula, lecturer in mental health nursing at Swansea University, Wales, UK and co-author of Chapter 12, who tragically lost his life to COVID-19.

Clinical Cases in Paramedicine

Edited by

Sam Willis

Lecturer in Paramedicine
Curtin University
Western Australia
Australia

Ian Peate

Head of School, School of Health Studies
Gibraltar Health Authority, St Bernard's Hospital
Gibraltar

Rod Hill

Head of Scool of Biomedical Sciences
Charles Sturt University
NSW, Australia

WILEY Blackwell

Registered Office(s)
John Wiley & Sons, Inc., 111 River Street, Hoboken, NJ 07030, USA
John Wiley & Sons Ltd, The Atrium, Southern Gate, Chichester, West Sussex, PO19 8SQ, UK

Editorial Office
9600 Garsington Road, Oxford, OX4 2DQ, UK

For details of our global editorial offices, customer services, and more information about
Wiley products visit us at www.wiley.com.

Wiley also publishes its books in a variety of electronic formats and by print-on-demand.
Some content that appears in standard print versions of this book may not be available in
other formats.

Library of Congress Cataloging-in-Publication Data

Names: Willis, Sam, 1978– editor. | Peate, Ian, editor. | Hill, Rod
   (Rodney), editor.
Title: Clinical cases in paramedicine / edited by Sam Willis, Ian Peate,
   Rod Hill.
Description: Hoboken, NJ : Wiley-Blackwell, 2021. | Includes
   bibliographical references and index.
Identifiers: LCCN 2020026984 (print) | LCCN 2020026985 (ebook) |
   ISBN 9781119619253 (paperback) | ISBN 9781119621041 (adobe pdf) |
   ISBN 9781119621034 (epub)
Subjects: MESH: Emergency Treatment | Emergency Medical Technicians |
   Emergencies | Problems and Exercises | Case Reports
Classification: LCC RC86.9 (print) | LCC RC86.9 (ebook) | NLM WB 18.2 |
   DDC 616.02/5076–dc23
LC record available at https://lccn.loc.gov/2020026984
LC ebook record available at https://lccn.loc.gov/2020026985

Cover Design: Wiley
Cover Image: Courtesy of Sarah Angelou

Set in 9/12pt Minion by SPi Global, Pondicherry, India
Printed and bound by CPI Group (UK) Ltd, Croydon, CR0 4YY

10 9 8 7 6 5 4 3 2 1

Contents

Preface

Paramedicine is a fast-paced, ever-changing profession and those who practise as paramedics must be able to keep up to date with changes using the latest evidence and expert opinion where evidence does not exist. Paramedic education precedes clinical practice and therefore high-quality learning materials are essential to prepare student paramedics for employment.

The case studies in this book bring together a diverse range of examples that accurately represent the caseload experienced by contemporary paramedics all in one place. They use a mix of evidence-based cases and expert opinion supplied by leaders in the industry.

Case-based learning (CBL) and problem-based learning (PBL) rely on high-quality, well-written case studies that paramedic educators, students and clinicians can use to aid their understanding of out-of-hospital care. Not only is the content contemporary, but the cases are structured in a manner that reflects a systematic approach to each scene, allowing students to develop a sense of structure to the way they proceed in each case. Each chapter has a range of interactive learning activities that allow students to stop and think about what is going on, and the questions throughout the cases provide students with additional learning opportunities.

List of contributors

Joel Beake
Registered Advanced Care Paramedic
Queensland Ambulance Service
Brisbane, QLD, Australia

Curtis Northcott
Registered Advanced Care Paramedic
RMA Medical Rescue and Registered Paramedic
Mount Isa, QLD, Australia

Fenella Corrick
GP Registrar
Western Isles, Scotland, UK

David Davis
College of Paramedics, Bridgewater, UK

Georgette Eaton
Clinical Practice Development Manager
Advanced Paramedic Practitioner (Urgent Care)
London Ambulance Service, NHS Trust, London, UK

Paul Grant
Registered Paramedic
Mines Emergency Rescue and Response (MERR)
QLD, Australia

Yasaru Gunaratne
Advanced Care Paramedic
Queensland Ambulance Service, Gold Coast, QLD
Australia

Alisha Hensby
Lecturer in Paramedicine
Charles Sturt University, Bathurst, NSW, Australia

Tom Hewes
Senior Lecturer and Programme Director of Paramedic
Sciences, Swansea University, Wales, UK

Mark Hobson
Clinical Practice Educator for Specialist Practice,
Paramedic
South Central Ambulance Service NHS Foundation
Trust, Bicester, UK

Tania Johnston
Lecturer in Paramedicine
Charles Sturt University, Bathurst, NSW, Australia

David Krygger
Advanced Care Paramedic with Specialist Training in
Low Acuity Referral Services
Queensland Ambulance Service
Gold Coast, QLD, Australia

Erica Ley
Senior HEMS Paramedic
Lincolnshire and Nottinghamshire Air Ambulance
Lincoln, UK
Associate Lecturer in Paramedic Science
University of East Anglia, Norwich, UK

Tom E. Mallinson
Rural GP & Paramedic
BASICS Scotland, Auchterarder, UK

Kristina Maximous
Lecturer in Paramedicine
Charles Sturt University, Bathurst, NSW, Australia

Brian Mfula
Lecturer in Mental Health Nursing
Swansea University, Wales, UK

Georgina Pickering
Lecturer in Paramedicine
Charles Sturt University, Bathurst, NSW, Australia

Michael Porter
Paramedic
Queensland Ambulance Service
Brisbane, QLD, Australia

Samantha Sheridan
Lecturer in Paramedicine
Charles Sturt University, Bathurst
NSW, Australia

Jennifer Stirling
Lecturer in Paramedicine
Charles Sturt University, Bathurst, NSW, Australia

Clare Sutton
Lecturer in Paramedicine, Discipline Group Leader
Charles Sturt University, Bathurst, NSW, Australia

Sam Taylor
HEMS Paramedic
Air Ambulance Kent Surrey Sussex, Chatham, UK

Ruth Townsend
Senior Lecturer in Paramedicine
Charles Sturt University, Bathurst, NSW, Australia

Lynne Walsh
Senior Lecturer in Mental Health/Public Health
Swansea University, Wales, UK

Steve Whitfield
Lecturer/Course Convenor
Griffith University, School of Medicine (Paramedicine), Gold Coast, QLD, Australia
Registered Paramedic
Queensland Ambulance Service
Brisbane, QLD, Australia

Kerryn Wratt
Registered Paramedic
President, Australasian Wilderness and Expedition Medicine Society (AWEMS), Omeo, VIC, Australia
CEO, RescueMED, Omeo, VIC, Australia

Aimee Yarrington
Registered Paramedic and Registered Midwife
Shropshire, UK

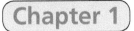 **Respiratory emergencies**

Jennifer Stirling, Clare Sutton and Georgina Pickering
Charles Sturt University, Bathurst, NSW, Australia

LEVEL 1 CASE STUDY
Asthma

Information type	Data
Time of origin	17:08
Time of dispatch	17:10
On-scene time	17:20
Day of the week	Friday
Nearest hospital	30 minutes
Nearest backup	15 minutes
Patient details	Name: Betsy Booper
	DOB:10/09/2002

CASE
You have been called to an outdoor running track for an 18-year-old female with shortness of breath. The caller states she has taken her inhaler to no effect.

Pre-arrival information
The patient is conscious and breathing. You can access the area via the back gate of the sports field and drive right up to the patient, who is sat down on the track.

Windscreen report
The location appears safe. Approx. 10 people around the patient. Environment – warm summer evening and good light.

Entering the location
The sports coach greets you as you get out of the ambulance and informs you that the patient suffers with exercise-induced asthma, but this is worse than normal and her inhaler has been ineffective.

Clinical Cases in Paramedicine, First Edition. Edited by Sam Willis, Ian Peate, and Rod Hill.
© 2021 John Wiley & Sons Ltd. Published 2021 by John Wiley & Sons Ltd.

On arrival with the patient

The patient is sat on a bench on the side of the track. She is leaning forward, resting her elbows on her thighs (tripodding). She says hello as you introduce yourself to her.

Patient assessment triangle

General appearance

Alert. Speaking in short sentences. She looks panicked.

Circulation to the skin

Flushed cheeks.

Work of breathing

Breathing appears rapid and shallow. An audible wheeze is noted.

SYSTEMATIC APPROACH

Danger

None at this time.

Response

Alert on the AVPU scale.

Airway

Clear.

Breathing

RR: 28. Regular and shallow. No accessory muscle use. Expiratory wheeze on auscultation.

Circulation

HR: 100. Regular and strong. Capillary refill time <2 seconds. Flushed cheeks and peripherally warm.

Disability

Moving all four limbs.
Pupils equal and reactive to light (PEARL).

Exposure

Bystanders have left. Next of kin are now on scene.
Temperature: warm summer evening – approx. 20 °C.

Vital signs

RR: 28 bpm
HR: 100 bpm
BP: 125/74 mmHg
SpO_2: 93%
Blood glucose: 5.2 mmol/L
Temperature: 36.9 °C
PEF: 300 L/min
GCS: 15/15
4 Lead ECG: sinus tachycardia

TASK

Look through the information provided in this case study and highlight all of the information that might concern you as a paramedic.

Aside from auscultation, which you have already done, what examination techniques should you incorporate into this patient assessment?

- Inspection – observe the chest for an abnormalities such as wounds, scars, bruising, asymmetry and recession.
- Palpation – feel for any asymmetry, vocal fremitus and tenderness.
- Percussion – hyper- or hypo-resonance.

What adventitious (added) sounds might indicate asthma and why?

Expiratory wheeze. This sound is made when air has a restricted path through the bronchi, due to inflammation and muscle spasm in the airways.

What medicine (pharmacology) is likely to relieve the patient's symptoms and why?

Nebulised salbutamol – it is a Beta2, adrenergic agonist that relaxes smooth muscle in the bronchi.

Case Progression

You treat the patient with 5 mg of nebulised salbutamol and 6 L of oxygen. The nebuliser finishes and you remove the mask.

Patient assessment triangle
General appearance
The patient is now speaking in full sentences.

Circulation to the skin
Flushed.

Work of breathing
Normal effort of breathing.

SYSTEMATIC APPROACH
Danger
None at this time.

Response
Alert.

Airway
Clear.

Breathing
RR:16. Regular. Normal depth. No accessory muscle use. No wheeze or adventitious sounds.

Circulation
HR: 105. Regular and strong. Capillary refill time <2 seconds. Flushed cheeks and peripherally warm.

Disability
No change.

Exposure
No change.

Vital signs
RR: 16 bpm
HR: 105 bpm
BP: 128/78 mmHg
SpO_2: 97%
Blood glucose: not repeated
Temperature: not repeated
PEF: 380 L/min
GCS: 15/15
4 lead ECG: sinus tachycardia

What kinds of questions would you ask this patient specifically related to asthma as part of the history-taking process?

See Table 1.1.

Table 1.1 History-taking questions

Asthma history
Does this feel like your normal asthma?
Is this the worst it's ever been?
What time did this episode start today?
Do you take your asthma medication regularly?
What were you doing when it started today?
What usually triggers your symptoms?
When was the last time your visited your GP and/or went to hospital with these symptoms?
Have you ever been intubated or been in ICU with these symptoms?

Medication history
What asthma medications do you take?
How frequently do you have to take your medication?
Do you usually have to take your inhaler while exercising?
When was the last time you had a medication review with your GP?
Have you had any recent changes in medication?
Do you take any other medications?
Have you had any coaching on the best way to take your inhaler?

F/SH (family and social history)
Does anyone else in your family experience asthma?
Do you smoke? If so, how frequently?
Do you drink or take any drugs recreationally?
Who do you live with?
What do you do for work?
Do you exercise regularly?
Are you under any particular stress at the moment?

Past medical history (PMH)
Do you have any other medical problems?
Do you have any allergies?
Have you had a cough or cold recently?

The patient is 160 cm tall, what should her predicted peak expiratory flow reading (PEFR) be? Her first reading was 300 – what percentage is that from predicted?

(Hint: you will be required to look this up using the Australian National Asthma Council chart found here: http://www.peakflow.com/pefr_normal_values.pdf or by doing an internet search.)

- 400 L/min.
- 75%.

LEVEL 1 CASE STUDY
Chronic obstructive pulmonary disease (COPD)

Information type	Data
Time of origin	07:09
Time of dispatch	07:12
On-scene time	07:30
Day of the week	Wednesday
Nearest hospital	15 minutes
Nearest backup	40 minutes
Patient details	Name: Dave Beater
	DOB: 21/09/1954

CASE
You have been called to a residential address for a 66-year-old male with difficulty in breathing. The caller states he has been breathless all night and has had a cough recently. He has seen his GP who prescribed antibiotics and steroids but he feels his breathing has got worse overnight.

Pre-arrival information
The patient is conscious and breathing and is in a first-floor flat/unit.

Windscreen report
The location appears safe. Greeted at the main door by the patient's wife.

Entering the location
Wife escorts you up in the lift to the patient's flat.

On arrival with the patient
Patient is sat in the tripod position and appears distressed. He makes eye contact when you arrive, but does not speak as is so short of breath. He has a productive cough that results in a string of green-looking sputum that he manages to capture in his handkerchief to show you.

Patient assessment triangle

General appearance
Alert, and makes eye contact, but is acutely distressed. Can only speak in single words and is reluctant to talk. In tripod position, coughing.

Circulation to the skin
Pink face, breathing through pursed lips.

Work of breathing
Increased work of breathing – rapid and shallow breaths with accessory muscle use.

SYSTEMATIC APPROACH

Danger
None at this time.

Response
Alert.

Airway
Clear.

Breathing
RR: 36. Rapid and shallow, with accessory muscle use. Widespread bilateral wheeze noted on auscultation.

Circulation
HR: 110. Radial palpable – irregular. Capillary refill time 2 seconds.

Disability
Pupils equal and reactive to light (PEARL).

Exposure
The patient is in his own home.

Vital signs
RR: 36 bpm
HR: 110 bpm
BP: 150/90 mmHg
SpO_2: 86%
Blood glucose: 4.5 mmol/L
Temperature: 37.8 °C
PEF: unable to record
GCS: 15/15
4 Lead ECG: atrial fibrillation
Allergies: nil

TASK
Look through the information provided in this case study and highlight all of the information that might concern you as a paramedic.

What is COPD?

COPD is a progressive disease and is characterized by air flow obstruction that is not fully reversible. The airway obstruction results from damage to alveoli, alveolar ducts and bronchioles due to chronic inflammation.

List the features of an acute exacerbation of COPD.

- Increased dyspnoea.
- Increased sputum production.
- Increased cough.
- Upper airway symptoms, such as a cold and sore throat.
- Increased wheeze.

- Reduced exercise tolerance.
- Fluid retention.
- Increased fatigue.
- Acute confusion.
- Worsening of previously stable condition.

Case Progression

After administration of 5 mg salbutamol via nebuliser, the patient's condition improves slightly and he hands you a medical card that his 'breathing doctor' gave to him. The card states the patient is at risk of retaining CO_2 and should only be administered with 28% oxygen to achieve saturations between 88 and 92%.

Patient assessment triangle
General appearance
Alert and more interactive.

Circulation to the skin
Pink.

Work of breathing
Increased work of breathing – breathing rapid, but not as shallow as before.

SYSTEMATIC APPROACH
Danger
None at this time.

Response
Alert.

Airway
Clear.

Breathing
RR: 30. Audible wheeze on auscultation.

Circulation
HR: 120. Palpable radial. Capillary refill time 2 seconds.

Disability
Moving all four limbs.

Exposure
Normal temperature in the ambulance.

Vital signs
RR: 30 bpm
HR: 120 bpm
BP: 148/78 mmHg
SpO_2: 90%
Blood glucose: not repeated
Temperature: not repeated
GCS: 15/15
4 lead ECG: atrial fibrillation
Allergies: nil

When the nebuliser has finished, you notice that the patient's SpO$_2$ is dropping so you decide to keep the patient on oxygen. What percentage of oxygen would you administer to this patient and why?

28% oxygen through a nasal cannula. The patient is at risk of developing hypercapnia respiratory failure, so it is important the oxygen is titrated to maintain saturations between 88 and 92%. Research suggests that over-oxygenation increases the mortality and morbidity of COPD patients and that titration of oxygen administration can reduce mortality.

What is meant by the term hypercapnia?

- 'A condition of abnormally elevated carbon dioxide (CO_2) levels in the blood, caused by hypoventilation, lung disease, or diminished consciousness' (NAEMT, 2015, p. 92).
- 'Alveolar hypoventilation with increased alveolar carbon dioxide limits the amount of oxygen available for diffusion into the blood, leading to secondary hypoxemia' (McCance et al., 2010, p. 1269).

LEVEL 2 CASE STUDY
Pulmonary embolism (PE)

Information type	Data
Time of origin	17:55
Time of dispatch	18:01
On-scene time	18:10
Day of the week	Friday
Nearest hospital	30 minutes
Nearest backup	15 minutes
Patient details	Name: Jasmine Wallis
	DOB: 27/12/2000

CASE
You have been called to a car park for a 20-year-old female who is complaining of feeling dizzy and faint.

Pre-arrival information
She is conscious and breathing.

Windscreen report
The car park is behind a row of shops and is poorly lit. The patient is hard to spot at first, as she is sitting on the metal fire escape steps with her head in her hands at the back of a building. She is alone. The car park is full, which prevents you parking near to the patient.

Entering the location
You park your ambulance as near as possible and cross the car park to get to your patient.

On arrival with the patient
The patient is able to raise her head and make eye contact.

Patient assessment triangle
General appearance
The patient looks at you when you speak and is able to speak in full sentences.

Circulation to the skin
Mildly pale.

Work of breathing
Increased. The patients looks mildly short of breath.

SYSTEMATIC APPROACH
Danger
None at this time.

Response
Alert.

Airway
Clear.

Breathing
RR: 26. Mildly increased effort, no accessory muscle use. Auscultation – clear.

Circulation
HR: 120. Tachycardic, weak and regular pulse. Capillary refill time >2 seconds.

Disability
Pupils equal and reactive to light (PEARL).

Exposure
The patient is sitting on metal fire escape stairs, in a dark, cold car park in an undesirable part of town.

Vital signs
RR: 26 bpm
HR: 120 bpm
BP: 90/60 mmHg
SpO_2: 90%
Blood glucose: 4.4 mmol/L
Temperature: 36.5 °C
ECG: sinus tachycardia
Allergies: nil

TASK
Look through the information provided in this case study and highlight all of the information that might concern you as a paramedic.

List your differential diagnoses for this patient.

- Musculoskeletal pain.
- Pericarditis.
- Hyperventilation.
- Chest infection.
- Syncope.
- Pneumothorax.

List as many predisposing factors associated with PE as you can. Which could assist you with working through your differential diagnosis and history taking?

See Table 1.2.

Table 1.2 Pulmonary embolism predisposing factors

Surgery, especially recent
Abdominal
Pelvic
Hip or knee
Post-operative intensive care

Obstetrics
Pregnancy

Cardiac
Recent acute myocardial infarction

Limb problems
Recent lower limb fractures
Varicose veins
Lower limb problems secondary to stroke or spinal cord injury

Malignancy
Abdominal and /or pelvic, in particular advanced metastatic disease
Concurrent chemotherapy

Other
Risk increases with age
>60 years of age
Previous proven deep vein thrombosis (DVT)/PE
Immobility
Thrombotic disorder
Neurological disease with extremity paresis
Thrombophilia
Hormone replacement therapy and oral contraception
Prolonged bed rest >3 days
Other recent trauma

Source: JRCALC (2019), p. 367.

What validated assessment tool could assist you with assessing the probability of PE in this patient?

See Table 1.3.

Table 1.3 Wells' criteria for PE

Criteria	Score
Clinical signs and symptoms of DVT (leg swelling and pain with palpation of the deep veins)	3
An alternative diagnosis is PE is less likely	3
Pulse rate >100 bpm	1.5
Immobilisation or surgery in the previous 4 weeks	1.5
Previous DVT/PE	1.5
Haemoptysis	1
Malignancy (treatment ongoing or within the last 6 months or palliative)	1
Clinical probability	
High	>6 points
Moderate	2–6 points
Low	<2 points

Source: JRCALC (2019), p. 368.
Note: When using the Wells' criteria, a low probability does not rule out PE.

Case Progression

You decide to move your patient to the back of the ambulance to continue the examination in a warm and private environment. On standing, the patient complains of feeling dizzy and faint and is unable to walk even a couple of steps. You instruct your crewmate to fetch the carry chair as you can't get the stretcher close enough to the patient.

Patient assessment triangle
General appearance
Patient feels better when lying flat.

Circulation to the skin
Normal.

Work of breathing
Increased. Patient complains of not being able to 'catch her breath'.

SYSTEMATIC APPROACH
Danger
None at this time.

Response
Alert.

Airway
Clear.

Breathing
RR: 30.

Circulation
HR: 128. Weak radial.

Disability
Moving all four limbs.

Exposure
Normal temperature in the ambulance.

Vital signs
RR: 30 bpm
HR: 128 bpm
BP: 88/60 mmHg
SpO_2: unable to obtain
Blood glucose: not repeated
Temperature: not repeated
GCS: 15/15
12 lead ECG: sinus tachycardia with right bundle branch block (RBBB)

What is the most common ECG finding in PE? What other ECG changes are associated with PE?

The most common ECG finding in PE is sinus tachycardia. PE can cause any of the following ECG changes:

- T-wave inversion.
- New-onset atrial fibrillation.
- Right bundle branch block.
- Right axis deviation.

- S1Q3T3 (this is a specific pattern that is seen rarely in PE):
  - S waves in lead I.
  - Q waves in lead III.
  - T-wave inversion in lead III.

Explain why females taking the oral contraceptive pill are at greater risk of developing a PE.

Virchow's triad explains the three broad categories that play a part in thrombus formation:

1. Hypercoagulability.
2. Hemodynamic changes (stasis, turbulence).
3. Endothelial injury/dysfunction.

Taking contraceptive drugs that contain oestrogen can actually change the constitution of the blood, increasing plasma and other clotting factors. This causes the woman to be in a hypercoagulative state, increasing the risk of developing DVT/PE.

LEVEL 2 CASE STUDY
Life-threatening asthma

Information type	Data
Time of origin	07:13
Time of dispatch	07:15
On-scene time	07:26
Day of the week	Monday
Nearest hospital	20 minutes
Nearest backup	10 minutes
Patient details	Name: Billy Bob
	DOB: 01/06/1995

CASE
You have been called to a residential address for a 25-year-old male with difficulty in breathing. Caller states he has been breathless all night and has had a cough recently.

Pre-arrival information
The patient is conscious and breathing and is located in a third-floor flat/unit – there is no lift.

Windscreen report
The location appears safe and you are greeted at the communal entrance by the patient's partner.

Entering the location
The partner appears agitated and hurries you up the stairs, stating that the patient was having his breakfast and his breathlessness got a lot worse.

On arrival with the patient
The patient is sat leaning forward and appears panicked. He does not say hello when you introduce yourself and states repeatedly that he cannot breathe, in short sharp breaths.

Patient assessment triangle
General appearance
Alert, but does not acknowledge your presence. Acutely distressed. Unable to speak in full sentences, leaning forward with clear dyspnoea.

Circulation to the skin
Pale and peripherally cyanosed.

Work of breathing
He has increased breathing effort and only giving 1 word answers.

SYSTEMATIC APPROACH

Danger
None at this time.

Response
Alert.

Airway
Clear.

Breathing
RR: 32. Rapid and shallow. No accessory muscle use. Minimal air movement bilaterally on auscultation.

Circulation
HR: 130. Radial weak and barely palpable, regular. Capillary refill time 3 seconds. Nail beds appear bluish.

Disability
Pupils equal and reactive to light (PEARL) – 5 mm.

Exposure
The chest is exposed to conduct an assessment. The patient is in a private residence and the unit has a warm temperature.

Vital signs
RR: 32 bpm
HR: 130 bpm
BP: 100/54 mmHg
SpO_2: 87%
Blood glucose: 4.3 mmol/L
Temperature: 37.2 °C
Peak expiratory flow reading (PEFR): unable to record
GCS: E4, Verbal – not complying with your questioning, only stating he cannot breathe, M6
4 Lead ECG: sinus tachycardia, regular
Allergies: nil

TASK
Look through the information provided in this case study and highlight all of the information that might concern you as a paramedic.

Using the latest guidelines from the Australia and New Zealand Thoracic Society (ANZTS), the British Thoracic Society (BTS) or a source that draws on these resources, compare and contrast the differences between life-threatening asthma and anaphylaxis, and explain why this is more likely to be asthma than any other differential diagnosis.

Similarities: asthma and anaphylaxis both present with respiratory distress and a wheeze. Both are due to an inflammatory response. And both may appear flushed – from exertion in asthma, and in anaphylaxis the skin's reaction to the allergen.

Differences: in anaphylaxis the whole airway can be affected, producing particular symptoms not associated with asthma, such as voice changes, stridor, inspiratory wheeze and tongue and lip swelling. Also asthma is predominantly a respiratory problem, whereas anaphylaxis can present with gastrointestinal problems and hypotension, which can lead to distributive shock.

Although this did occur after eating, the patient seems to be presenting with symptoms limited purely to the respiratory system. There are no dermatological, gastrointestinal or cardiovascular changes that would indicate anaphylaxis.

Is this patient suffering from moderate, severe or life-threatening asthma, and why?

Life-threatening asthma. See Table 1.4.

Table 1.4 Comparison of asthma severity

Near-fatal asthma	Raised $PaCO_2$ and/or requiring mechanical ventilation with raised inflation pressures
Life-threatening asthma	In a patient with severe asthma any one of:
	PEF <33% best or predicted
	SpO_2 <92%
	PaO_2 <8 Kpa
	'Normal' $PaCO_2$ (4.6–6.0 Kpa)
	Altered conscious level
	Exhaustion
	Arrhythmia
	Hypotension
	Cyanosis
	Silent chest
	Poor respiratory effort
Acute severe asthma	Any one of:
	PEF 33–50% best or predicted
	Respiratory rate ≥25/min
	Heart rate ≥110/min
	Inability to complete sentences in one breath
Moderate acute asthma	Increasing symptoms
	PEF >50–75% best or predicted
	No features of acute severe asthma

Source: British Thoracic Society (2019).

List your treatment, route and dosages.

- Adrenaline – 500 µg IM.
- Salbutamol – 5 mg nebulised.
- Ipatropium bromide – 500 µg nebulised.
- Oxygen – 6/8 L.
- Hydrocortisone – 100 mg IV (IM possible if unable to gain IV access).

Case Progression

You treat this patient rapidly with 500 µg of intramuscular (IM) adrenaline while your crewmate administers 5 mg of salbutamol and ipratropium bromide via a nebulizer, on 6 L of oxygen. After nebuliser therapy and 1 dose of IM Adrenaline, you rapidly extricate your patient to the ambulance. You deliver a pre-alert to the nearest emergency department.

Patient assessment triangle
General appearance
Alert and now looking at you and nodding or shaking his head in response to your questions.

Circulation to the skin
Pale.

Work of breathing
Increased work of breathing – breathing still rapid, but less shallow.

SYSTEMATIC APPROACH

Danger
None at this time.

Response
Alert.

Airway
Clear and peripherally cyanosed.

Breathing
RR:28. Audible wheeze on auscultation.

Circulation
HR: 128. Palpable radial. Capillary refill time 2 seconds. Nail beds appear bluish.

Disability
Moving all four limbs.

Exposure
Normal temperature in the ambulance.

Vital signs
RR: 28 bpm
HR: 128 bpm
BP: 110/78 mmHg
SpO_2: 91%
Blood glucose: not repeated
Temperature: not repeated
GCS: 15/15
4 lead ECG: sinus tachycardia

This type of incident may lead to high levels of stress during the time you are with the patient. Name at least four short-term effects of stress.

- Increased heart rate
- Increased blood pressure
- Pupil dilation
- Sweating
- Increased blood sugar levels
- Inhibitions of digestive secretions
- Peripheral vasoconstriction
- Bronchodilation

Source: ANZ (2015).

It is important to recognise symptoms of long-term (chronic) stress in yourself or others. Name at least two long-term effects of stress.

- Behaviour changes:
  - Difficulty sleeping.
  - Altered eating habits.
  - Smoking/drinking more.
  - Avoiding friends and family.
  - Sexual problems.
- Physical responses:
  - Tiredness.
  - Indigestion and nausea.
  - Headaches.
  - Aching muscles.
  - Palpitations.
- Mental responses:
  - Increased indecision.
  - Difficulty concentrating.
  - Poor memory.
  - Feeling inadequate.
  - Low self-esteem.
- Emotional responses:
  - Mood swings, becoming irritable or angry.
  - Increased anxiety.
  - Feeling numb.
  - Hypersensitivity.
  - Feeling drained and listless.

Source: Ambulance care practice (2019).

LEVEL 3 CASE STUDY
Respiratory sepsis

Information type	Data
Time of origin	09:15
Time of dispatch	09:30
On-scene time	09:43
Day of the week	Sunday
Nearest hospital	20 minutes
Nearest backup	40 minutes
Patient details	Name: Nicholas Beaumont DOB: 01/01/1947

CASE

You have been called to a residential address for a 73-year-old male complaining of weakness and shortness of breath.

Pre-arrival information

Patient is conscious and breathing. Upstairs in bed.

Windscreen report

The scene is safe. You are met at the door by the patient's wife.

Entering the location

The wife tells you her husband has had a productive cough for 3 days and is now unable to get out of bed.

On arrival with the patient

The patient is lying in bed and appears lethargic.

Patient assessment triangle

General appearance

Alert but lethargic.

Circulation to the skin

Flushed, warm to touch and clammy.

Work of breathing

Increased work of breathing.

SYSTEMATIC APPROACH

Danger

None at this time.

Response

Alert on the AVPU scale.

Airway

Clear.

Breathing

RR: 34. Rapid. Mild accessory muscle use. Right basal crackles on auscultation.

Circulation

HR: 130. Radial palpable but weak – regular. Capillary refill time 3 seconds.

Disability

Pupils equal and reactive to light (PEARL).

Exposure

The patient is in his own bed and the ambient temperature is warm.

Vital signs

RR: 34 bpm
HR: 130 bpm
BP: 108/54 mmHg
SpO_2: 87%
Blood glucose: 8.3 mmol/L
Temperature: 38.4 °C
GCS: 15/15
4 lead ECG: sinus tachycardia
Allergies: nil

TASK

Look through the information provided in this case study and highlight all of the information that might concern you as a paramedic.

Case Progression

You administer high-flow oxygen titrated to maintain an SpO_2 of 94–98%. Fluid is not indicated at this time and your local guidelines do not allow for the administration of prehospital antibiotics. You commence rapid transport to the Emergency Department with a sepsis pre-alert.

Patient assessment triangle
General appearance
Alert.

Circulation to the skin
Flushed.

Work of breathing
Increased work of breathing.

SYSTEMATIC APPROACH
Danger
None at this time.

Response
Alert.

Airway
Clear.

Breathing
RR: 30. Right basal crackles.

Circulation
HR: 126. Weak radial. Capillary refill time 3 seconds.

Disability
Moving all four limbs.

Exposure
Normal temperature in the ambulance. Patient covered with sheet not blanket to assist with ambient cooling.

Vital signs
RR: 30 bpm
HR: 126 bpm
BP: 100/58 mmHg
SpO_2: 90%
Blood glucose: not repeated
Temperature: 38.3 °C
GCS: 15/15
4 lead ECG: sinus tachycardia

What is sepsis?

'Sepsis is characterised by a life-threatening organ dysfunction due to a dysregulated host response to infection' (UKST, 2019, p. 14).

Outline the pathophysiology of sepsis.

Sepsis is when the body's natural inflammatory immune response to a localised infection becomes systemic, setting off a chain of physiological responses that quickly become life-threatening. It is an exaggerated response involving both the complement system (immune response) and the coagulation cascades.

The body tries to keep up with the increased demand for oxygen by raising the respiratory rate (RR) to increase the level of oxygen in the blood and to oxygenate the extra blood flow through the lungs. The heart rate (HR) and stroke volume (SV) are raised, leading to an increased cardiac output (CO). Vasodilation occurs, allowing the blood vessels to transport a greater blood volume, which eventually leads to reduced preload and reduced SV. The HR increases further to compensate, resulting in tachycardia. Some patients may be on medications that mask tachycardia (e.g. betablockers).

Profound vasodilation leads to a 'relative loss' in circulating volume and the increased permeability of the blood vessels following the release of histamine results in an 'absolute loss' as fluid escapes into the extravascular space. 25% of patients with septic shock present with a normal BP (cryptic shock or occult hypoperfusion) and others may present with relative hypotension (systolic BP >40 mmHg lower than normal systolic BP).

In the early stages patients may be warm and flushed as vasodilation leads to an increased blood volume in the peripheries. Heat generated soon becomes lost through the skin, reducing the temperature. In the later stages, the patient begins to peripherally shut down as the body attempts to redirect the blood to its core organs, which results in a further cooling of the skin. Hypothermia/cold sepsis occurs in 10–20% of patients and is more common in elderly patients. The mortality rate for these patients is double that of those with pyrexia.

Which groups are most at risk of developing sepsis?

- Elderly patients (>75 years or frail).
- Young patients (under 1 year).
- Immunocompromised patients whose immune system is impaired by medication or illness (e.g. chemotherapy patients) or where immune function is impaired due to medical conditions (diabetes and sickle cell) or medications (immunosuppressants or steroids).
- Post-surgery (within the last 6 weeks).
- Open wounds.
- Patients with indwelling medical devices (catheters or cannulas).
- Intravenous drug users.
- Pregnant women with recent history of miscarriage or termination and post-delivery.

What prompts or tools are used to determine when to screen for sepsis?

Guidelines used to recommend use of the modified systemic inflammatory response syndrome (SIRS) criteria, whereby patients presenting with two of more SIRS criteria with a confirmed or suspected infection were deemed to require further investigation to confirm or exclude a diagnosis of sepsis. This screening tool captured those patients presenting with 'uncomplicated' sepsis who were otherwise well and were at low risk for clinical deterioration. The definition of sepsis has now been updated so only those with a degree of organ dysfunction or clinical compromise are included. The SIRS criteria are no longer used as a screening tool.

The red flag system was developed to be used in conjunction with the SIRS criteria as a guide to which patients needed early intervention. This was to ensure responsible antibiotic stewardship due to the sensitivity of the SIRS criteria. The red flag system is quick to apply and is used by over 90% of UK hospitals.

The revised version of the National Early Warning Score (NEWS2) track and trigger system has been shown to be the most effective screening tool for predicting adverse outcomes for patients presenting with sepsis. This has now been incorporated into many systems, where screening is recommended for those with a NEWS2 of greater than 5 with identified risk factors or clinician concerns.

Which components of the Sepsis Six apply to the prehospital environment?

- Oxygen: titrate to maintain SpO_2 at 94–98%.
- Fluids: bolus of 500 mL over 15 minutes if indicated (systolic BP <90 mmHg).
- Antibiotics: benzylpenicillin for meningococcal septicaemia. Refer to local guidelines regarding the use of broad-spectrum antibiotics. Not routinely recommended.
- Lactate: measure lactate if indicated by local guidelines. Not routinely recommended.

LEVEL 3 CASE STUDY
Smoke inhalation

Information type	Data
Time of origin	02:24
Time of dispatch	02:25
On-scene time	02:30
Day of the week	Friday
Nearest hospital	15 minutes
Nearest backup	10 minutes
Patient details	Name: Sam Bryant
	DOB: 09/09/1990

CASE
You have been called to a fire at a residential address for a 30-year-old male with smoke inhalation.

Pre-arrival information
The patient is conscious and breathing and has extricated himself from the fire. He is at the neighbour's house when you arrive.

Windscreen report
Fire and police units are on scene. The incident has been contained.

Entering the location
The patient is sat on the couch at a neighbour's house.

On arrival with the patient
The patient is talking to a police officer and appears distressed.

Patient assessment triangle
General appearance
He is alert and has soot around his mouth and nose. He is coughing quite badly.

Circulation to the skin
Normal skin colour.

Work of breathing
Increased work of breathing.

SYSTEMATIC APPROACH
Danger
None at this time – the hazard has been contained.

Response
Alert on the AVPU scale.

Airway
Clear. Soot is noted in the mouth and nose. Singed nasal hairs and hoarse voice.

Breathing
RR: 28. No accessory muscle use. Equal air entry in both lungs, no adventitious (added) sounds on auscultation.

Circulation
HR: 106. The radial pulse is palpable – regular. Capillary refill time 1 second.

Disability
Pupils equal and reactive to light (PEARL), 4 mm.

Exposure
The chest is exposed in a private dwelling to undertake a physical exam – the ambient temperature is warm.

Vital signs
RR: 28 bpm
HR: 106 bpm
BP: 125/82 mmHg
SpO_2: 97%
Blood glucose: 5.1 mmol/L
Temperature: 36.6 °C
GCS: 15/15
4 lead ECG: sinus tachycardia

TASK

Look through the information provided in this case study and highlight all of the information that might concern you as a paramedic.

Case Progression

En route to hospital, the patient starts to become lethargic and complains of a headache and dizziness. On checking the patients carbon monoxide (CO) level, you notice it is much higher than expected. You administer high-flow oxygen through a non-rebreathe mask using 15 L of oxygen and transport the patient to the nearest Emergency Department with a pre-alert call due to the smoke inhalation and potential for CO poisoning.

Patient assessment triangle
General appearance
Alert but no longer meeting gaze.

Circulation to the skin
Normal.

Work of breathing
Increased work of breathing – but improved since treatment provided.

SYSTEMATIC APPROACH
Danger
None at this time.

Response
Alert but becoming lethargic.

Airway
Clear.

Breathing
RR: 28. Wheeze resolving following interventions.

Circulation
HR: 128. Palpable radial. Capillary refill time 1 second.

Disability
Moving all four limbs.

Exposure
Normal temperature in the ambulance.

Vital signs
RR: 28 bpm
HR: 128 bpm
BP: 130/78 mmHg
SpO_2: 97%
CO: 25 ppm
Blood glucose: not repeated
Temperature: not repeated
GCS: E3, V6, M5, 14/15
4 lead ECG: sinus tachycardia

Explain the significance of the soot in and around the mouth and nose.

Soot in mouth and nose is suggestive of inhalation injury. The patient also has singed nasal hair and a hoarse voice, so there is the potential for airway burns that may lead to further complications as the airway starts to swell. The cough indicates the patient may have inhaled irritants, so be aware for signs of toxicity as well. Inhalation injury is the main cause of mortality in burn patients.

Why might SpO_2 monitoring be unreliable in this patient? What else could you measure?

Pulse oximetry measures peripheral capillary oxygen saturation (SpO_2) and the percentage of haemoglobin (oxygenated haemoglobin) compared to the total amount of haemoglobin. Carbon monoxide is one of the products of combustion and can affect patients exposed to smoke-filled environments. CO diffuses across the alveoli in a similar way to oxygen, creating carboxyhaemoglobin, which has a much greater affinity with haemoglobin than oxygen (approx. 250 times greater). This reduces the ability of the haemoglobin to transport oxygen around the body. Pulse oximetry cannot distinguish between oxyhaemoglobin and carboxyhaemoglobin and SpO_2 readings may be falsely elevated, making it challenging to accurately determine the severity of the patient. Some non-invasive pulse oximetry devices can measure carboxyhaemoglobin saturation (SpCO) levels, although most are not validated and should be used as an adjunct to clinical decision making.

End-tidal carbon dioxide ($EtCO_2$) would be another useful addition, as it would help detect any bronchospasm that may not be noted on auscultation.

What are the signs and symptoms of carbon monoxide poisoning?

See Table 1.5.

Table 1.5 Signs and symptoms related to carboxyhaemoglobin (COHb) level at time of exposure to carbon monoxide

COHb level %	Signs and symptoms
0	None
10	Frontal headache
20	Throbbing headache, shortness of breath on exertion
30	Impaired judgement, nausea, fatigue, visual disturbances, dizziness
40	Confusion, loss of consciousness
50	Seizures, coma
60	Hypotension, respiratory failure
70	Death

Source: Adapted from Curtis et al. (2019), p. 535.

What additional questions might help you to determine the severity?

- Duration of time in the smoke-filled room?
- Any prior history of respiratory problems, especially asthma?
- Any action taken to prevent inhalation (cloth or towel across mouth and nose, stayed low to floor to avoid fumes, etc.)?
- Any signs and symptoms associated with CO poisoning?
- Does patient smoke (smokers have a higher baseline reading of CO)?

References and further reading

Austin, M., Wills, K., Blizzard, L. et al. (2010) Effect of high flow oxygen on mortality in COPD patients in prehospital setting: Randomised controlled trial. *BMJ*, 341: c5462.

Australian Medicines Handbook (2020) Salbutamol. Adelaide: Australian Medicines Handbook Pty Ltd. https://amhonline. amh.net.au/chapters/respiratory-drugs/drugs-asthma-chronic-obstructive-pulmonary-disease/beta2-agonists/salbutamol (accessed 14 January 2020).

Bendall, J. & Middleton, P. (2015) Pulmonary embolism. In *Paramedic Principles and Practice ANZ: A Clinical Reasoning Approach* (eds M. Johnson, L. Boyd, H. Grantham & K. Eastwood), Chatswood: Elsevier Australia, p. 313.

British Thoracic Society (2019) *BTS/SIGN Guideline for the Management of Asthma*. https://www.brit-thoracic.org.uk/quality-improvement/guidelines/asthma/ (accessed 29 June 2020).

Burns, E. (2019) ECG changes in pulmonary embolism, *Life in the Fast Lane*, 9 May. https://litfl.com/ecg-changes-in-pulmonary-embolism/ (accessed 30 January 2020).

Busti, A. (2015) The mechanism of oral contraceptive (birth control pill) induced clot or thrombus formation (DVT, VTE, PE). *Evidence-Based Medicine Consult*. https://www.ebmconsult.com/articles/oral-contraceptive-clotting-factors-thrombosis-dvt-pe (accessed 15 January 2020).

Camilleri, T. (2020) Medical emergencies. In *Fundamentals of Paramedic Practice,* 2nd edn (eds S. Willis & R. Dalrymple), Hoboken, NJ: Wiley-Blackwell, pp. 347–348.

Curtis, K., Ramsden, C., Shaban, R. et al. (2019) *Emergency and Trauma Care*, 3rd edn. Chatswood: Elsevier.

Hampson, N. (2012) Non-invasive pulse CO-oximetry expedites evaluation and management of patients with carbon monoxide poisoning. *American Journal of Emergency Medicine*, 30(9): 2021–2024.

Johnson, M. (2015) The inflammatory response. In *Paramedic Principles and Practice ANZ: A Clinical Reasoning Approach* (eds M. Johnson, L. Boyd, H. Grantham & K. Eastwood), Chatswood: Elsevier Australia, pp. 993–1000.

Joint Royal Colleges Ambulance Liaison Committee (2019) *JRCALC Clinical Guidelines 2019*. Bridgwater: Class Professional Publishing.

McCance, K., Huether, S., Brashers, V. & Rote, N. (2010) *Pathophysiology: The Biologic Basis for Disease in Adults and Children*. Toronto: Mosby Elsevier.

McManamny, T. (2015) Paramedic health and wellbeing. In *Paramedic Principles and Practice ANZ: A Clinical Reasoning Approach* (eds M. Johnson, L. Boyd, H. Grantham & K. Eastwood), Chatswood: Elsevier Australia, pp. 88–102.

Meadley, B. (2015) Sepsis. In *Paramedic Principles and Practice ANZ: A Clinical Reasoning Approach* (eds M. Johnson, L. Boyd, H. Grantham & K. Eastwood), Chatswood: Elsevier Australia, pp. 778–796.

NAEMT (2010). *AMLS: Advanced Medical Life Support*, 2nd edn. Burlington, MA: Jones & Bartlett.

Olivera, P. & Johnson, M. (2015) Asthma. In *Paramedic Principles and Practice ANZ: A Clinical Reasoning Approach* (eds M. Johnson, L. Boyd, H. Grantham & K. Eastwood), Chatswood: Elsevier Australia, pp. 240–259.

Pilbery, R. & Lethbridge, K. (2019) *Ambulance Care Practice*, 2nd edn. Bridgwater: Class Professional Publishing.

Staines, D., Sheridan, S. & Pickering, G. (2020), Respiratory assessment. In *Fundamentals of Paramedic Practice*, 2nd edn (eds S. Willis & R. Dalrymple), Hoboken, NJ: Wiley-Blackwell, p. 269.

Talley, N.J. & O'Conner, S. (2020) *Clinical Examination Essentials*, 5th edn. Chatswood: Elsevier.

Tintinalli, J. (2016) *Tintinalli's Emergency Medicine: A Comprehensive Study Guide*, 8th edn. New York: McGraw-Hill Education.

Toon, M., Maybauer, M., Greenwood, J. et al. (2010) Management of acute smoke inhalation injury. *Critical Care and Resuscitation: Journal of the Australasian Academy of Critical Care Medicine*, 12(1): 53–61.

United Kingdom Sepsis Trust (UKST) (2019) *The Sepsis* Manual, 5th edn. https://sepsistrust.org/wp-content/uploads/2020/01/5th-Edition-manual-080120.pdf (accessed 1 February 2020).

Wilcox, S.R., Aydin, A. & Marcolini, E.G. (2019) Specific circumstances: Asthma and COPD. In *Mechanical Ventilation in Emergency Medicine* (eds S.R. Wilcox, A. Aydin & E.G. Marcolini, Cham: Springer Nature, pp. 79–88.

Wyatt, A. & Mulholland, S. (2015) Chronic obstructive pulmonary disease. In *Paramedic Principles and Practice ANZ: A Clinical Reasoning Approach* (eds M. Johnson, L. Boyd, H. Grantham & K. Eastwood), Chatswood: Elsevier Australia, ch. 19.

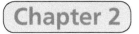 **Cardiac emergencies**

Michael Porter and Joel Beake
Queensland Ambulance Service, Brisbane, QLD, Australia

LEVEL 1 CASE STUDY
Cardiac arrest

Information type	Data
Time of origin	07:15
Time of dispatch	07:30
On-scene time	07:39
Day of the week	Tuesday
Nearest hospital	15 minutes
Nearest backup	Critical care paramedic (CCP), 15 minutes
Patient details	Name: Robert Drury DOB: 12/09/1946

CASE

You have been dispatched code 1 (the most urgent response) to a residence of a 74-year-old male who has woken with chest pain and collapsed.

Pre-arrival information

The male is unconscious and not breathing effectively. CPR instructions are being given over the phone to a female on scene.

Windscreen report

The house is low set and appears to be neat, nil signs of any danger. You can see through the window that the patient is in the bedroom on the bed, with CPR being performed by a neighbour.

Clinical Cases in Paramedicine, First Edition. Edited by Sam Willis, Ian Peate, and Rod Hill.
© 2021 John Wiley & Sons Ltd. Published 2021 by John Wiley & Sons Ltd.

Entering the property

You are met at the door by an elderly woman, visibly distressed. She states that the patient is in the bedroom with the neighbour, also stating that he woke up and did not look well and collapsed onto the bed. You walk through the large, spacious lounge room into a small, cramped bedroom where the patient is located.

On arrival with the patient

The male patient is lying on the bed with a neighbour performing ineffective CPR. The patient is in his pyjamas, but his exposed limbs look grey in colour. You notice some saliva coming out of his mouth and he is not responding to the CPR being provided.

Patient assessment triangle

General appearance

The patient is unresponsive, lying across the bed.

Circulation to the skin

Grey in colour and is the same temperature as the bedroom.

Work of breathing

The patient took an agonal breath as you walked in the room, but no other breaths have been noted.

SYSTEMATIC APPROACH

Danger

Nil.

Response

No response.

Airway

Some saliva noted in the airway.

Breathing

One deep breath on arrival, no more breaths witnessed.

Circulation

No pulse.

Disability

GCS 3/15.

Exposure

Nil signs of trauma, The patient has central cyanosis.

Case history

The partner states that the patient slept in this morning and when he awoke he screamed that he had the worst chest pain he has ever experienced, then he went to get out of bed and groaned and collapsed onto the bed. He was unresponsive, so the partner screamed out and the neighbour heard and came to help. When they rang the ambulance the dispatcher asked them to commence CPR. The partner stated that she could not do such a task, but the neighbour had begun CPR when the ambulance arrived.

TASK

Look through the information provided in this case study and highlight all of the information that might concern you as a paramedic.

Given the chain of survival, high-quality compressions are urgently required for this patient. What is your next move? Consider what you have just walked through.

Moving the patient to the spacious lounge room you have just walked through is ideal. This will provide a better working area and ensure that good-quality uninterrupted compressions can be achieved.

You have moved the patient out to the lounge room to a large area. Your partner is a qualified advanced care paramedic. What are the first steps you are going to take with this patient?

If there are no signs of life, e.g. no pulse, or no normal breathing, chest compressions need to be started and continued while the patient's chest is exposed by removing his pyjama top (cutting it off). The defibrillation pads can then be attached to the patient.

Case Progression

An automatic rhythm check is immediately performed and the patient is found to be in ventricular tachycardia (VT), so a direct current countershock (DCCS) is advised and delivered.

Vital signs
Defibrillation pads: ventricular tachycardia at a rate of 180 bpm
RR: 0
BP: unrecordable
SPO_2: unrecordable
Blood glucose: 5.1 mmol/L
GCS: 3/15
Pupils: fixed, 3 mm
Colour/appearance: grey
Respiratory effort/rhythm: no effort, irregular
Pulses: absent
Head to toe: reveals nil obvious injuries, deformities, scarring and nil medical alerts

---

The person performing chest compressions asks you where their hands should be positioned on the patient's chest and how to best perform compressions. What would you say?

Kneel down to the side of the patient. Place the heel of your hand in the centre of the patient's chest this should be on the lower half of the sternum, roughly between the nipples (ANZCOR, 2016). Ensure that it is not placed over ribs or the upper abdomen. Their other hand is then placed on top of this hand and the fingers may be interlocked. Keep your arms straight and position yourself vertically above the patient's chest and press down on the sternum at least one-third the depth of the chest (5–6 cm). Ensure that pressure is released after each compression and that you don't lean on the chest wall, allowing recoil.

Your partner is continuing chest compressions and the neighbour will assist them. You are positioned at the head of the patient. What actions will you take next?

By positioning yourself at the head of the patient you are in an ideal position to manage the airway. First check the airway for any obstructions, suction the saliva out of the patient's mouth and check for any foreign bodies. Next an oropharyngeal (OP) tube needs to be correctly sized to the patient and inserted. The sizing is important, as inappropriate size will be ineffective and can be detrimental to the patient by not sitting in the correct position and causing trauma. Size the airway by measuring from the middle of the front teeth to the angle of the jaw.

After an oropharyngeal (OP) tube has been inserted, what ratio of compressions to ventilations will be used?

The ratio is 30 : 2. Perform 30 compressions to every 2 ventilations, with compressions at a rate of 100–120 per minute.

How often should the person performing compressions change over?

The person performing compressions should be changed every 2 minutes to prevent fatigue and ensure that good-quality compressions are been delivered.

Case Progression

Your partner and the neighbour are delivering good-quality compressions and swapping every 2 minutes. You have inserted an OP tube and you are delivering 2 breaths after pausing briefly (2 breaths in 1 second) following every 30 compressions. You have completed your rhythm checks every 2 minutes, delivering 1 shock when the patient was in VT, but now on your last rhythm check the patient was in asystole. You have completed 6 minutes of basic life support (BLS).

Patient assessment triangle
General appearance
The patient is unresponsive.

Circulation to the skin
Grey in colour.

Work of breathing
Nil

SYSTEMATIC APPROACH
Danger
Nil.

Response
None.

Airway
Clear, pale.

Breathing
Nil.

Circulation
Asystole, 0 heart rate.

Disability
As stated previously.

You have completed 6 minutes of BLS and another crew arrive to assist. The patient is now is asystole and you are completing rhythm checks every 2 minutes. What other interventions could now be considered?

An advanced airway can now be inserted: a supraglottic airway device (SAD) can be correctly sized and inserted to ensure effective ventilations. Once this is inserted and confirmed in position, compressions can become continuous and the patient can be ventilated at a rate of 6–10 bpm (approx. 1 every 6 seconds).

An IV line can be inserted, or an intra-osseous (IO) infusion if your skill set allows, with adrenaline administration commenced.

LEVEL 1 CASE STUDY
Acute coronary syndrome (ACS)

Information type	Data
Time of origin	10:00
Time of dispatch	10:01
On-scene time	10:06
Weather	21 °C, blue skies
Nearest hospital	10 minutes
Nearest backup	CCP, 15 minutes
Patient details	Name: Georgia Perry
	DOB: 14/02/1941

CASE

You have been dispatched code 1 to the residence of a 79-year-old female who has had an onset of chest pain while gardening.

Pre-arrival information

The female is conscious and breathing, and states she developed central chest and abdominal pain while gardening.

Windscreen report

The house is low set and appears to have neat gardens, nil signs of any danger. The patient is sat under a tree with a lawn mower nearby and you can see that it has been turned off.

Entering the property

You are met at your vehicle by the patient's neighbour, who is concerned as he witnessed the patient mowing her lawn and then suddenly stop and appear to hold her chest. He immediately ran to her assistance and sat her on a chair, where she is located now. The lawn mower is turned off and there are no dangers in the garden.

On arrival with the patient

The female patient is sitting on a chair, holding her chest. She is alert to your presence and orientated to time and place. There are no obvious injuries or major haemorrhage.

Patient assessment triangle

General appearance

The patient appears in mild distress, pink in colour, alert to your presence and speaking in full sentences.

Circulation to the skin

Well perfused, mildly pink to her face and sweaty, but it is a warm day.

Work of breathing

Occasional sighing.

SYSTEMATIC APPROACH

Danger

Nil.

Response

Alert and orientated.

Airway

Clear.

Breathing

Appears to be slightly short of breath.

Circulation

Slow strong radial pulse palpable, normal rate, regular, capillary refill time <2 seconds, skin appears pink and warm.

Disability

Reveals nil obvious injuries or deformities, no loss of sensation in any limbs, no loss of sensation, normal skin turgor, dry mucosa, nil medical alerts, and see vital signs. Nil allergies noted.

Exposure

Not necessary on this patient.

Vital signs

RR: 21 bpm
BP: 129/80 mmHg
SPO_2: 98%
Blood glucose: 5.1 mmol/L
GCS: 15/15
4 lead ECG: Sinus rhythm at a rate of 75, regular
Pupils equal and reactive to light (PEARL)
Colour/appearance: Pink colour to the skin, sweaty forehead and warm to touch
Respiratory effort/rhythm: Normal effort, regular
Auscultate: Clear air entry both sides
Pulses: strong radial pulses both sides, rate of approximately 100 bpm and regular
Head to toe: The patient has not reported any trauma, so no head to toe conducted

Case history

The patient states that she was gardening when she felt a sudden chest pain in the middle of her chest, radiating to her left arm, described as heavy in nature. She felt quite short of breath and then her neighbour arrived and called the ambulance. She normally uses a spray under her tongue, but hasn't refilled her prescription.

TASK

Look through the information provided in this case study and highlight all of the information that might concern you as a paramedic.

Given the initial vital signs, what further assessment needs to be acquired as soon as possible?

A 12 lead ECG.

What history would you like from the patient?

A systematic approach should be utilised when assessing your patient. The pneumonic SAMPLE is widely used and provides the treating paramedic with the vital patient information (see Table 2.1). For this patient we have her signs and symptoms, next we need to enquire about any medical allergies, what medications she is currently taking, what is her past medical history, her last ins and outs and what the events leading up to today were.

The patient's pain also needs to be assessed, and there are many methods for doing so. One common method is using OPQRST (Table 2.2).

Table 2.1 SAMPLE mnemonic

S	Central chest pain, described as heavy, short of breath
A	No known allergies
M	GTN, clopidogrel
P	Suffers from angina, hypertension and high cholesterol
L	Had normal breakfast at 07:00 and moved her bowels this morning
E	Gardening when experienced sudden central chest pain

Table 2.2 OPQRST mnemonic

O	Onset of pain	Sudden onset while gardening
P	Provocation	Sitting makes it a little better
Q	Quality	It's a heavy pain, like someone sitting on her chest
R	Radiating	To left arm and initially jaw
S	Severity	7/10
T	Time of onset	Begun at 09:50 and has remained constant

What would be your treatment plan be for this patient, given that she has not taken any medications and she has no known allergies?

- 300 mg aspirin PO.
- 400 μg sublingual glyceryl trinitrate (GTN) every 5 minutes if not contraindicated.
- IV access and administer opioid medication, commonly 25 μg fentanyl or low-dosage morphine.
- Treat any hypoxia with oxygen. If no signs of hypoxia then oxygen is not indicated.

Case Progression

300 mg oral aspirin has been administered, the patient has also received 2 sprays of sublingual GTN across a 10-minute time frame and 25 μg fentanyl.

Patient Assessment Triangle
General appearance
The patient is less distressed, speaking in full sentences and not holding her chest any more.

Circulation to the skin
Normal.

Work of breathing
Normal.

SYSTEMATIC APPROACH
Danger
Nil.

Response
Alert.

Airway
Clear.

Breathing
RR: 18 bpm.

Circulation
HR: 70 bpm. Effort: strong. Heart regularity: regular.

Vital signs
RR: 18 bpm
HR: 70 bpm
BP: 125/85 mmHg
SPO_2: 98%
Blood glucose: 5 mmol/L
Temperature: 37 °C
12 lead ECG: Sinus rhythm

The patient is still complaining of 2/10 pain. What treatment plans would you advise for this case?

- The patient should be given sublingual GTN and IV pain relief.
- We are treating this patient as having acute coronary syndrome (ACS), therefore we need to reduce her pain to salvage myocardial tissue.
- As long as GTN is not contraindicated, this should be continued and IV pain relief continued.
- A 12 lead ECG should be continued while the patient is transported to hospital, looking for any ischemic changes.
- The patient should remain monitored during transport and until handed over.
- Consider transporting to an ACS facility if recommended in a local protocol.

What are some risk factors for ACS that should be addressed in your questioning?

- Family history of ACS.
- Stress levels, e.g. work type, work/life balance, diet, exercise.
- Advancing age.
- Male.
- Smoking.
- Diabetes mellitus.
- History of prior ischemic heart disease.

LEVEL 2 CASE STUDY
Pericarditis and pericardial tamponade

Information type	Data
Time of origin	20:58
Time of dispatch	21:00
On-scene time	21:10
Day of the week	Tuesday
Nearest hospital	25 minutes
Nearest backup	CCP, 15 minutes
Patient details	Name: David Bryant DOB: 27/12/1994

CASE

You are called to a 26-year-old male complaining of retrosternal chest pain and shortness of breath.

Pre-arrival information

Patient is conscious and breathing, with severe sharp chest pain with no known cardiac history.

Windscreen report

On arrival on scene, no obvious dangers observed. Lights are on inside the house. Weather is fine, no rain, you consider nearest hospital and confirm if backup is available.

On arrival with the patient

On arrival on scene, you are able to gain access to the house and find the patient sitting upright on a dining-room chair, clutching at his chest.

Patient assessment triangle

General appearance

The patient is alert and he looks at you as you approach. He is sitting upright on a chair. Patient presentation is flushed and sweaty, and he is able to speak in full sentences.

Circulation to the skin

Patient appears well perfused. Skin pink, warm and dry.

Work of breathing

Nil increased work of breathing, air entry = L/R clear, nil adventitious sounds.

SYSTEMATIC APPROACH

Danger

No danger, scene feels safe and controlled.

Response

Patient is alert. He looks at you and acknowledges you as you approach. Patient says hello after you introduce yourself and partner.

Airway

The airway is clear. The patient is able to speak in full sentences. Nil blood or secretions coming from airway.

Breathing

There is breathing with spontaneous effort, equal rise and fall of chest, nil difficulty in breathing (DIB), some increased effort and work of breathing observed. Respiratory rate 26 respirations per minute – adequate ventilation.

Circulation

Strong, regular, palpable radial pulses felt.

Exposure

Nil evidence of trauma on head-to-toe assessment, patient denies trauma to chest. He is able to take a deep breath, but reports it increases the pain in his chest when he does so.

O (onset): patient states pain suddenly increased 4 hours prior to calling ambulance and has been gradually increasing in severity.

P (provocation): Pain is worse upon laying supine/flat, but is relieved by sitting upright.

Q (quality): The pain is described as a sharp, burning and at times stabbing pain that is isolated to behind the sternum.

R (relieving factors): Pain is not relieved by anything, but is improved by sitting forward/upright.

S (severity): Pain is described as an 8/10 severe pain.

T (time): Patient reports sudden sharp pain developed 2 weeks ago, but he didn't think it was enough to seek medical attention. Approximately 4 hours ago pain suddenly increased to severe.

Vital signs

RR: 26 bpm

HR: 120 bpm

BP: 126/78 mmHg

SpO$_2$: 98%

Blood glucose: 6.2 mmol/L

Temperature: 38.4 °C (tympanic thermometer) – warm to touch

12-lead ECG: Sinus tachycardia at a rate of 120 with global ST elevation. QRS width = 0.12 seconds, no further abnormalities detected

Allergies: Benzylpenicillin

TASK

Look through the information provided in this case study and highlight all of the information that might concern you as a paramedic.

CHAPTER 2: CARDIAC
EMERGENCIES

What is your initial diagnosis for this patient?

The clinical presentation is suggestive of pericarditis. The patient has ECG changes indicative of pericarditis. Patient is febrile with recent viral illness. The 12 LEAD ECG = global or widespread ST elevation and PR depression throughout most of the limb leads (1, 2, 3 and aVL) and reciprocal ST depression and PR elevation in lead aVR.

What are some differential diagnoses that you may be considering?

Differential diagnoses: myocarditis, benign early repolarisation, STEMI (occlusive myocardial infarction, OMI), pleurisy, chest infection, pleural effusion, pericardial tamponade, pneumothorax (spontaneous/tension), gastric reflux, recent chest trauma, pulmonary embolus (PE), muscle strain, abdominal aortic aneurysm.

Identify several causes of pericarditis. (Look up and list as many as you can.)

- Infections (mainly viral).
- Immunological – SLE, rheumatic fever.
- Uraemia.
- Dressler's syndrome.
- Trauma.
- Following cardiac surgery.
- Drug induced.
- Illicit drug use.
- Post-radiotherapy.

From the following, which best identifies pericarditis?

a. Retrosternal chest pain (generally sharp/burning and often exacerbated by lying supine).

b. Signs of infection (fever, rigors, rash, diarrhoea, vomiting, malaise).

c. Shortness of breathing (particularly when lying flat).

d. ECG changes (specifically PR depression, Spodick's sign, global ST elevation).

e. All of the above.

e. All of the above (these signs can be found in isolation or can all be present during assessment).

Which of the following is your treatment goal for this patient?

a. Reassurance, keep the patient in a position of comfort. Adequate analgesia, using paracetamol and opioids if required. Keep patient monitored. AJPIR (assessment, judgement, planning, implementation, reassessment).
b. Non-steroidal anti-inflammatory drugs (NSAIDs) – aspirin, ibuprofen etc.
c. Rapid removal to hospital.
d. IV access, 12 lead ECG, oxygen and elevate legs.

a. Reassurance, keep the patient in a position of comfort. Adequate analgesia, using paracetamol and opioids if required. Keep patient monitored. AJPIR (assessment, judgement, planning, implementation, reassessment).

Case Progression

Your patient states he is now feeling tired and is finding it hard to breathe. He feels dizzy and nauseated. You notice that he wants to lie down and appears pale. He is now cool to touch and clammy.

Patient assessment triangle
General appearance
The patient is alert but confused, he looks anxious and wants to lay supine. He is pale and clammy, but is able to speak in full sentences.

Circulation to the skin
Slightly pale and clammy. Cool to touch. Weak radial pulses palpated.

Work of breathing
Increased work of breathing. Air entry = L/R clear, nil adventitious sounds. Respiratory rate is now 30.

SYSTEMATIC APPROACH
Danger
The scene is still safe.

Response
Patients is alert but is now confused.

Airway
The airway is clear. The patient is able to speak in full sentences. Nil blood or secretions coming from airway.

Breathing
There is breathing with spontaneous effort, equal rise and fall of chest, some DIB observed, respiratory rate increased to 30 respirations per minute – adequate ventilation.

Circulation
The circulation is weak with regular palpable radial pulses, nil obvious signs of haemorrhage.

Exposure
Increased respiratory effort, but talking in full sentences – mild shortness of breath (dyspnoea).

Vital signs
RR: 30 bpm
HR: 150 bpm
BP: 90/62 mmHg
SpO$_2$: 88% on room air
Temperature: warm to touch
12 lead ECG = Sinus tachycardia at a rate of 150 with S-T segment elevation in all leads. QRS width = 0.12 seconds, QRS appears to be half the amplitude of the original ECG.

It is apparent that the patient is deteriorating. What type of shock is the patient in?

a. Distributive.
b. Hypovolemic.
c. Cardiogenic.
d. Obstructive.

d. Obstructive. Pericardial tamponade causes an obstructive shock, as the myocardium can no longer adequately pump blood due to being restricted by an excessive build-up of fluid in the pericardial sac surrounding the heart.

LEVEL 2 CASE STUDY
Narrow complex tachycardia

Information type	Data
Time of origin	16:55
Time of dispatch	17:00
On-scene time	17:08
Day of the week	Friday
Nearest hospital	20 minutes
Nearest backup	CCP, 15 minutes
Patient details	Name: Steve Whitefield
	DOB: 05/09/1982

CASE
You have been called to a public address for a 38-year-old male who was witnessed to be running along a footpath when he suddenly collapsed.

Pre-arrival information
The patient is now conscious and breathing, complaining of palpitations and shortness of breath (SOB).

Windscreen report
On arrival on scene, the patient is found to be lying supine on the footpath with three bystanders standing around him. The scene appears safe to approach and the patient seems to be alert.

On arrival with the patient
You remove yourself from the ambulance, acquire the oxygen and airway kit, primary response kit (drug kit) and defibrillation monitor, and undertake an observational assessment. After identifying the patient has no physical injuries, you place him on the ambulance stretcher and remove him to the ambulance to maintain confidentiality. You are greeted by a female who states she is an off-duty Registered Nurse and advises how the patient was witnessed to be jogging along the footpath and suddenly 'collapsed' or 'fell'. The patient was unresponsive for 1 minute before regaining consciousness and was placed in the recovery position.

Patient assessment triangle
General appearance
The patient is alert and he looks at you as you approach. The patient was lying in the right lateral position prior to placing him on the ambulance stretcher. The patient is pale and clammy, but is able to speak in full sentences.

Circulation to the skin
Slightly pale and clammy.

Work of breathing:
Nil increased work of breathing, air entry = L/R clear, nil adventitious sounds.

SYSTEMATIC APPROACH

Danger

You are in a public place, you observe bystanders, but the scene appears safe to proceed.

Response

The patient is alert on the AVPU scale. He looks at you and acknowledges you as you approach. Patient says hello after you introduce yourself and partner.

Airway

The airway is clear. The patient is able to speak in full sentences. Nil blood or secretions coming from airway.

Breathing

There is breathing with spontaneous effort, equal rise and fall of chest with asymmetry, nil DIB, respiratory rate 22 respirations per minute – adequate ventilation.

Circulation

The circulation is weak with regular palpable radial pulses, nil obvious signs of haemorrhage and nil C-spine pain on palpation, with nil report of focal neurological deficits (nil paraesthesia reported).

Exposure

Nil evidence of trauma on head-to-toe assessment, patient able to move all limbs freely, nil evidence of head strike. Nil obvious bleeding. Patient states 0/10 pain, but says he has palpitations/fluttery feeling in his chest.

Vital signs

RR: 22 bpm
HR: 180 bpm
BP: 90/68 mmHg
SpO$_2$: 97%
Blood glucose: 5.0 mmol/L
Temperature: 36.3 °C
12 lead ECG: Narrow complex tachycardia with nil discernible P wave and nil apparent ST/T wave abnormalities

> ### TASK
>
> Look through the information provided in this case study and highlight all of the information that might concern you as a paramedic.

What are some differential diagnoses for this patient? (Consider both regular and irregular rhythms.)

- Regular: Physiological sinus tachycardia, inappropriate sinus tachycardia, sinus nodal re-entrant tachycardia, focal atrial tachycardia, atrial flutter with fixed AV conduction, AV-nodal reentrant tachycardia (AVNRT), orthodromic AVRT, idiopathic VT, Wolff–Parkinson–White syndrome.
- Irregular: Atrial fibrillation, focal atrial tachycardia or atrial flutter with varying AV block, multifocal atrial tachycardia (MATT).

What are your treatment priorities for this patient?

The 12 lead ECG has become one of the most important prehospital diagnostic tools. In cases such as this where a patient has suddenly collapsed, an early 12 lead ECG is required. If the patient is haemodynamically stable, conduct modified Valsalva manoeuvres (vagal manoeuvres).

What is your plan if the patient begins to deteriorate?

Request intensive care paramedic backup, prepare for synchronised cardioversion, position patient appropriately, oxygen if hypoperfused/hypoxemic, place defibrillation pads on patient, IV access, crystalloid fluids.

Case Progression

You manage to complete primary and secondary surveys, including early 12 lead ECG acquisition, which identifies a regular narrow complex tachycardia. The patient continues to complain of shortness of breath, palpitations and dizziness, but is haemodynamically stable and maintaining a perfusing blood pressure.

Patient assessment triangle
General appearance
Patient is alert and orientated, sitting upright and speaking in full sentences.

Circulation to the skin
Well perfused, skin is pink, warm and dry.

Work of breathing
Increased work of breathing noted, with increased respiratory effort. Nil intercostal recession or supraclavicular retractions seen, patient airway is patent and he is able to speak in full sentences.

SYSTEMATIC APPROACH

Danger
The scene is still safe.

Response
Patient is alert and orientated.

Airway
The airway is clear. The patient is able to speak in full sentences. Nil blood or secretions coming from airway.

Breathing
There is breathing with spontaneous effort, equal rise and fall of chest, nil DIB, respiratory rate 28 respirations per minute – adequate ventilation.

Circulation
The circulation is weak with regular palpable radial pulses, nil obvious signs of haemorrhage.

Exposure
Increased respiratory effort, but talking in full sentences – mild shortness of breath (dyspnoea).

What is your treatment goal for this patient now? What hospital would you ideally like to transport the patient to?

To successfully revert patient into normal sinus rhythm, improving cardiac output and subsequent perfusion. This can be achieved by attempting vagal manoeuvres. Should this fail, transport to hospital for further medical care is required. It would be expected that the patient be transported to a hospital with a cardiac unit/cardiology capabilities.

What types of questions would you ask this patient as part of your history-taking process?

See Table 2.3.

Table 2.3 History-taking questions

Signs and symptoms: Rapid pulse, pale, clammy, increased work of breathing, complains of mild nausea, palpitations (fluttering feeling in chest)
Allergies: NSAIDs
Medications: Nil reported
Previous medical history: Nil reported
Last meal: Breakfast at 07:00 – oats
Events leading up to today: Witnessed collapse while running, normal water intake

Additional questioning
Does the patient remember falling? If so, what caused the fall?
Can the patient retain new information? Is there retrograde amnesia?
Does the patient have a cardiac history (Hx)?
What is your full name and DOB?
Is there any family or emergency contact you'd like us to call?

Case Progression

Despite two attempts at a modified Valsalva, the patient is now feeling short of breath, dizzy, nauseated, has chest pains and palpitations, and states he feels like he is going to pass out. You are unable to palpate a radial pulse and blood pressure is unrecordable.

What are your treatment priorities now and what interventions may be required to prevent further deterioration and cardiovascular collapse?

In-hospital treatments may include antiarrhythmic drugs such as betablockers or adenosine, which are often used to try to slow AVN conduction and induction of an intermittent AV block. Adenosine also has a short half-life and works within 6–10 seconds, so its effects are short term. However, in this case the patient has no other treatments available pre-hospital, so DC cardioversion should be initiated.

LEVEL 3 CASE STUDY
S-T segment elevation myocardial infarction (STEMI)

Information type	Data
Time of origin	12:30
Time of dispatch	12:32
On-scene time	12:40
Weather	24 °C, blue skies
Nearest hospital	15 minutes (no cath lab)
Nearest backup	CCP, 10 minutes
Patient details	Name: Robert Henson DOB: 12/02/1950

CASE
You have been dispatched code 1 to a GP clinic to attend a 70-year-old male who has presented with chest pain.

Pre-arrival information
The male is not a patient of the GP clinic, he is travelling through town and developed chest pain this morning and presented to the clinic. The clinic called 000 straight away as the patient does not look well.

Windscreen report
You know the GP clinic, it is well respected in your area.

Entering the location
You are greeted by the practice nurse, who states the male is not a patient of the practice, they do not have any records as he is from interstate. He walked into the practice holding his chest and looked very pale, so they called immediately. She has put him on their bed, she attempted to gain a history but he is in a lot of pain. The doctor has come in but is in the middle of an important patient procedure so has been unable to assess the patient. They attempted a 12 lead ECG but he won't sit still.

On arrival with the patient
The patient is lying on a bed in some distress, his friend is next to him looking concerned.

Patient assessment triangle
General appearance
The patient is very pale in colour, diaphoretic, alert to you walking in the room, able to speak in sentences, holding his chest, unable to sit still.

Circulation to the skin
Very pale, almost ashen in colour.

Work of breathing
Slightly increased with the patient 'puffing' in pain every third breath.

SYSTEMATIC APPROACH
Danger
Nil.

Response
Alert and orientated.

Airway
Clear.

Breathing
Increased rate and effort, no accessory muscle use.

Circulation
Slow strong radial pulse palpable, regular, capillary refill time <2 seconds.

Vital Signs
RR: 24 bpm
BP: 135/75 mmHg
SpO_2: 93%
Blood glucose: 5.1 mmol/L
GCS: 15/15
Pupils equal and reactive to light (PEARL)
Colour/appearance: Pale, diaphoretic, almost grey/ashen in colour
Respiratory effort/rhythm: Increased effort, regular
Auscultate: Clear air entry both sides
Pulses: Strong radial pulses both sides
4 lead ECG: Sinus bradycardia at a rate of 40 (undiagnostic ST changes)

Exposure
Head-to-toe survey reveals no obvious injuries/deformities, no loss of sensation, poor skin turgor, dry mucosa, nil medical alerts.

CHAPTER 2: CARDIAC EMERGENCIES

> **TASK**
> Look through the information provided in this case study and highlight all of the information that might concern you as a paramedic.

Given the patient's presentation and initial observation, what is a critical vital sign that assists in the diagnosis of the condition and needs to be acquired as soon as possible?

A 12 lead ECG.

The patient is rolling in pain and unable to respond to the nurse's questions. What strategies could you incorporate in your practice to ensure you gather all relevant information?

Reassurance, the importance of which is often underestimated. This patient appears to be very unwell and it is vital that he is assessed thoroughly. This requires good communication and plenty of reassurance, while at the same time treating the underlying problem. Remember the patient is scared, he has never had chest pain before and is frightened of what might happen.

What history would you like from the patient?

The patient appears to be having chest pain, so it is important to ascertain what type of chest pain this is. Cardiac chest pain can be fatal and needs to be treated and assessed appropriately. In this case we need to find out when the pain began, does anything make it better or worse, what it feels like, does it radiate anywhere, what is the quality of the pain, has he ever experienced this pain before and if so does he know what it was. Use the OPQRST mnemonic:

Onset: What were you doing when the pain came on?
Provocation: Does anything make the pain better or worse?
Quality: How do you describe the pain?
Radiation: Does the pain move anywhere?
Severity: On a scale of 1–10, what number would you give the pain?
Timing: How long have you had it?

What are some of the differential diagnoses for this patient?

- Trauma to the area – broken ribs, pneumothorax (tension).
- Pulmonary embolus.
- Muscle strain.
- Pericarditis.
- Myocarditis.
- Abdominal aortic aneurysm (AAA).
- Aortic dissection.

How would you treat this patient? (Use a bulleted list.)

- Pharmacology:
  - Aspirin.
  - GTN.
  - Oxygen (to treat hypoxia).
  - Antiemetic (anti-sickness).
  - Pain relief.
- Make the patient as comfortable as possible.
- Rapid removal to a cardiac cath lab.
- Lots of reassurance.
- Close monitoring for deterioration.

- Prepare for cardiac arrest.
- Thorough history taking.

LEVEL 3 CASE STUDY
Hyperkalemia

Information type	Data
Time of origin	14:30
Time of dispatch	14:31
On-scene time	14:39
Weather	34 °C, very humid
Nearest hospital	15 minutes
Nearest backup	CCP, 15 minutes
Patient details	Name: Steve Roberto
	DOB: 09/09/1965

CASE
You have been dispatched code 1 to the residence of a 55-year-old male who has been unwell for several days. He has collapsed and is not breathing.

Pre-arrival information
The male is unconscious and his breathing is absent. CPR instructions are currently being provided over the phone.

Windscreen report
The house is a located in a low socioeconomic neighbourhood that is well known by your ambulance service for many different calls, including a fatal stabbing on your last run of shifts. There are several people gathering outside the house due to the commotion occurring inside. You are advised that the police have also been dispatched due to the location.

Entering the location
The residence appears safe, with no pets in the yard and a large driveway to the side of the house. You are met at the door by a very distressed female. She states that the patient is in the bedroom and their 18-year-old son is performing CPR. She is extremely anxious and yelling at you to 'hurry up and do something'. She states that the patient has been very unwell for 5 days and has missed his appointments at the renal centre. You walk through a well-kept house into the bedroom.

On arrival with the patient
The male patient has been moved to the floor, where the son is performing good-quality CPR. You note the patient has significant swollen lower peripheries and scratch marks on his lower limbs.

Patient assessment triangle
General appearance
The patient is unresponsive, lying on the floor.

Circulation to the skin
Pale in colour, cool to touch.

Work of breathing
The patient does not appear to be breathing.

SYSTEMATIC APPROACH
Danger
Nil.

Response
No response.

Airway
Vomit in the airway.

Breathing
Nil.

Circulation
No pulse.

TASK
Look through the information provided in this case study and highlight all of the information that might concern you as a paramedic.

Think about the location you have been dispatched to. Discuss, as you would with your partner, what actions you may take to ensure your safety prior to arriving on scene.

Often we attend areas where police assistance is required for our safety. Discussion should include early activation of police (if this has not already been arranged), staging prior to arrival and awaiting police attendance to ensure scene safety, utilising prior history you or comms have on the location, parking your vehicle in a position that would allow for a quick egress if required (this may involve backing into a driveway or ensuring you are not facing a dead-end street), identifying risks as they arise and using your 'gut instinct' to assess the scene. These are just a few to mention. Utilise other paramedics' experiences to gain knowledge into how others approach these scenes.

Case Progression

History taking
You ask the patient's partner what has occurred and she does not directly respond to your questions, continually yelling 'Fix him, fix him, hurry up and do something to fix him'. She is visibly distressed and emotional despite your attempts to calm her.

TASK
What must you do in this situation where an accurate/thorough history cannot be gained quickly from the patient's partner due to her emotive state? Discuss/write down what options you have.

   Consider the utilisation of others on scene – the patient's son may be of benefit and could possibly be a source of information. Other family members or neighbours who are present may assist with information and/or reassurance to the patient's wife.

   Look for other information on scene such as medications, doctor's letters, medical aids or medical bracelets. You notice leftover boxes of dialysis solution in the hallway as you walk in – what does this tell you?

Case Progression

History taking (cont.)
The son states that the patient has not been well lately. His medical history includes diabetes, hypertension, hypercholesterolemia and end-stage renal failure. They used to use home dialysis, but for the last two months he has had to go to hospital as his condition has worsened. For the last week he has not been to the hospital as he has been too unwell and hates hospitals. Last night he was not well and had a restless sleep. He said his heart was racing, but didn't tell anyone until this morning. He has been in bed since as he told them his muscles were aching and tingling. When they checked on him they found him unconscious with vomit in the bed.

Describe your primary survey for this patient.

- Danger: No danger.
- Response: None.
- Circulation: No pulse, commence CPR and remove any clothing on patient's thorax area and place the defibrillation pads and analyse rhythm, shock if advised.
- Airway: vomit is present, requires suctioning that clears airway.
- Breathing: No breaths.

Describe how you would manage your crew and others on scene. What roles would you allocate and would an early sit rep be of benefit?

As lead paramedic you should allocate roles and ensure they are maintained. As airway clinician you should assist with removal of clothing and placement of the defibrillation pads onto the patient's chest to ensure quick automatic analysis of the rhythm. The son is performing quality compressions, so asking him to assist and continue would be appropriate if he is willing. Compressions can then be managed by your partner.

The airway then needs to be cleared with suctioning and a correctly sized OPA placed (describe your sizing technique). Then you need to ensure the ratio of 30 compressions to every 2 breaths is maintained and the rate is between 100 and 120 bpm, with appropriate compression depth (1/3 of chest wall). Rhythm checks completed every 2 minutes.

An early sit rep is vital in any high-acuity case. In this case a request for another crew to assist with resuscitation would be appropriate, as would a request for an intensive care paramedic.

Case Progression

You continue your resuscitation to plan and there is no change in the patient's condition despite defibrillating the patient three times. You are coming up to 6 minutes.

Patient assessment triangle

General appearance

Patient is unresponsive.

Circulation to the skin

Pale in colour.

Work of breathing

Nil.

SYSTEMATIC APPROACH

Danger

Nil.

Response

None.

Airway

Clear.

Breathing

Nil intrinsic.

Circulation

Ventricular tachycardia at a rate of 180 bpm (after three shocks delivered).

Vital signs

Defibrillation pads: Ventricular tachycardia at a rate of 180 bpm

RR: 0

BP: Unrecordable

SpO$_2$: Unrecordable

Blood glucose: 16.2 mmol/L

GCS: 3/15

Pupils: Size 3, reactive

Colour/appearance: Pale

Respiratory effort/rhythm: No effort

Pulses: Absent

Head to toe: Reveals nil obvious injuries/deformities, nil medical alerts

Discuss other interventions that could be considered after 6 minutes.

Other interventions include gaining IV or IO access and adrenaline administration (after second unsuccessful shock) every 3–5 minutes. The placement of an advanced airway should not interrupt CPR, with waveform capnography being considered.

List the reversible causes of cardiac arrests. Taking into account the history, what is the reversible cause that is most likely to be causing the patient's condition and what additional treatment could be considered? (Think of a higher scope of practice.)

Cardiac arrest caused by hyperkalemia is most likely. Other reversible causes (see Table 2.4) include a build-up of potassium, which can cause suppression of electrical activity of the heart and can cause the heart to stop beating. This patient has renal failure and has missed his dialysis appointments, indicating that this is the likely cause. To treat a suspected hyperkalemia we need to shift the potassium back into the cell and protect the myocardium. This is achieved by administering calcium gluconate, which will stabilise the myocardium. Sodium bicarbonate 8.4% should be considered as a buffer to treat the metabolic acidosis. These interventions often require the presence of critical care paramedics, so early identification and activation are vital and it helps to think ahead.

Table 2.4 The 4 Hs and 4Ts – reversible causes of cardiac arrest

Hypoxia	Tension pneumothorax
Hypovolemia	Cardiac tamponade
Hyper/hypokalemia/metabolic causes	Thrombus
Hyper/hypothermia	Toxins

TASK

You have completed 30 minutes of CPR, for the last 20 minutes of which the patient has been in asystole. Discuss with your peers, or make notes on, the discussion that you would be having with the patient's family around terminating resuscitation.

References and further reading

Australian and New Zealand Committee on Resuscitation (2016) *ANZCOR Guideline 6 – Compressions.* https://resus.org.au/guidelines/ (accessed 8 December 2019).

Australian and New Zealand Committee on Resuscitation (2016) ANZCOR guideline 8 – Cardiopulmonary resuscitation. ANZCOR. https://www.hpw.qld.gov.au/__data/assets/pdf_file/0010/5203/anzcorguideline8cprjan16.pdf (accessed 30 June 2020).

CHAPTER 2: CARDIAC EMERGENCIES

Australian and New Zealand Committee on Resuscitation (2017) ANZCOR Guideline 11.2 – Protocols for adult advanced life support. https://www.nzrc.org.nz/assets/Guidelines/Adult-ALS/ANZCOR-Guideline-11.2-Protocols-June17.pdf (accessed 30 June 2020).

Brugada, J., Katritsis, D.G., Arbelo, E. et al. (2020) 2019 ESC Guidelines for the management of patients with supraventricular tachycardia. *European Heart Journal*, 41(5): 655–720. doi: 10.1093/eurheartj/ehz467

Burns, E. (2019) ECG findings in massive pericardial effusion. *Life in the Fast Lane*, 16 March. https://litfl.com/ecg-findings-in-massive-pericardial-effusion/ (accessed 30 June 2020).

Burns, E. (2019) Pericarditis. *Life in the Fast Lane*, 16 March. https://litfl.com/pericarditis-ecg-library/ (accessed 30 June 2020).

Burns, E. (2019) Superventricular tachycardia (SVT). *Life in the Fast Lane*, 30 March. https://litfl.com/supraventricular-tachycardia-svt-ecg-library/ (accessed 30 June 2020).

Chaubey, V.K. (2014) Spodick's sign: A helpful electrocardiographic clue to the diagnosis of acute pericarditis. *Permanente Journal*, 18(1): e122. doi: 10.7812/TPP/14-001

Deakin, C., Brown, S., Jewkes, F. et al. (2015) Prehospital resuscitation. Resuscitation Council (UK). https://www.resus.org.uk/resuscitation-guidelines/prehospital-resuscitation/ (accessed 30 June 2020).

Jensen, J.K., Poulson, S.H. & Molgaard, H. (2017) Cardiac tamponade: A clinical challenge. *E-Journal of Cardiology Practice*, 15(17). https://www.escardio.org/Journals/E-Journal-of-Cardiology-Practice/Volume-15/Cardiac-tamponade-a-clinical-challenge (accessed 30 June 2020).

Queensland Ambulance Service (2018) Clinical practice guidelines: Cardiac/tachycardia – narrow complex. https://www.ambulance.qld.gov.au/docs/clinical/cpg/CPG_Tachycardia_narrow%20complex.pdf (accessed 30 June 2020).

Resuscitation Council (UK) (2014) Treatment of hyperkalaemic cardiac arrest. Renal Association. https://renal.org/wp-content/uploads/2017/10/HYPERKALAEMIA-CARDIAC-ARREST-ALGORITHM-MARCH-2014.pdf (accessed 30 June 2020).

Stoppler, M. (2019) Hyperkalemia (high blood potassium). *MedicineNet*. https://www.medicinenet.com/hyperkalemia/article.htm (accessed 30 June 2020).

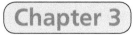 **Neurological emergencies**

Kristina Maximous
Charles Sturt University, Bathurst, NSW, Australia

CHAPTER CONTENTS

LEVEL 1 CASE STUDY
Transient ischaemic attack (TIA)

Information type	Data
Time of origin	06:59
Time of dispatch	07:00
On-scene time	07:12
Day of the week	Friday
Nearest hospital	20 minutes
Nearest backup	None available at present
Patient details	Name: Bob Robertson
	DOB:12/04/1950

CASE

You have been called to a nursing home for a 70-year-old male who is having difficulty in speaking.

Pre-arrival information

The patient is conscious and breathing.

Windscreen report

The area outside the nursing home appears to be safe, with an ambulance bay parking spot available close to the main access door.

Entering the location

As you arrive, a staff member of the nursing home greets you at the door. She tells you that the patient was struggling to swallow his breakfast and suddenly dropped his spoon. She informs you that this is unusual for the patient, as he normally enjoys his breakfast and eats autonomously.

Clinical Cases in Paramedicine, First Edition. Edited by Sam Willis, Ian Peate, and Rod Hill.
© 2021 John Wiley & Sons Ltd. Published 2021 by John Wiley & Sons Ltd.

On arrival with the patient
The male patient is sitting in a chair in the communal dining area.

Patient assessment triangle
General appearance
The patient is alert, conscious and appears to be slumped to the left-hand side.

Circulation to the skin
Pale.

Work of breathing
Normal.

SYSTEMATIC APPROACH
Danger
Nil.

Response
Alert on the AVPU scale.

Airway
Open, clear and patent.

Breathing
Rate: appears normal rate (3 RR in 10 second check x 6 = 18 RR). Rhythm: regular. Quality: bilateral equal air entry and chest rise and fall.

Circulation
Heart rate: feels slightly fast. Rhythm: irregular. Quality: palpable radial pulse. Skin: normal skin temperature. Capillary refill time: 2 seconds.

Disability
PEARL: normal pupil size. GCS: E4, V3, M6 = 13/15. Grip strength: weakness in left-hand side. Allergies: ibuprofen.

Exposure
Exposure appropriate for vital signs.

Environment
There is a chair and ` by patient's front door. Safety reassessed – nil danger.

TASK
Look through the information provided in this case study and highlight all of the information that might concern you as a paramedic.

Using the basic history, general impression and thorough primary survey results, which vital signs should you undertake first and why? And what other information would be valuable?

As the patient is presenting with an irregular heart rate and an altered level of consciousness, the vital assessments to be undertaken should be oxygen saturation, heart rate and blood glucose level (BGL). As the primary survey has identified neurological deficit, patient presentation alongside oxygen saturation reading must be considered and treated accordingly. Identifying a new onset or existing irregular heart rate can provide a valuable red flag.

The BGL testing will enable the paramedic to rule hypoglycaemia in or out as a potential cause or mimic for patient presentation. You would then continue to take the rest of your vitals, including blood pressure, temperature, respiration rate, pupil reassessment and a pain score.

Case Progression

Vital signs
RR: 18 bpm
HR: 95 bpm
BP: 159/82 mmHg
SpO$_2$: 96%
Blood glucose: 4.4 mmol/L
Temperature: 36.7 °C
Pupils: PEARL
Pain score: unable to obtain

Once you have undertaken the essential vital signs, what would your next action be?

Focused neurological assessment (see Table 3.1).

Table 3.1 Focused neurological assessment

Fast test examination

Face: LHS facial droop
Arm: Unilateral weakness on LHS
Speech: Slurred speech and excessive facial drooling
Time: Review the onset of symptoms and time spent on scene

Is the patient FAST test positive or negative?

Positive. Tip: It is important always to identify whether the patient has any previous deficits prior to examination (Table 3.2). This will give you a baseline for identifying whether the presentation is a new onset or has changed in severity.

Table 3.2 AEIOUTIPS results (causes of unconsciousness)

A: No **alcohol** consumption
E: No history of **epilepsy** (seizures)
I: No history of diabetes or **insulin** intake
O: No indication of **overdose** (patient is given his medication by nurses on site)
U: No history of **uraemia** (renal failure)
T: No recent **trauma**
I: No clinical indication of **infection** (sepsis)
P: No history of **psychiatric** conditions
S: **Stroke** possibility due to neurological deficit. No clinical signs of **shock**

What kinds of questions would be important to cover in the history-taking process?

See Table 3.3.

Table 3.3 History-taking questions

What were the signs and symptoms leading up to this event?

Do you have any allergies?

Have you ever had a stroke?

Do you have any cardiac (heart) problems?

Do you have high cholesterol?

Do you have diabetes?

Do you have high blood pressure?

Do you have atrial fibrillation?

Answers to past medical history (PMH)

Atrial fibrillation (AF).

Hypertension (HTN).

Cholesterol.

Medication history questions

What medications are you on for AF, HTN and cholesterol?

How frequently do you take them?

Are they working?

Have there been any changes to the way they work?

Has your prescription changed at all?

Do you take any medications for any other condition?

F/SH (family and social history) questions

Does anyone in your family have a history of stroke, heart disease, high cholesterol or high blood pressure?

Are you a smoker? If so, how often do you smoke and how many a day?

Do you consume alcohol on a regular basis? If so, how often?

Would you consider yourself to be alcohol dependent?

Have you been under stress recently?

How is your general diet?

Do you exercise on a regular basis?

How long have you been in this nursing home for?

Do you have family or friends who visit on a regular basis? If so, how often?

Which of the following non-technical skills do you think are important to be able to treat this patient safely?
a. Compassion.
b. Reassurance.
c. Excellent verbal and non-verbal communication.
d. Empathy.
e. All the above.

e. All the above.

Case Progression

While working through your assessment, you see that the patient's clinical symptoms have started to improve. The patient's speech has begun to return to normal and he is now able to hold his position without being slumped to one side. You rapidly reassess the primary survey and a FAST test and notice that the patient's symptoms have completely resolved.

What is your working diagnosis?

Transient ischaemic attack.

Differential diagnosis (DDx) – what else could this be?

- Seizure disorder.
- Hypoglycaemia.
- Multiple sclerosis.

Given the patient's improvement as listed in the case progression, and the patient's responses, which of the following would you choose to do next?

a. Wait on scene for another half hour to see if the patient's condition stabilizes and then leave the patient in the nursing home because they are in good care.
b. Refer the patient to his GP.
c. Leave the patient on scene, but inform the nursing staff of your findings and worsening care advice.
d. Take the patient to hospital and monitor thoroughly en route.

d. Take the patient to hospital and monitor thoroughly en route.

LEVEL 1 CASE STUDY
Dementia: Delirium

Information type	Data
Time of origin	15:30
Time of dispatch	15:31
On-scene time	16:12
Day of the week	Wednesday
Nearest hospital	45 minutes
Nearest backup	None available at present
Patient details	Name: Joyce Summerscales DOB: 04/07/1942

CASE
You have been called to a care home for a 78-year-old female who has become acutely agitated. The patient is known to have dementia.

Pre-arrival information
The patient is conscious and breathing.

Windscreen report
The area outside the care home appears to be safe, with an ambulance bay available close to the main access door.

Entering the location
As you arrive on scene, a healthcare staff member greets you and informs you that the patient's behaviour has become erratic and out of character since yesterday. She informs you that they were going to call for help much earlier, but the patient appeared to be making progress; however, the disturbance of behaviour seems to be fluctuating since yesterday.

On arrival with the patient
The patient is in her living room and is mobilizing on her Zimmer frame. She appears to be disorientated and off balance.

Patient assessment triangle

General appearance

The patient is alert and conscious.

Circulation to the skin

Pale.

Work of breathing

Normal.

SYSTEMATIC APPROACH

Danger

Nil.

Response

Alert on the AVPU scale.

Airway

Open, clear and patent.

Breathing

Rate: normal rate (3 RR in 10 second check x 6 = 18 RR). Rhythm: regular. Quality: bilateral equal air entry and chest rise and fall.

Circulation

Heart rate: tachycardia. Rhythm: regular. Quality: palpable radial pulse. Skin: slightly warm. Capillary refill time: 2 seconds.

Disability

PEARL: normal pupil size. GCS: E4, V3, M6 = 13/15. Grip strength: equal strength.

Exposure

Exposure appropriate for vital signs.

Environment

Overall a safe and clean room.

TASK

Look through the information provided in this case study and highlight all of the information that might concern you as a paramedic.

Which of the following non-technical skills do you think are important to be able to safely treat this patient?

a. Compassion.

b. Reassurance.

c. Excellent verbal and non-verbal communication.

d. Empathy.

e. All the above.

e. All the above.

At this stage of the case study, what neurological-related questions would you ask the healthcare worker on scene? And why are these important?

What are the patient's communication, mood and behaviour usually like? And how have they differed in the past 24 hours?

Identifying the patient's neurological baseline is important because it enables the clinician to detect neurological changes, which can be either evidently present or subtle. The Glasgow Coma Scale can also be used to identify these changes.

Case Progression

Vital signs
RR: 18 bpm
HR: 106 bpm
BP: 110/72 mmHg
SpO_2: 96%
Blood glucose: 4.9 mmol/L
Temperature: 37.7 °C
GCS: 4, 3, 6 = 13/15
Pupils: PEARL, 5 mm
Pain score: unable to obtain
Allergies: penicillin

History taking
Presenting complaint
Acute change in behaviour and increased confusion.

History of presenting complaint
1/7 Hx fluctuating confusion and erratic behaviour. Patient has also had a 2/7 Hx of abdominal pain, increased frequency of urination, pain during urination and loss of appetite. No recent falls or trauma.

Past medical history
Dementia, HTN, frequent urinary tract infection, frequent falls.

Medications
Memantine, ramipril.

Social history
Lives in care home (healthcare workers on site 24/7). Daughter lives locally.

Family history
Cardiovascular disease.

Read through the history-taking answers and highlight all the red flags that may be a potential cause of the patient's acute change in behaviour.

- Acute change in behaviour and increased confusion.
- 1/7 Hx fluctuating confusion and erratic behaviour. Patient has also had a 2/7 Hx of abdominal pain, increased frequency of urination, pain during urination and loss of appetite.
- Dementia, frequent urinary tract infection.

What is the connection between a urinary tract infection (UTI) and the patient's clinical presentation?

UTI could be a potential cause of the delirium.

What is delirium?

Delirium is an acute medical emergency and condition that causes sudden confusion, subsequently impacting a person's mental abilities and safety. Delirium can start within hours or days, with fluctuating symptoms.

What are the three types of delirium?

- Hyperactive delirium.
- Hypoactive delirium.
- Mixed delirium.

Which of the following groups is most at risk of developing delirium?
a. Everyone.
b. Individuals with pre-existing cognitive impairment and older age.
c. Elderly.
d. Children.

b. Individuals with pre-existing cognitive impairment and older age.

Why are dementia patients at risk of delirium?

Patients with dementia become more susceptible and vulnerable to developing delirium. Both disorders can occur at separate times or at the same time, resulting in significant cognitive impairment, which can have an impact on quality of life, health and wellbeing, and mental abilities. Therefore, as a paramedic it is imperative to know the neurological disorders and risk factors associated with delirium.

What is your provisional diagnosis?

Delirium secondary to UTI, as patient has the risk factor of an infection and also falls within a high-risk category for developing delirium due to dementia. The history and clinical presentation support the provisional diagnosis.

Name two other risk factors that can cause delirium.

- Severe illness.
- Dehydration.

Given the clinical presentation, history information and social setting, which of the following would be your disposition be for this patient?
a. Ask the healthcare staff member to arrange a GP appointment.
b. Contact the GP yourself and make a referral.
c. Transport the patient to the Emergency Department, as her condition could deteriorate further and may require the IV route of medication.
d. Contact the daughter to take the patient up to the Emergency Department.

c. Transport the patient to the Emergency Department, as her condition could deteriorate further and may require the IV route of medication.

LEVEL 2 CASE STUDY
Haemorrhagic stroke

Information type	Data
Time of origin	02:59
Time of dispatch	03:00
On-scene time	03:41

Information type	Data
Day of the week	Saturday
Nearest hospital	35 minutes
Nearest backup	1 hour
Patient details	Name: Jeanette Sanders DOB: 20/08/1952

CASE

You have been called to a private address for a 68-year-old female complaining of a headache with multiple episodes of vomiting.

Pre-arrival information

The patient is conscious and alert.

Windscreen report

The private address appears to be a block of apartments and there are no immediate safety concerns. However, the ambulance will be parked in the middle of the road as there is no parking outside the patient's house.

Entering the location

It is a single-storey house that appears to be well kept and clean.

On arrival with the patient

The husband greets you at the door and informs you that his wife was awoken at 01:00 with a sudden headache and has vomited multiple times since. They had gone out to dinner last night for their daughter's birthday

Patient triangle assessment

General appearance

The patient is in a dark living room, sitting in a corner chair, complaining of a severe headache and nausea.

Circulation to the skin

Flushed.

Work of breathing

Normal.

SYSTEMATIC APPROACH

Danger

Nil.

Response

Alert on the AVPU scale.

Airway

Open, clear and patent (however, you notice dentures appear loose).

Breathing

Rate: appears normal (3 RR in 10 second check x 6 = 18 RR). Rhythm: regular. Quality: bilateral equal air entry and chest rise and fall.

Circulation

Heart rate: tachycardia. Rhythm: regular. Quality: palpable radial pulse. Skin: flushed. Capillary refill time: 2 seconds.

Disability

PEARL: normal pupil size, slow on reaction. GCS: E4, V4, M6 = 14/15. Grip strength: unable.

Exposure
Exposure appropriate for vital signs.

Environment
Broken lift in apartment block and access and egress not suitable for stretcher.

Vital signs
HR: 99 bpm
BP: 180/130 mmHg
SpO_2: 95%
Blood glucose: 4.8 mmol/L
Temperature: 36.5 °C
Pupils: reactive, slow and normal size
GCS: E4, V4, M6 = 14/15

TASK
Look through the information provided in this case study and highlight all of the information that might concern you as a paramedic.

What kinds of questions would it be important to cover in the history-taking process?

See Table 3.4.

Table 3.4 History-taking questions

What were the signs and symptoms leading up to this event?
Do you have any allergies?
Have you ever had a stroke?
Do you have any cardiac (heart) problems?
Do you have high cholesterol?
Do you have diabetes?
Do you have high blood pressure?
Do you have atrial fibrillation?

Medication history questions
What medications are you on for HTN and cholesterol?
How frequently do you take them?
Are they working?
Have there been any changes to the way they work?
Has your prescription changed at all?
Do you take any medications for any other condition?

F/SH (family and social history)
Does anyone in your family have a history of stroke, heart disease, high cholesterol or high blood pressure?
Are you a smoker? If so, how often do you smoke and how many a day?
Do you consume alcohol on a regular basis? If so, how often?
Would you consider yourself to be alcohol dependent?
Have you been under stress recently?
How is your general diet?
Do you exercise on a regular basis?

Additional questions:
When was your last oral intake?
What were the events leading up to this case?
Use AEIOUTIPS.

Case Progression

Answers gathered from history taking

Signs and symptoms: Awoken by sudden onset of a headache associated with nausea, vomiting, progressive sensitivity to light and confusion.

Allergic to penicillin and ibuprofen.

Medications: Ramipril, simvastatin, eye drops.

Past medical history: Hypertension, cholesterol, constipation and glaucoma.

Surgical history: No surgical history.

Family history of hypertension.

Social history: Patient and husband live independently and have a daughter who lives locally.

Last oral intake: Dinner around 19:30 and a glass of water at 03:10.

Events: Patient felt generally unwell last night and was awoken by a sudden headache.

Pain assessment questions

Onset: Patient was asleep when the headache occurred at around 02:00.

Palliation or provocation: Pain is not provoked or alleviated by anything.

Quality: Pain is described as severe and explosive.

Radiation: Pain all over the head.

Severity: Pain score 9/10.

Time: Awakening pain was 10/10, however has reduced to 9/10.

FAST test examination

Face: Negative.

Arm: Unable to complete due to patients altered level of consciousness (ALOC).

Speech: Speech not slurred, however inappropriate responses and words dissemble.

Time: Review time on scene.

Has there been any significant change in patient presentation during the FAST test?

Yes, the patient's GCS has now deteriorated from 14 to 13 as the verbal response has declined from confused to inappropriate response and words dissemble.

Case Progression

As you look at your patient, you notice her eyes roll back and then she starts to have a tonic-clonic seizure lasting 1 minute and a half. Following the seizure you manage the airway and undertake primary and secondary surveys.

Vital signs

HR: 99 bpm

BP: 192/138 mmHg

SpO_2: 92% (oxygen administered to reach target of 94–98%)

Blood glucose: 4.8 mmol/L

Temperature: 36.7 °C

Pupils: reactive, slow and normal size.

GCS: 4, 4, 6 = 14/15

Which of the following classes of drugs would be used to stop the seizure?

a. Betablockers.

b. Benzodiazepines.

c. Anti-coagulants
d. Narcotics.

b. Benzodiazepines.

Can you identify all the clinical red flags presented within this case study?

- Age >50 years.
- Sudden onset of headache.
- Nausea and vomiting.
- Light sensitivity.
- ALOC.
- FAST test positive.
- Deteriorating LOC.
- History of HTN and cholesterol.
- Family history of HTN.
- Seizure.

Which of the following is your provisional diagnosis for this patient?
a. Subdural haematoma.
b. Subarachnoid haemorrhage secondary to aneurysm.
c. Transient ischaemic attack.
d. Ischaemic stroke.

b. Subarachnoid haemorrhage secondary to aneurysm.

What is a subarachnoid haemorrhage?

A subarachnoid haemorrhage is a bleed that occurs below the arachnoid layer of the brain. The arachnoid layer is the middle layer of the meninges that covers the brain and spinal cord. Subarachnoid haemorrhage poses significant risk of secondary strokes due to vasospasm caused by blood pooling and blood breakdown products irritating neighbouring blood vessels.

What is your management plan for this patient?

Management of the ABCs (don't forgot to keep a close eye on the loose dentures you identified in your primary survey and consider removing them if they block the airway). Administration of oxygen therapy aiming to achieve a saturation of 94–98% (refer to your service or local and national oxygen guidelines) and administration of anticonvulsant medication.

Which of the following non-technical skills do you think are important to be able to safely treat this patient?
a. Compassion.
b. Reassurance.
c. Excellent verbal and non-verbal communication.
d. Empathy.
e. All the above.

e. All the above.

Differential diagnosis (DDx) – what else could this be?

- Epilepsy.
- Ischaemic stroke.
- Migraine.

Given the patient's deterioration listed in the case progression, which of the following is your choice now for what to do next?

a. Wait on scene for another half hour to see if the patient's condition stabilises and then leave the patient at home and give worsening care advice to the husband.

b. Call the daughter to transport the patient to hospital.

c. Refer the patient to her GP.

d. Rapidly transport the patient to hospital with a call alert ahead for a possible subarachnoid stroke.

d. Rapidly transport the patient to hospital with a call alert ahead for a possible subarachnoid stroke.

Patients suffering from a subarachnoid haemorrhage require rapid transport to hospital. It is imperative that paramedics alert the hospital prior to arrival, giving clinicians on the receiving end enough time to contact the stroke team and to ensure scanning facilities are immediately available for this patient.

En route to hospital, the paramedic must ensure that they are reassessing the primary survey and managing the patient according to their presentation and managing life-threatening presentations. It is important that IV access has been acquired and the patient is monitored en route using an ECG device. Paramedics should not remain on scene any longer than necessary.

LEVEL 2 CASE STUDY
Seizure

Information type	Data
Time of origin	19:01
Time of dispatch	19:02
On-scene time	19:12
Day of the week	Saturday
Nearest hospital	25 minutes
Nearest backup	50 minutes
Patient details	Name: Rob Nashville
	DOB: 03/03/1975

CASE
You have been called to a private address for a 45-year-old male witnessed to have a seizure.

Pre-arrival information
The patient is in and out of consciousness.

Windscreen report
The private address appears to be a house in a built-up residential area and there is no concern with scene safety. However, continuous dynamic risk assessment is imperative.

Entering the location
The house has two storeys with the patient's bedroom situated upstairs. The house appears to be unkempt, with empty bottles of alcohol around. The mother of the patient has greeted you at the door and takes you upstairs to the patient.

On arrival with the patient
The patient's mother informs you that he has had a seizure and appears to be confused and agitated. She informs you that her son consumes a lot of alcohol and they are worried about him, and that his last seizure was approximately 4 months ago.

Patient Triangle Assessment
General appearance
The patient is lying on his back on his bedroom floor. The mother informs you that the patient was sitting on the floor prior to having the seizure.

Circulation to the skin
Pale.

Work of breathing
Regular with prolonged inspiratory and expiratory phase.

SYSTEMATIC APPROACH
Danger
Nil.

Response
Alert on the AVPU scale.

Airway
Open, clear and patent. You move the patient from his back to the recovery position to assist with maintaining an open and clear airway.

Breathing
Rate: 3 RR in 10 second check x 6 = 18 RR. Rhythm: regular. Quality: bilateral equal air entry and chest rise and fall.

Circulation
Heart rate: tachycardia. Rhythm: regular. Quality: palpable radial pulse. Skin: pale. Capillary refill time: 2 seconds.

Disability
PEARL: normal pupil size, slow on reaction. GCS: E3, V4, M5 = 12/15. Grip strength: unable.

Exposure
Exposure appropriate for vital signs.

Environment
The bedroom is on the second floor of the house, and there are bottles of alcohol around the patient.

TASK
Look through the information provided in this case study and highlight all of the information that might concern you as a paramedic.

Having highlighted your concerns, as a paramedic what would your next action be?

As the patient has an altered mental state and has not fully recovered, it is important to ensure that you have 360° access around the patient and the airway is accessible at all times. The patient will then require supplementary oxygen therapy to reach 94–98%.

Case Progression

Vital signs
HR: 109 bpm
BP: 134/89 mmHg
SpO$_2$: 92%
Blood glucose: 4.8 mmol/L
Temperature: 37.0 °C
Pupils: reactive, slow and normal size
GCS: E3, V4, M5 = 13/15

Which of the following non-technical skills do you think are important to be able to safely treat this patient?
a. Compassion.
b. Reassurance.
c. Excellent verbal and non-verbal communication.
d. Empathy.
e. All the above.

e. All the above.

Case Progression

As you start to undertake a set of observations, the patient's muscles become stiff and flexed, followed by violent muscle contractions. The seizure lasts for approximately 90 seconds.

What is your medical management plan for this patient?

Management of the ABCs. Administration of oxygen therapy aiming to achieve a saturation of 94–98% and gaining IV access for administration of anti-convulsant medication should the seizure occur again.

Which of the following pieces of equipment should always be set up alongside airway management adjuncts or devices?
a. Cervical collar.
b. Suction unit.
c. Head blocks.
d. Spinal board.

b. Suction unit.

Which of the following types of seizure is this?
a. Myoclonic.
b. Complex partial.
c. Tonic-clonic.
d. Simple partial.

c. Tonic-clonic.

Which of the following classes of drugs would be used to stop the seizure?
a. Betablockers.
b. Benzodiazepines.
c. Anti-coagulants.
d. Narcotics.

b. Benzodiazepines.

What are the mechanism of action of benzodiazepines?

Benzodiazepines work by slowing down the activity of the central nervous system and are considered a depressant drug. Benzodiazepines bind to benzodiazepine receptors located on the allosteric site of the gamma-aminobutyric acid (GABA)-A receptor on the post-synaptic neuron. The allosteric site can be located between alpha and gamma subunits of the GABA-A receptor. The result of this is an increase of frequency of chloride channels opening, as a result increasing the inhibitory effect of GABA and decreasing neuronal excitation.

What kinds of questions would it be important to cover in the history-taking process?

See Table 3.5.

Table 3.5 History-taking questions

What were the signs and symptoms leading up to this event?
Do you have any allergies?
Alcohol consumption/how often/have you withdrawn from alcohol?
Epilepsy, electrolytes or encephalopathy
Insulin/diabetes
Overdose or opiates
Uraemia
Trauma to the head, toxins and temperature
Infection
Psychiatric conditions or medications
Stroke, seizures, shock, subarachnoid haemorrhage or space-occupying lesion
Medications Past medical history Social history Last oral intake Events to present

Assessment questions
Onset, palliation or provocation, quality, radiation and time

Clinical considerations
From arriving on scene, has the patient shown signs of stability, deteriorating or improvement?

How does alcohol consumption increase the risk of seizure activity?

During small to moderate amounts of alcohol consumption, seizures are less likely to occur. However, too much alcohol raises the seizure threshold. Commonly between 6 and 48 hours after cessation of consuming alcohol, an individual is at risk of seizures because the intoxicating drink can bind to the GABA receptor and inhibit neuronal signals, as a result increasing the ratio of the excitatory neurotransmitter glutamate, resulting in neuronal excitability.

As a paramedic, what is the major concern for this patient? And why are prompt management and treatment important?

The major concern for this patient would be status epilepticus, as the patient has had two seizures and remained postictal without full recovery.

What is your provisional diagnosis for this patient?

Tonic-clonic seizure secondary to alcohol consumption.

What is a tonic-clonic seizure?

A tonic-clonic seizure is a convulsion that occurs when there is a sudden, uncontrolled electrical disturbance in both hemispheres of the brain, which results in complete loss of consciousness.

Differential diagnosis (DDx) – what else could this be?

- Stroke.
- Transient global amnesia.

In consideration of all your findings and the clinical presentation of the patient, which of the following is the final disposition?
a. Refer the patient to his GP for follow-up.
b. Transport the patient to the Emergency Department due to concerns for potential alcohol-induced seizures and for further monitoring and treatment.
c. Assist the patient back into bed until he recovers, with worsening care advice.
d. Ask the mother to make an appointment with the patient's GP.

b. Transport the patient to the Emergency Department due to concerns for potential alcohol-induced seizures and for further monitoring and treatment.

LEVEL 3 CASE STUDY
Epidural Haematoma

Information type	Data
Time of origin	04:00
Time of dispatch	04:01
On-scene time	04:38
Day of the week	Saturday
Nearest hospital	90 minutes
Nearest backup	12 minutes
Patient details	Name: Roger Dalrymple DOB: 02/02/1975

CASE
You have been called to a night club for a 45-year-old male who has been struck on the side of the head with an unknown object following an altercation that occurred at 02:00. The patient is now sitting outside the nightclub with a friend.

Pre-arrival information
Police on scene called for an ambulance and state that the patient was unconscious, but is now conscious.

Windscreen report
Police are managing the scene and have evacuated a parking spot for the ambulance.

Entering the location
This incident is located outside the nightclub.

On arrival with the patient

A female who identifies herself as a close friend informs you that the patient had lost consciousness, but is now coherent. She states that he has been complaining of a headache and has vomited multiple times. She also informs you that the patient is an exchange student and that English is not his first language.

Patient assessment triangle

General appearance

The patient is sat outside on the floor, appears conscious, but holding his head and is looking down.

Circulation to the skin

Flushed.

Work of breathing

Normal.

SYSTEMATIC APPROACH

Danger

There are crowds of people nearby, but controlled by the police.

Response

Alert on the AVPU scale.

Catastrophic haemorrhage

Nil.

Airway

Open, clear and patent (however, patient has a cut lip, which is bleeding).

Breathing

Respiration rate: 3 in 10 second check x 6 = 18 RR. Rhythm: regular. Quality: bilateral equal air entry and chest rise and fall.

Circulation

Heart rate: slow. Rhythm: regular. Quality: palpable radial pulse. Skin: flushed. Capillary refill time: 2 seconds.

Disability

PEARL: slow on reaction. GCS: E4, V5, M6 = 15/15. Grip strength: equal strength.

Exposure

Appropriate for vital signs.

Environment

There are lots of people around under the influence of alcohol and possibly other substances.

Vital signs

RR: 18 bpm
HR: 58 bpm
BP: 170/90 mmHg
SpO_2: 96%
Blood glucose: 6.0 mmol/L
Temperature: 36.5 °C
Pupils: PEARL – slow
GCS: E4, V5, M6 = 15/15
Pain score: 8/10, headache

> **TASK**
> Look through the information provided in this case study and highlight all of the information that might concern you as a paramedic.

What clinical significance do the first three vital signs have in relation to head injuries?

Blood pressure, heart rate and breathing patterns are three vitals used to identify increased intracranial pressure (ICP). Hypertension, resulting in widening pulse pressures, bradycardia and Cheyne–Stokes breathing, make up Cushing's triad, a clinical triad tool used to recognize increased ICP.

What causes ICP?

The cranium is a rigid structure that contains three elements: blood, brain and cerebral spinal fluid. The rigidity of the cranium means that the total volume of all three components is fixed. An increase in one element will increase the pressure within the cranium, and if it persists can be a threat to life.

Which two of the following are the implications of increased ICP due to change in volume of one component?
a. Decrease in cerebral blood flow.
b. Cranium adjusts and expands accordingly.
c. Intracranial pressure will reduce within 48 hours.
d. Herniation of the brain.

a. Decrease in cerebral blood flow, and d. Herniation of the brain.

Case Progression

You undertake a neurological assessment and in consideration of your findings and appreciation of the force and location of impact, you request intensive care paramedic backup and ask your paramedic colleague to get the immobilisation equipment. During this time you reassure the patient and undertake another set of observations and start to think about undertaking a thorough secondary survey.

Vital Signs
RR: 16 bpm
HR: 50 bpm
BP: 192/104 mmHg
SpO_2: 94%
Response: alert on the AVPU scale
Pupils: PEARL – slow
GCS: E4, V4, M6 = 14/15

Cranial nerve examination
Disturbance in eye movement.

Motor function
Weaker in strength on one side.
Poor coordination.
No obvious facial weakness.
No history or evidence of a seizure.

Sensory
Hearing intact.
Superficial sensation intact.

Symptoms
Nausea and vomiting.
Confusion.
Drowsiness.
Severe headache.
Amnesia.

What are the benefits of requesting intensive care support for this patient?

Patients with traumatic brain injury pose a high risk of mortality, disability and secondary brain injury, which can be managed using sedation, rapid sequence intubation, paralysis and ventilation by intensive care paramedics or doctors.

Early request for backup is imperative, as paramedics should take into account type and time of injury, distance travelled, backup distance and distance to hospital.

What head injury signs would you be actively looking for in the secondary survey?

1. Skull fractures (gently palpate).
2. Haemotympanum.
3. Periorbital ecchymosis (raccoon eyes).
4. Battle's sign.
5. Facial oedema.
6. Cerebral spinal fluid rhinorrhoea.
7. Cerebral spinal fluid otorrhoea.

What kind of questions would be important to cover in the history-taking process for this patient?

See Table 3.6.

Table 3.6 History-taking questions

Have any of the following been present or are present?
• Loss of or impaired consciousness – if so, duration
• Confusion or irritation
• Nausea and vomiting
• Poor coordination
• Dizziness
• Severe headache
• Visual disturbances
• Unequal pupil size, equality and reactivity

Time and date of injury
Mechanism of action
Incidence: accident, inflicted by others, medical event, trauma etc.
Are there any distracting injuries?
Any evidence of or history of seizure activity?
Other injuries sustained?
History of bleeding or coagulation disorders
Presence of amnesia? If so, which type, e.g. retrograde
Glasgow coma scale prior to arrival

Table 3.6 (Continued)

AEIOUTIPS

Medications
Past medical history/social history
Last oral intake
Events to present

Assessment questions
Onset, palliation or provocation, quality, radiation and time

Clinical considerations
From arriving on scene has the patient shown signs of stability, deterioration or improvement?

Case Progression

You have pre-alerted and are en route to your nearest major trauma hospital. The deteriorating patient has been immobilised, cannulated and, alongside continuous monitoring of ABCs, is being monitored using ECG and capnography.

While on the way to hospital, the patient's level of consciousness has rapidly declined accompanied by deterioration of vital signs. You promptly undertake C-ABC management and ventilate the patient with a high concentration of oxygen, aiming to achieve a target saturation of 94–98%.

Vital signs
RR: Cheyne–Stokes breathing
HR: 42 bpm
BP: 200/120 mmHg
SpO_2: 87% (pre-oxygenation), 97% (post-oxygenation)
Pupils: unequal, L is dilated and fixed, R is slow on reaction
GCS: E1, V2, M4 = 7/15
Decorticate positioning

Why is monitoring oxygenation and end-tidal CO2 important in traumatic brain injury (TBI)? What role does ventilation play in this?

Monitoring oxygen saturation and capnography can reduce the risk of hypoxemia or changes in ventilation in patients with TBI.

An increase in the partial pressure of carbon dioxide ($PaCO_2$) in the arterial blood results in vasodilation, subsequently increasing blood volume within the cranial volt and resulting in an increase of ICP. Hyperventilation decreases the level of $PaCO_2$, causing vasoconstriction and therefore lowering blood volume and ICP. This is a commonly used method to control ICP in patients with TBI. However, it is not without risk, as prolonged hypocapnia increases the risk of disability and mortality in patients with TBI.

How does increased intracranial pressure from a TBI affect cerebral perfusion pressure? How does this connect with Cushing's triad?

Cerebral perfusion pressure is the net pressure gradient that permits cerebral blood flow to the brain. As ICP increases from a TBI, the mean arterial pressure (MAP) must increase to compensate for the lack of perfusion to the brain. This will also result in peripheral vasoconstriction, causing a further increase in ICP and MAP. Eventually as bleeding continues and blood volume increases within the rigid structure of the cranium, the brain will start to herniate, triggering the signs in Cushing's triad.

How does herniation of the brain cause the signs in Cushing's triad?

In Cushing's triad, the blood pressure increases as the brain starts to herniate. The herniation of the brain compresses the vagus nerve, causing bradycardia and an irregular breathing pattern commonly known as Cheyne–Stokes breathing.

Which of the following non-technical skills do you think are important to be able to treat this patient safely?
a. Compassion.
b. Reassurance.
c. Excellent verbal and non-verbal communication.
d. Empathy.
e. All the above.

e. All the above.

Which of the following is your provisional diagnosis?
a. Subdural haematoma.
b. Epidural haematoma.
c. Subarachnoid haemorrhage.
d. Ischaemic stroke.

b. Epidural haematoma.

Differential diagnosis (DDx) – what else could this be?

- Subdural haematoma.
- Intracranial mass.
- Brain abscess.

LEVEL 3 CASE STUDY
Meningococcal septicaemia

Information type	Data
Time of origin	01:30
Time of dispatch	01:31
On-scene time	01:58
Day of the week	Tuesday
Nearest hospital	30 minutes
Nearest backup	20 minutes
Patient details	Name: Nicholas Taylor
	DOB: 12/12/2001

CASE
You have been called to a university campus for a 19-year-old male complaining of flu-like symptoms and severe aches in his muscles and joints.

Pre-arrival information
Security to meet ambulance at university entrance to provide directions of patient location.

Windscreen report
The scene appears to be safe. The campus has students milling around.

Entering the location

The room appears dark, but clean, with clear access and egress route.

On arrival with the patient

As you enter the room, a friend greets you at the door to inform you that he is concerned about his friend who has vomited a couple of times and states that the light in his room is too bright.

Patient assessment triangle

General appearance

The patient is in his dorm room, lying in bed with the lights switched off.

Circulation to the skin

Pale.

Work of breathing

Normal.

SYSTEMATIC APPROACH

Danger

No immediate danger. Security with ambulance.

Response

Alert on the AVPU scale.

Airway

Open, clear and patent.

Breathing

Rate: tachypnoea (5 RR in 10 second check x 6 = 30 RR). Rhythm: regular. Quality: bilateral equal air entry and chest rise and fall.

Circulation

Heart rate: tachycardia. Rhythm: regular. Quality: detectable pulse. Skin: pale. Capillary refill time: >2 seconds.

Disability

PEARL: slow on reaction. GCS: E4, V5, M6 = 15/15. Grip strength: equal strength

Exposure

Exposure appropriate for vital signs. Patient appears to have red spots on hands and feet.

Environment

The dorm room appears clean.

Vital signs

RR: 28 bpm

HR: 130 bpm

BP: 97/64 mmHg

SpO_2: 92%

Blood glucose: 4.5 mmol/L

Temperature: 38 °C

Pupils: PEARL – slow

GCS: E4, V5, M6 = 15/15

Pain score 8/10, generalised aches and headache

TASK

Look through the information provided in this case study and highlight all of the information that might concern you as a paramedic.

You decide to rapidly undertake a set of vital observations and gain a history of events. What sort of questions would it be imperative to ask?

See Table 3.7.

Table 3.7 History-taking questions

History of events
Signs and symptoms
   Nausea and vomiting
   Headache
   Neck stiffness
   Photophobia
   Fever and chills
   Tachypnoea
   Fatigue
   Diarrhoea
   Severe aches or pains to muscles, joints, chest or abdomen
   Blanching, non-blanching or maculopapular rash
Past medical history
Medications
Family history
Social history
Last oral intake

Pain assessment questions
Onset, palliation or provocation, quality, radiation and time

Clinical considerations
From arriving on scene has the patient shown signs of stability, deteriorating or improvement?

Case Progression

Summary of history-taking answers
19-year-old male has had a 4/7 Hx of flu-like symptoms, which had progressed in the past 48 hours to generalized body aches, neck stiffness and a headache (8/10) not relived by paracetamol. Patient also states ongoing nausea with 4 episodes of vomiting in the past 24 hours. Progressive photophobia and evidence of red spots in hands and feet in the past 24 hours.
   Last food oral intake was 2/7 ago, with sips of water since. Patient is usually well and fit with no significant past medical history.

Given the information, clinical presentation and history, which of the following is your provisional diagnosis of this patient?
a. Meningitis.
b. Meningococcal meningitis.
c. Meningococcal septicaemia (meningococcaemia).
d. Viral meningitis.

c. Meningococcal septicaemia (meningococcaemia).

Having identified a provisional diagnosis, what should you and your colleague do? And why?

Meningococcal bacteria can spread through close contact and therefore protection for those on scene is imperative. PPE such as protective eye wear, gloves, gown and face mask should be used.

What is the name of the bacteria that causes meningococcal septicaemia?

Neisseria meningitidis.

What is the difference between meningococcal septicaemia and meningococcal meningitis?

Meningitis is inflammation of the meninges, which can be caused by infection, autoimmune diseases or adverse reaction to medication. Meningococcal meningitis is caused by the bacteria *Neisseria meningitidis*, which multiplies and infects the brain and the spinal cord, causing swelling; whereas in meningococcal septicaemia, the bacteria has also infected the bloodstream, resulting in damaged blood vessels, which leak into tissue and cause further damage.

What are the names of the two common tests undertaken when querying meningitis?

- Kernig's sign.
- Brudzinski's sign.

Which of the following is your next treatment plan?
a. Oxygen therapy, fluids, benzyl penicillin, paracetamol and ondansetron.
b. Oxygen therapy, paracetamol, hydrocortisone and chlorphenamine.
c. Oxygen, glucose, chlorphenamine, fluids.
d. Benzyl penicillin, salbutamol, paracetamol and fluids.

a. Oxygen therapy, fluids, benzyl penicillin, paracetamol and ondansetron.

Case Progression

You have cannulated the patient and started your treatment plan. You have also transferred the patient onto the stretcher and already alerted the local hospital. You take a second set of observations on route.

Vital signs
RR: 30 bpm
HR: 135 bpm
BP: 89/60 mmHg
SpO$_2$: 94%
Blood glucose: 4.5 mmol/L
Temperature: 38.1 °C
Pupils: PEARL – slow
GCS: E4, V5, M6 = 14/15
Pain score 8/10, generalised aches and headache

Exposure
Non-blanching rash on chest
Kernig's sign: Positive
Brudzinski's sign: Positive

Can meningitis cause a patient to suffer from a seizure?

Yes. Meningitis causes brain swelling or pressure due to toxin release from the infection alongside a response from inflammatory mediators. The combination can result in neuronal irritation and excitability, causing a disruption to normal brain activity resulting in a seizure.

Does meningitis always present as a non-blanching rash?

No. In the early stages a rash can present as blanching, however it usually develops into a non-blanching petechial rash that does not disappear when pressed.

Who else do you need to consider in this case study and why?

The patient's friend, security guard and anyone else who has come into contact with the patient. Those in close contact will need to be assessed and may be treated with prophylactic antibiotics, therefore they should be referred and the university-associated doctors will need to be informed.

Which of the following non-technical skills do you think are important to be able to safely treat this patient?
a. Compassion.
b. Reassurance.
c. Excellent verbal and non-verbal communication.
d. Empathy.
e. All the above.

e. All the above.

What are your differential diagnoses?

- Meningococcal meningitis.
- Encephalitis.
- Encephalopathy.

References and further reading

Agata, E.D., Loeb, M.B. & Mitchell, S.L. (2013) Challenges in assessing nursing home residents with advanced dementia for suspected urinary tract infections. *Journal of the American Geriatrics Society*, 61(1): 62–66.

Ala'Aldeen, D.A., Oldfield, N.J., Bidmos, F.A. et al. (2011) Carriage of meningococci by university students, United Kingdom. *Emerging Infectious Diseases*, 17(9): 1762.

Alcohol and Drug Foundation (2020) Benzodiazepines. https://adf.org.au/drug-facts/benzodiazepines/ (accessed 30 June 2020).

Alcohol.org (2020) Alcohol and seizures. https://www.alcohol.org/effects/epilepsy-and-seizures/ (accessed 30 June 2020).

Avner, J.R. (2006) Altered states of consciousness. *Pediatrics in Review*, 27(9): 331.

Balestreri, M., Czosnyka, M., Hutchinson, P. et al. (2006) Impact of intracranial pressure and cerebral perfusion pressure on severe disability and mortality after head injury. *Neurocritical Care*, 4(1): 8–13.

Brain Foundation (2020) Subarachnoid haemorrhage. https://brainfoundation.org.au/disorders/subarachnoid-haemorrhage/ (accessed 30 June 2020).

Cahill, J. & Zhang, J.H. (2009) Subarachnoid hemorrhage: Is it time for a new direction? *Stroke*, 40(3, suppl 1): S86–S87.

Dementia Australia (2015) Delirium and dementia. https://www.dementia.org.au/files/helpsheets/Helpsheet-Dementia QandA21_Delirium_english.pdf (accessed 30 June 2020).

Dementia Australia (2020) What is dementia? https://www.dementia.org.au/about-dementia/what-is-dementia (accessed 30 June 2020).

Department of Health (2020) Meningococcal disease. https://www.health.gov.au/health-topics/meningococcal-disease (accessed 2 July 2020).

Fick, D., Kolanowski, A., Waller, J., & Maclean, R. (2002) Dementia and delirium: Prevalence and resource utilization. *Gerontologist*, 42: 14–14.

Harvard Health Online (2018) Subarachnoid hemorrage. https://www.health.harvard.edu/a_to_z/subarachnoid-hemorrhage-a-to-z (accessed 30 June 2020).

Kim, S., McNames, J. & Goldstein, B. (2006) Intracranial pressure variation associated with changes in end-tidal CO_2. In *2006 International Conference of the IEEE Engineering in Medicine and Biology Society*. New York: IEEE, pp. 9–12.

Lawton, M.T. & Vates, G.E. (2017) Subarachnoid hemorrhage. *New England Journal of Medicine*, 377(3): 257–266.

Melillo, K.D. (1991) Mnemonics: Use in gerontological nursing practice. *Journal of Gerontological Nursing*, 17(7): 40–43.

Möhler, H., Fritschy, J.M. & Rudolph, U. (2002) A new benzodiazepine pharmacology. *Journal of Pharmacology and Experimental Therapeutics*, 300(1): 2–8.

Nagel, F.W., Ezeoke, I., Antwi, M. et al. (2016) Delayed recognition of fatal invasive meningococcal disease in adults. *JMM Case Reports*, 3(3): e005027. doi: 10.1099/jmmcr.0.005027

Nimmo, G., Howie, A. & Grant, I. (2009) Effects of mechanical ventilation on Cushing's triad. *Critical Care*, 13(suppl 1): P77.

Nor, A.M., McAllister, C., Louw, S.J. et al. (2004) Agreement between ambulance paramedic- and physician-recorded neurological signs with Face Arm Speech Test (FAST) in acute stroke patients. *Stroke*, 35(6): 1355–1359.

Panuganti, K.K. & Dulebohn, S.C. (2017) Transient ischemic attack. In *StatPearls*. Treasure Island, FL: StatPearls Publishing.

Pathan, N., Faust, S.N. & Levin, M. (2003) Pathophysiology of meningococcal meningitis and septicaemia. *Archives of Disease in Childhood*, 88(7): 601–607.

Perth Children's Hospital (2017) Status epilepticus. https://pch.health.wa.gov.au/For-health-professionals/Emergency-Department-Guidelines/Status-epilepticus (accessed 30 June 2020).

Pinto, V.L. & Adeyinka, A. (2019). Increased intracranial pressure. *StatPearls*. Treasure Island, FL: StatPearls Publishing.

Rangel-Castilla, L., Lara, L.R., Gopinath, S. et al. (2010) Cerebral hemodynamic effects of acute hyperoxia and hyperventilation after severe traumatic brain injury. *Journal of Neurotrauma*, 27(10): 1853–1863.

Robertsson, B., Blennow, K., Gottfries, C.G. & Wallin, A. (1998) Delirium in dementia. *International Journal of Geriatric Psychiatry*, 13(1): 49–56.

Rockwood, K., Cosway, S., Carver, D. et al. (1999) The risk of dementia and death after delirium. *Age and Ageing*, 28(6): 551–556.

Samokhvalov, A.V., Irving, H., Mohapatra, S. & Rehm, J. (2010) Alcohol consumption, unprovoked seizures, and epilepsy: A systematic review and meta-analysis. *Epilepsia*, 51(7): 1177–1184.

Sanders, M.J., Lewis, L.M. & Quick, G. (2012) *Mosby's Paramedic Textbook*. Boston, MA: Jones & Bartlett.

Shields, A. & Flin, R. (2013) Paramedics' non-technical skills: A literature review. *Emergency Medicine Journal*, 30(5): 350–354.

Stephen, K.N., Hauser, W.A., Brust, J.C. & Susser, M. (1988) Alcohol consumption and withdrawal in new-onset seizures. *New England Journal of Medicine*, 319(11): 666–673.

Stephens, D.S., Greenwood, B. & Brandtzaeg, P. (2007) Epidemic meningitis, meningococcaemia, and Neisseria meningitidis. *The Lancet*, 369(9580): 2196–2210.

Stroke Foundation (2020) Transient ischaemic attack (TIA). https://strokefoundation.org.au/About-Stroke/Types-of-stroke/Transient-Ischaemic-Attack-TIA (accessed 30 June 2020).

Suarez, J.I., Tarr, R.W. & Selman, W.R. (2006) Aneurysmal subarachnoid hemorrhage. *New England Journal of Medicine*, 354(4): 387–396.

Taussky, P. (2008) Outcome after acute traumatic subdural and epidural hematoma in Switzerland: A single center experience. *Swiss Medical Weekly*, 138(19–20): 281–285.

Thomas, K.E., Hasbun, R., Jekel, J. & Quagliarello, V.J. (2002) The diagnostic accuracy of Kernig's sign, Brudzinski's sign, and nuchal rigidity in adults with suspected meningitis. *Clinical Infectious Diseases*, 35(1): 46–52.

Vroomen, P.C., Buddingh, M.K., Luijckx, G.J. & De Keyser, J. (2008) The incidence of stroke mimics among stroke department admissions in relation to age group. *Journal of Stroke and Cerebrovascular Diseases*, 17(6): 418–422.

Chapter 4

Abdominal emergencies

Tania Johnston[1] and Mark Hobson[2]

[1] Lecturer in Paramedicine, Charles Sturt University, Bathurst, NSW, Australia

[2] South Central Ambulance Service NHS Foundation Trust, Bicester, UK

CHAPTER CONTENTS

LEVEL 1 CASE STUDY
Acute appendicitis

Information type	Data
Time of origin	11:20
Time of dispatch	11:27
On-scene time	11:52
Day of the week	Saturday
Nearest hospital	25 minutes
Nearest backup	Intensive care crew, 15 minutes
Patient details	Name: Jane Ayre
	DOB: 01/09/2000

CASE

You have been called to a yoga studio for a 20-year-old female who is having abdominal pain. The caller states the patient began vomiting during the session and is in a lot of pain.

Pre-arrival information

The patient is conscious and breathing.

Windscreen report

The yoga studio is in a converted warehouse and situated on the second floor of a building with no lift. You can see that there are multiple people in the studio attending classes. There are no apparent hazards.

Entering the location

There is a small group of young women waiting for the ambulance at the entrance to the building. They are anxious and want you to hurry upstairs. On the way up they tell you that the patient was feeling unwell this morning with some nausea.

On arrival with the patient

The female patient is lying on her side on a yoga mat with the instructor sitting next to her. There is evidence that she vomited into a plastic bag.

Patient assessment triangle

General appearance

The patient is alert and crying

Circulation to the skin

Moderately pale.

Work of breathing

No evidence of shortness of breath.

SYSTEMATIC APPROACH

Danger

Nil.

Response

Alert on the AVPU scale.

Airway

Clear, recently vomited.

Breathing

Rate: 14 bpm. Effort: no increased effort. Accessory muscle use: no. Auscultation: clear air entry throughout.

Circulation

Heart rate: 108 bpm. Strength: strong. Heart regularity: regular. Capillary refill time: 2 seconds, pale.

Vital signs

RR: 14 bpm

HR: 108 bpm

BP: 132/76 mmHg

SpO_2: 99%

Blood sugar: 4.3 mmol/L

Temperature: 38.2 °C

Lead II ECG: sinus tachycardia

Exposure

9/10 right lower quadrant (RLQ) abdominal pain described as stabbing and coming in waves with nausea/vomiting. Pain present at McBurney's point between the umbilicus and iliac crest. She also has an increase in RLQ pain when the left is palpated, suggesting a positive Rovsing's sign.

TASK

Look through the information provided in this case study and highlight all of the information that might concern you as a paramedic.

Using what you currently know about the case at this point, including what you may have seen and how the patient is presenting to you, which vital signs and assessment should you prioritise?

The airway is clear and the patient is not short of breath, so SpO_2 is not an immediate priority, though it can be used to assist with determining the pulse rate. As the patient is pale, it would be important to assess circulation with a heart rate and blood pressure reading. A temperature is also useful to help with differential diagnoses of abdominal pain and to identify if the patient may have an infection. The paramedic will prioritise a focused abdominal exam, including inspection, auscultation, palpation and percussion. It is important to look for red flags that can indicate a life-threatening emergency while assessing the PQRST of the pain (provocation, quality, radiation, severity, time).

Once you have undertaken the essential vital signs and performed a general and focused assessment, what would your next action be?

The patient is experiencing severe pain and vomiting. The paramedic would initiate IV access in order to provide pain relief and to give an anti-emetic. Analgesia options can include one or more doses of morphine 2.5–5 mg IV/IM or fentanyl 25–50 µg IV. Anti-emetic options can include ondansetron 4 mg IV/PO/SL or metoclopramide 10 mg IV/IM. If no allergies or contraindications are present, medications can be given IM. The patient requires transport for investigations and a surgical consultation.

In order to determine what might be causing her abdominal pain, you will need to develop a good rapport with this patient. What are some of the potential barriers that could make it challenging to obtain a thorough history?

- The type of pain – there are many different potential causes of abdominal pain, making it more difficult to determine what the underlying problem is.
- Her age – it can be difficult to ask sensitive questions that will help to determine, for example, if the abdominal pain is related to obstetric/gynaecological issues or sexually transmitted infections.
- The scene – there are quite a few people around, including her friends. This can make it difficult to obtain a history while maintaining confidentiality.
- Her current pain score – she is in a lot of discomfort and may be too distracted to answer questions.

Case Progression

You have inserted an IV and after clarifying that the patient has no allergies, you administered 2.5 mg morphine IV and 4 mg ondansetron IV.

Patient assessment triangle:
General appearance
The patient is alert and calm.

Circulation to the skin
Moderately pale.

Work of breathing
No evidence of shortness of breath.

SYSTEMATIC APPROACH
Danger
Nil.

Response
Alert on the AVPU scale.

Airway
Clear, nausea has decreased.

Breathing

Rate: 14 bpm. Effort: no increased effort. Accessory muscle use: no. Auscultation: clear air entry throughout on auscultation.

Circulation

Heart rate: 92 bpm. Strength: strong. Heart regularity: regular. Capillary refill time: 2 seconds, pale.

Vital signs

RR: 14 bpm

HR: 92 bpm

BP: 110/68 mmHg

SpO_2: 99%

Blood sugar: 4.3 mmol/L

Temperature: 38.2 °C

Lead II ECG: sinus rhythm

Exposure

4/10 RLQ abdominal pain described as a dull ache. Pain remains at McBurney's point between the umbilicus and iliac crest.

What questions would you ask this patient specifically related to appendicitis as part of the history-taking process?

See Table 4.1.

Table 4.1 History-taking questions

Appendicitis

Did the pain originate anywhere else (i.e. periumbilicus) before it moved to the RLQ?

When did the pain start and have you had this pain before?

Is the pain constant or does it come and go?

Did you develop vomiting before or after the pain started?

Is there any chance you could be pregnant?

When was your last period and was it normal?

Have you had normal bowel motion and normal urination?

Medication history

Do you take any medications?

Have you taken anything for pain or nausea?

F/SH (family and social history)

Do you drink alcohol? If so, how much and how often?

Do you use recreational substances?

Who do you live with?

Past medical history (PMH)

Do you have any past medical conditions?

Have you had any abdominal surgery, including having your appendix removed?

Differential diagnosis (DDx) – what else could this be?

Ovarian cyst

Ectopic pregnancy

Cholecystitis (gallstones)

Urinary tract infection

Your patient appears more comfortable now and asks you if you know with certainty that she is having an episode of acute appendicitis.

It is not possible to diagnose appendicitis in the out-of-hospital environment. There are many differential diagnoses associated with abdominal pain and the patient will require further investigations in the Emergency Department before a diagnosis can be made. This includes but is not limited to urinalysis (including pregnancy test), blood work (including WBC), and abdominal CT or ultrasound. The patient will also likely receive a surgical consultation.

LEVEL 1 CASE STUDY
Gastroenteritis

Information type	Data
Time of origin	16:42
Time of dispatch	16:50
On-scene time	16:58
Day of the week	Friday
Nearest hospital	20 minutes
Nearest backup	25 minutes
Patient details	Name: Cassandra Johnson
	DOB: 07/09/1934

CASE
You have been called to a residential care home to see an 86-year-old female who has been vomiting all day. The call has originated from care staff on duty.

Pre-arrival information
The patient is conscious and breathing.

Windscreen report
You park up outside the residential care home and a care staff member opens the front door to greet you.

Entering the location
You are shown through the building and head upstairs to the patient's bedroom. The carer hands you a care file containing a summary of the patient's care needs, past medical history and medication administration sheet.

On arrival with the patient
An elderly female patient is sitting upright in bed with a carer by her side. The patient smiles and thanks you for coming to see her as you enter the room.

Patient assessment triangle
General appearance
Looks well and does not appear to be in pain.

Circulation to the skin
Well-perfused pink skin colour.

Work of breathing
Normal work of breathing.

SYSTEMATIC APPROACH
Danger
Infection prevention control risk, but not a dangerous scene.

Response
The patient is alert and fully orientated.

Airway
Clear, but has been vomiting.

Breathing
Rate: 16 bpm. Effort: no increased effort. Accessory muscle use: no. Auscultation: clear air entry throughout on auscultation.

Circulation
Heart rate: 64 bpm. Strength: strong radial pulse palpable. Heart regularity: regular. Capillary refill time: 2 seconds, good colour.

Vital signs
RR: 16 bpm
HR: 64 bpm
BP: 140/76 mmHg
SpO_2: 98%
Blood sugar: 6.1 mmol/L
Temperature: 37.8 °C
Lead II ECG: normal sinus rhythm

Exposure
Elderly woman with a normal BMI. There are no scars or skin signs on the abdomen. The abdomen is not distended.

TASK
Look through the information provided in this case study and highlight all of the information that might concern you as a paramedic.

Using what you currently know about the case at this point, including what you may have seen and how the patient is presenting to you, what questions will you ask the patient and carers during your history taking?

The airway, breathing, circulation and disability are all normal and the patient does not appear to be in a 'time-critical' condition, therefore there is time to take a thorough patient history. It is important to focus questions on establishing the patient's hydration and nutritional status and to identify any medical conditions and medications that can affect hydration and electrolyte balance. Also note any risk factors for acquiring gastroenteritis and for requiring hospital admission (Table 4.2).

What physical examination findings should you look for to assess the patient's hydration status?

The hands, arms, face and neck all contain helpful clues in examining for dehydration or hypovolaemia (Table 4.3). An easy method of remembering this is to start by examining the face, then find the jugular venous pressure (JVP) in the neck, then move downwards to the arms, testing blood pressure (including standing the patient, which would affect your JVP measurement if not performed in this order), then finally examine the hands.

Very few examination findings are entirely accurate and they are highly variable in specificity and sensitivity. Therefore it is important to examine the patient thoroughly by not relying on any single physical sign and to use all your findings together to guide your judgement.

Table 4.2 Focused history taking in gastroenteritis

Hydration and nutritional status
Frequency and amount of vomiting
Frequency and amount of diarrhoea
Both overweight and underweight patients are at increased risk of hospital admission
Fevers and sweating increase fluid loss
Colour, quantity and frequency of urine output
Is there thirst and are they able to drink without vomiting?
Postural lightheadedness indicates fluid depletion

Risk factors for acquiring gastroenteritis
Living in residential care
Inadequate handwashing
Contact with other people suffering from gastroenteritis
Diet that includes chicken, seafood or eggs

Risk factors for requiring hospital admission
Need for hospital admission closely linked to increasing age in the elderly
Overweight and underweight patients also have higher incidence of hospital admission
Heart and renal failure both affect the body's fluid balance – is the patient on a fluid restriction for either of these?
Does the patient have any chronic bowel disorders or invasive enteric organisms such as *Clostridium difficile*?
Is there a history of immunosuppression by cancer, HIV, long-term steroid use or systemic lupus erythematosus?

Table 4.3 Examining the patient to establish hydration status

Face
Sunken or withdrawn eyes and dry mouth and dry mucosal membranes should be observed. Pale conjunctivae are associated with anaemia.

Neck
JVP should be less than 3 cm above the sternal angle when the patient is laid at a 45° angle. The presence of reduced JVP is linked to hypovolaemia.

Arms/postural blood pressure
Take lying and standing blood pressure – a systolic drop greater than 20 mmHg after standing indicates postural hypotension. The systolic blood pressure should be found, then the cuff rapidly deflated. Then inflate the cuff again to re-find the systolic reading. This can be repeated to 'track' the systolic blood pressure constantly to ensure a drop in pressure is not missed. Many medications (not limited to antihypertensives) can also cause a postural blood pressure drop.

Hands
Peripheral and central capillary refill time.
Skin temperature, warm or cool peripheries.
Noting reduced skin turgor is useful, but this is less reliable in elderly patients as the skin ages.

To ensure that you are assessing the patient comprehensively, you decide to perform a urine dip test/urinalysis. How could this test the patient's hydration status and what other conditions could it help to detect?

Performing a urine dip test or urinalysis would be beneficial. Before a urine sample is tested, the clinician should note the colour, transparency and volume, as well as looking for visible (macroscopic) blood, sedimentation and froth, which could indicate proteinuria.

On the test strip, the urine specific gravity (SG) tells us the concentration of urine. A low SG tells us that the urine has a density close to that of water and therefore the patient likely has enough water within the body. An acidic urine pH is associated with dehydration, metabolic activity and renal tubular acidosis. The presence of ketones in urine warrants hospitalisation, as it indicates that the body is breaking down muscle mass for hydration and nutrition. A by-product of muscle breakdown is ketones, which are excreted via the renal system. Proteinuria can indicate kidney disease, acute kidney injury or pre-eclampsia in pregnant women. Nitrites and leukocytes are seen in urinary tract infections (UTIs); however, a common diagnostic pitfall is that these are often present even in the absence of a UTI, and therefore should not be used to diagnose a UTI in the absence of urinary symptoms. Glucose indicates diabetes or poorly controlled diabetes. A positive test for blood can indicate either haematuria or myoglobinuria from muscle breakdown or rhabdomyolysis. Blood could also indicate kidney stones or malignancy.

Case Progression

You have finished your patient history taking, physical examination and bedside testing. Your findings are as follows.

History taking
Following 5–6 episodes of vomiting since the early hours of the morning, the quantity of vomit has reduced but the patient remains nauseous. She also reports passing three episodes of watery stools this morning, of a moderate quantity each time. Describes 'cramping' generalised abdominal discomfort prior to passing stools, which is relieved by passing stools. No PR bleeding, no haematemesis, non-bilious vomiting. Has been able to drink approximately 50 mL of water at a time and has drank 600 mL since a new 1 L jug was placed at the bedside at 08:00. Has passed urine twice throughout the day and then a third time to provide a urine sample. Low-grade fever, but not sweating and no rigors. Complains of mild thirst.

No history of colitis, diverticula disease, cancer or immunosuppression, no cardiac or renal failure and is not diabetic. She has severe osteoarthritis and a malunion of a complex neck of femur fracture has left her with poor mobility. She was thereafter unable to cope at home after the death of her husband and this led to her move into residential care. She also has stable type 2 diabetes mellitus. One other resident has been unwell with similar symptoms this week and one carer phoned in unwell yesterday. Medications are metformin, enalapril, codeine phosphate and paracetamol.

Examination findings
Eyes are not sunken. No conjunctival pallor. JVP is 3 cm above the sternal angle. Mouth and mucosal membranes are not dry. There is a postural blood pressure drop of 6 mmHg, which is asymptomatic. Capillary refill time of 2 seconds. Hands are warm to touch. Skin turgor is slow, but the skin is a good colour, slightly shiny and not papery or dry appearing.

Normal BMI. There are no scars or skin signs on the abdomen. The abdomen is not distended. Bowel sounds are present. The abdomen is soft and non-tender to palpation. Flanks are non-tender.

Vital signs
RR: 16 bpm
HR: 58 bpm
BP (supine): 148/82 mmHg
BP (standing): 142/76 mmHg
SpO$_2$: 98%
Blood sugar: 6.1 mmol/L
Temperature: 37.8 °C
Lead II ECG: normal sinus rhythm

Urinalysis
Urine is straw coloured and clear. No sediment. No visible blood.
Specific gravity: 1.005 (1.000–1.025)
pH: 6.0 (5.0–9.0)
Glucose: neg
Ketones: neg
Protein: neg
Blood: neg
Nitrites: neg
Leukocytes: neg

What is your management plan for this patient?

The patient is elderly and living in residential care, is thirsty and has some poor skin turgor. However, by evaluating the rest of the clinical assessment and weighing up the findings as a whole, this patient does not require hospital admission at present. If the patient's vomiting is persisting, an anti-emetic could be administered and an anti-diarrheal such as loperamide obtained from the local pharmacy. All staff, residents and visitors to the care home must follow hand-washing procedures at all times and should be reminded of the importance of this.

The patient, carers and family should be counselled so that they are aware of the 'red flags' to watch out for. Dehydration red flags should include inability to drink, unquenchable thirst, persisting vomiting or diarrhoea for more than 48 hours, low urine output, dark urine colour, lightheadedness when standing and carer or familial concern. Sepsis red flags should also be given, to include severe abdominal pain, breathlessness, rapid heart rate, lightheadedness, high fever and rigors.

You should also be sure that the care staff have the ability and willingness to cope with her illness. The patient's primary care doctor should be informed of your visit and it is good practice to refer the patient's care back to him or her directly to allow a handover of your clinical findings to take place.

As part of your management plan, you telephone the patient's primary care doctor. The doctor kindly provides you with some medical teaching and asks you which of the patient's prescribed medications he should temporarily withhold to prevent an acute kidney injury (AKI).

How would you answer the doctor's question?

If this patient were to deteriorate in the community, then it would most likely be due to dehydration and an associated AKI. An AKI can be exacerbated or even caused by angiotensin-converting enzyme inhibitors due to their effect on normal renal haemodynamics. Metformin should also be withheld for two reasons: first, it predisposes patients with reduced fluid volume to an AKI; second, it can induce metformin lactic acidosis, which can in itself be life threatening. The patient's codeine is likely to prevent diarrhoea to some extent and her paracetamol should be effective in treating the low-grade fever. Of course, all prescribed medications should be discussed with a doctor prior to advising a patient to stop them.

Other medications at risk for causing AKI can be remembered by the mnemonic DAMN: Diuretics, Angiotensin-converting enzyme inhibitors/angiotensin II receptor blockers (ACEi/ARBs), metformin and non-steroidal anti-inflammatory drugs (NSAIDs).

LEVEL 2 CASE STUDY
Ectopic pregnancy

Information type	Data
Time of origin	15:00
Time of dispatch	15:40
On-scene time	15:51
Day of the week	Thursday
Nearest hospital	15 minutes
Nearest backup	Intensive care paramedic crew, 5 minutes
Patient details	Name: Julie Bishops DOB: 12/08/1985

CASE
You have been called to a local bank where a 35-year-old female has had a syncopal episode and is now complaining of abdominal pain.

Pre-arrival information
The patient is conscious and breathing and in the staff lunchroom with her supervisor, who knows first aid.

Windscreen report

You can park your ambulance outside the bank, which is on a busy metro street. There are no apparent dangers.

Entering the location

The bank is busy with a large number of customers and you are led by an administrative assistant to the rear of the main floor, where there is a small staff lunchroom. You find the patient lying on the floor, her feet elevated on a chair. The supervisor tells you that the patient had been complaining of right-sided abdominal pain for the last few hours, but didn't want to say anything since she is new to her position. Approximately 10 minutes ago she had a fainting episode while behind the counter, lasting 10 seconds. When she awoke, the staff assisted her to the lunchroom, where they laid her on the floor with her feet elevated.

On arrival with the patient

The patient is awake and in discomfort, with her hands placed on her lower abdomen. She weighs approximately 55 kg. She reports one episode of vomiting. Her abdominal pain has been steady and she is in obvious discomfort.

Patient assessment triangle

General appearance

The patient is alert and in moderate discomfort with abdominal pain.

Circulation to the skin

Slightly pale.

Work of breathing

No evidence of shortness of breath.

SYSTEMATIC APPROACH

Danger

Nil.

Response

Alert on the AVPU scale.

Airway

Clear.

Breathing

Rate: 18 bpm. Effort: no increased effort. Accessory muscle use: no. Auscultation: clear air entry throughout on auscultation.

Circulation

Heart rate: 108 bpm. Heart regularity: regular. Radial pulses strong bilaterally. Capillary refill time: 2 seconds.

Vital signs

RR: 18 bpm

HR: 108 bpm

BP: 104/60 mmHg

SpO_2: 99%

Blood sugar: 5.2 mmol/L

Temperature: 37.1 °C

Lead II ECG: sinus tachycardia

Exposure

6/10 dull right lower abdominal pain, non-radiating.

TASK

Look through the information provided in this case study and highlight all of the information that might concern you as a paramedic.

You now have a brief history of events and some assessment findings. There are a number of possible differential diagnoses for a female patient of maternal age with RLQ pain, including ectopic pregnancy. Knowing the risk factors for ectopic pregnancy is useful to assist in determining a working diagnosis.

What are the risk factors associated with ectopic pregnancy?

Maternal age 35–44, history of tubal surgery, previous ectopic pregnancy, history of pelvic inflammatory disease, history of sexually transmitted infections, current use of intrauterine device (IUD), assisted reproductive techniques, smoking, prior pharmacologically induced abortion.

Once you have undertaken the essential vital signs and performed a general and focused assessment, what would your next action be?

The patient is in significant discomfort, but is presenting stable at this point. You will want to complete a thorough history as well as initiate a treatment plan to address her symptoms. You would initiate IV access to give medications and, if needed, to give IV fluids. It would be important to administer analgesia such as an opioid (morphine or fentanyl) to help manage her pain. You would also want to address the vomiting with an anti-emetic such as ondansetron.

In addition to questions related to risk factors, what questions would you ask this patient specifically related to abdominal pain and possible ectopic pregnancy?

See Table 4.4.

Table 4.4 History-taking questions

Ectopic pregnancy
When did the pain start, and have you had this pain before?
Was it a sudden or gradual onset?
Can you specifically describe the nature of the pain?
Does it move anywhere else?
Is the pain constant or does it come and go?

Medication history
Do you take any medications?
Specifically, are you taking contraceptives, including the use of an IUD?

F/SH (family and social history)
Do you drink alcohol? If so, how much and how often?
Do you use recreational substances?
Do you smoke?

Past medical history (PMH)
Do you have any past medical conditions?
Is there a possibility you could be pregnant?
When was your last normal menstrual period? Have you missed a period?
How would you describe your menses? Heavy, normal, light?
Have you had any previous pregnancies? Pregnancy problems or abortions?
Have you had any abdominal surgery?

Differential diagnosis (DDx) – what else could this be?
Appendicitis
Renal colic
Ovarian cyst
Crohn's disease

You continue to question the patient to develop and explore a list of differential diagnoses. The signs and symptoms of an ectopic pregnancy are highly variable and in many cases the vital signs can be completely normal.

Assuming you suspect an ectopic pregnancy, what is your primary concern regarding the possible progression of this condition?

The ectopic pregnancy may progress to a ruptured ectopic, with the risk of internal bleeding and hypovolaemic shock.

Case Progression

Your partner is organising the cot and preparing for extrication. You have inserted an IV and after clarifying that the patient has no allergies, you prepare to administer analgesia. Approximately 10 minutes after your arrival, the patient experiences a sudden worsening of pain in the RLQ and appears in severe distress due to the pain.

Patient assessment triangle
General appearance
The patient is alert and now has severe distress with pain.

Circulation to the skin
Slightly pale.

Work of breathing
No evidence of shortness of breath.

SYSTEMATIC APPROACH
Danger
Nil.

Response
Alert on the AVPU scale, but anxious.

Airway
Clear.

Breathing
Rate: 22 bpm. Effort: no increased effort. Accessory muscle use: no. Auscultation: clear air entry throughout on auscultation.

Circulation
Heart rate: 122 bpm. Heart regularity: regular. Radial pulses strong bilaterally. Capillary refill time: 2 seconds.

Vital signs
RR: 22 bpm
HR: 122 bpm
BP: 102/58 mmHg
SpO$_2$: 98% on room air
Temperature: 37.1 °C
Lead II ECG: sinus tachycardia

Exposure
10/10 sharp right lower abdominal pain, now radiating to the right shoulder tip.

Though you can't be certain without further investigations (i.e. beta-hCG serum blood test and pelvic ultrasound), you suspect that the patient may have progressed to a ruptured ectopic pregnancy.

What would your treatment priority be at this time?

You would prioritise rapid transport to the nearest hospital. It would still be important to treat the patient's pain, keeping in mind that she may have the potential for shock. If she does develop shock, you would follow your medical control guidelines to administer a bolus of isotonic crystalloid IV fluid, such as normal saline or lactated Ringer's. You would also treat for shock using basic measures such as oxygen, posturing and keeping the patient warm.

For many women, experiencing an ectopic pregnancy represents the loss of a pregnancy much like a miscarriage. This can elicit feelings of loss and sadness.

As a paramedic, you are taking measures to provide the necessary emergency care. How would you also address the emotional needs of this patient?

As appropriate to the specific situation, you would determine if the patient was experiencing an emotional response and, if so, acknowledge the situation. You would attempt to validate the patient's feelings and demonstrate empathy towards her. You would be sensitive in your approach and try to provide as much information as possible. Since she is alone in her workplace, you could facilitate contacting someone to support her and perhaps ask if she wants a co-worker to accompany her to the hospital.

LEVEL 2 CASE STUDY
Portal hypertension

Information type	Data
Time of origin	11:09
Time of dispatch	11:12
On-scene time	11:50
Day of the week	Tuesday
Nearest hospital	50 minutes
Nearest backup	Air ambulance service response car, parked at the nearest hospital, 50 minutes
Patient details	Name: Geoff Winehead DOB: 04/10/1960

CASE

You have been called to a hostel to a 60-year-old male who is a high-frequency user of your ambulance service. Normally your visits are due to alcohol abuse and he has shown aggression towards you in the past. The hostel where he lives is rural and out of town.

Pre-arrival information

The patient is unconscious and breathing. There is some vague information suggesting bleeding.

Windscreen report

The building is in a state of disrepair. There are people loitering and drinking alcohol in an overgrown front garden who glance at you as you arrive. They don't approach you and appear disinterested in your arrival.

Entering the location

You call inside the building and there is no reply. You enter and walk along a corridor to the patient's room, which you remember from prior visits.

On arrival with the patient

You recognise the patient, who is sitting upright with his back against a wall. A bucket between his legs contains at least one litre of red blood. There are further bloodstains on the floor. You attach automatic monitoring to the patient as you perform the patient assessment triangle.

Patient assessment triangle
General appearance
Drowsy and weak appearance.

Circulation to the skin
Grey colour and sweating profusely.

Work of breathing
Increased respiratory rate, but not laboured.

SYSTEMATIC APPROACH

Danger
Bodily fluids splash risk. Alcohol intoxication in other residents and prior aggression at the same address.

Response
The patient is drowsy, but responds to your voice.

Airway
Clear, has been vomiting blood.

Breathing
Rate: 26 bpm. Effort: no increased effort. Accessory muscle use: no. Auscultation: clear air entry throughout on auscultation.

Circulation
Heart rate: 160 bpm. Strength: no radial pulse palpable, weak carotid pulse. Heart regularity: regular. Capillary refill time: 6 seconds, very pale.

Vital signs
RR: 26 bpm
HR: 160 bpm
Automatic BP: 244/160 mmHg
SpO$_2$: 93%
Blood sugar: 8.1 mmol/L
Temperature: 34.8 °C
Lead II ECG: sinus tachycardia

Exposure
Thin-appearing male with little body fat or muscle mass; the ribcage is easily visible. Abdomen is large, distended with periumbilical bruising; other small bruising exists on the patient's limbs. No jaundice.

TASK
Look through the information provided in this case study and highlight all of the information that might concern you as a paramedic.

Using what you currently know about the case at this point, including what you may have seen and how the patient is presenting to you, what do the vital signs and assessment findings indicate?

The airway is clear, although the patient could be at risk from vomiting, particularly as he is drowsy. Increased breathing effort appears to be a compensatory mechanism. Circulatory assessment and obvious blood loss appear to point towards hypovolaemic shock. However, the blood pressure reads very high, which confuses the presentation. The patient has a decreased conscious level and reduced temperature, which are symptoms of clinical shock.

You know that your patient is critically ill with hypovolaemic shock that can only be stopped by a surgeon.

Considering your location, what will your next actions be?

You realise that time is critical here and ask your crewmate to fetch the stretcher immediately. While your crewmate is returning, you apply oxygen titrated to hold the SpO$_2$ at normal oxygen levels and lay the patient on his side flat on the floor to improve blood pressure. Then you prioritise inserting a large-bore IV line. It is vital not to be misled by the fallibility of automatic monitoring that can occur with any patient, but is more common at the extremes of monitoring ranges and with irregular heartbeats. Using a manual sphygmomanometer you hear faint Korotkoff sounds begin at 62 mmHg and discount the automatic reading.

You are a great distance from both the nearest hospital and backup. However, you contact ambulance control requesting backup from the air ambulance car. Arranging to rendezvous with the air ambulance car at a location halfway between your locations is usually feasible and will halve the timeframe to receive critical care backup. Most air ambulance services carry packed red blood cells and/or fresh frozen plasma, which will be of great benefit to this patient, but it is equally important not to wait on scene for it in this situation.

You leave the scene and administer 250 mL boluses of sodium chloride 0.9% while allowing the patient to be permissively hypotensive at 90 mmHg systolic. Removing clothing saturated with sweat and wrapping in dry blankets will warm the patient, which will also prevent a coagulopathy developing. An anti-emetic could be considered to help protect the airway, but is unlikely to provide a mortality benefit.

How does alcoholism relate to the pathophysiology of gastrointestinal (GI) bleeding and what is this patient's long-term prognosis?

Alcohol abuse predisposes patients to a number of causes of GI bleeding, of which two are the most common. First, alcohol leads to gastric and duodenal ulceration, which is the commonest cause of serious GI bleeding. In all patients (including alcoholics) 50% of all upper GI bleeding will be caused by ulceration. Second, alcohol-related liver disease and ascites cause raised portal pressures within the hepatic venous system. At the gastro-oesophageal junction there are superficially positioned veins known as varices that are prone to rupture if their pressure gradients increase beyond their normally low tolerances of 5–8 mmHg. After rupture, venous bleeding into the gastro-oesophageal junction then ensues, depleting blood volume and causing life-threatening hypovolaemic shock. Liver failure also causes a reduction in blood platelets and clotting factors.

Alcoholic cirrhosis carries a 5-year survival of 90% if the patient manages to remain sober, but with drinking this falls to 60%. If jaundice, ascites or haematemesis occurs, then survival falls to 35% and the majority of fatalities occur within a year. The following risk factors increase the odds of re-bleeding after hospitalisation: old age, chronic liver disease, heart failure, ischaemic heart disease, renal disease, malignancy or a patient presenting with clinical shock.

Case Progression

After meeting with the air ambulance response car doctor and paramedic, you continue the journey to hospital. They administered packed red blood cells and fresh frozen plasma. The patient has vomited twice more after you administered ondansetron 4 mg IV.

Patient assessment triangle
General appearance
The patient remains drowsy and weak.

Circulation to the skin
Very pale.

Work of breathing
Mildly breathless.

SYSTEMATIC APPROACH
Danger
Nil.

Response
Voice on the AVPU scale.

Airway
Clear, nauseous.

Breathing
Rate: 24 bpm. Effort: no increased effort. Accessory muscle use: no. Auscultation: clear air entry throughout on auscultation.

Circulation
Heart rate: 156 bpm. Strength: weak radial pulse, strong carotid pulse. Heart regularity: regular. Capillary refill time: 5 seconds, pale.

Vital signs
RR: 24 bpm
HR: 156 bpm
BP: 86/38 mmHg
SoO_2: 95%
Blood sugar: 7.9 mmol/L
Temperature: 35.2 °C
Lead II ECG: sinus rhythm

Exposure
The skin is not jaundiced, but the eye sclera is yellowed. Striae are noted. The abdomen is distended, but non-tender to palpation. The liver is palpable. There is a fluid wave present with shifting areas of dullness when the patient rolls onto each side.

You reflect on previous visits to this patient for his alcoholism. What physical examination findings might you have found previously that could suggest advanced alcoholic liver disease? Also, what six Fs are causes of abdominal distension?

See Table 4.5.

Table 4.5 Examination findings suggestive of liver disease

Skin findings
Jaundice, pruritus, purpura, spider angiomas, telangiectasias, loss of muscle and fat bulk

Hand findings
Terry's nails, leukonychia, Muehrcke's lines, palmar erythema, hepatic flap (asterixis)

Abdominal findings
Palpable hypertrophic liver, fluid wave, shifting areas of percussive dullness

Six Fs causing abdominal distension
Fluid (ascites), foetus, flatus, faeces, fat, fatal tumour

You dislike this patient, he has been aggressive towards you in the past and you have heard of violence towards ambulance staff occurring at the hostel. You also feel that he uses the ambulance service too much. How can you prevent your feelings from having a negatively impact on his treatment?

Clearly, it would be completely unacceptable for any patient to receive substandard care because of your feelings, and it is important to understand that this patient's past negative behaviours are likely to be symptomatic of his alcoholism and socio-economic struggles. You have a professional relationship with this patient and your profession requires positive behaviours from you as a paramedic that are recognised by your registering body. However, it could be difficult to be professional when treating a patient who has previously been aggressive towards you. The situation is challenging, but can be much more difficult if other 'human factors' are present that increase psychological stress. Examples of these could be high workload, severity of situation, perceived consequences of your actions, environmental conditions, team support, fatigue and hunger. Human factors can usually be prevented or mitigated. This makes positive thinking in situations much easier. As a professional, it is vital that you 'rise above' any personal feelings you have towards a patient and a good attitude from you will go a long way towards preventing aggression occurring again.

LEVEL 3 CASE STUDY
Abdominal aortic aneurysm

Information type	Data
Time of origin	02:10
Time of dispatch	02:30
On-scene time	03:18
Day of the week	Sunday
Nearest hospital	45 minutes
Nearest backup	HEMS crew, 20 minutes
Patient details	Name: George Grewin
	DOB: 12/09/1942

CASE
You have been called to a rural property for a 78-year-old male with abdominal pain. The caller, the patient's wife, states the patient has high blood pressure and was seen by his family physician earlier today.

Pre-arrival information
The patient is conscious and breathing and reportedly 'changing colour'.

Windscreen report
The large property is remote and accessible by a 1 km long driveway. There is a two-storey farmhouse and a number of sheds in the yard. The wife is holding a phone and waving from the front door. Two large dogs are barking from a fenced enclosure.

Entering the location
You are led inside by the patient's wife, who is alone with her husband. She takes you upstairs in a house that is crowded with antique furniture and various collector's items cluttering every available surface. The wife is crying and tells you that they were at the doctor's earlier today to manage her husband's blood pressure. There is a walker at the entrance to the patient's bedroom.

On arrival with the patient
The male patient is supine and lying in the middle of a large bed. He is awake and in a significant amount of distress, moaning in pain. He weighs approximately 90 kg.

Patient assessment triangle
General appearance
The patient is alert, anxious and moaning in pain, and shifting positions on the bed.

Circulation to the skin
Significantly pale, evidence of diaphoresis.

Work of breathing
No evidence of shortness of breath.

SYSTEMATIC APPROACH
Danger
Nil.

Response
Alert on the AVPU scale, but anxious.

Airway
Clear.

Breathing
Rate: 20 bpm. Effort: no increased effort. Accessory muscle use: no. Auscultation: clear air entry throughout on auscultation.

Circulation
Heart rate: 62 bpm. Heart regularity: irregular. Radial pulses strong bilaterally. Capillary refill time: 2 seconds.

Vital signs
RR: 20 bpm
HR: 62 bpm
BP: 188/104 mmHg
SpO_2: 92%
Blood sugar: 11.7 mmol/L
Temperature: 36.3 °C
Lead II ECG: sinus rhythm with occasional PVCs

Exposure
10/10 lower abdominal pain radiating to left flank and hip described only as 'severe'. Patient unable to lay still for assessment. Left leg mottled and cool to touch.

TASK
Look through the information provided in this case study and highlight all of the information that might concern you as a paramedic.

Using what you currently know about the case at this point, including what you may have seen and how the patient is presenting to you, what additional vital signs and assessments would you want to perform?

The airway is clear and the patient is breathing, with no evidence of respiratory distress. With the pain description and location, it would be prudent to perform bilateral blood pressures, assess the quality of the patient's radial and pedal pulses bilaterally, and compare capillary refill time in each limb. The paramedic would carefully perform a focused abdominal exam to determine if the patient has evidence of a pulsatile mass and if bowel sounds are present and normal. It would also be important to explore whether the patient is having concurrent chest pain, as this will assist with differential diagnoses. The paramedic would also perform a 12 lead ECG.

Once you have undertaken the essential vital signs and performed a general and focused assessment, what would your next action be?

The patient is experiencing severe pain and is potentially very unstable. There are two priorities: determining a strategy to manage the patient's symptoms; and organising cautious yet swift extrication and rapid transport to the hospital. The key priority would be to decide how best to extricate the patient, ideally with additional assistance, and then to arrange rapid transport to a tertiary hospital where vascular surgery is available. You anticipate that extrication will be a challenge since the patient is unstable, weighs 90 kg, uses a walker, and you need to get him down the stairs. You also have to move him as cautiously as possible to avoid unnecessary movement.

You continue to question the patient to develop and explore a list of differential diagnoses and to help you understand your assessment findings.

What are your thoughts about the patient's heart rate? Is it consistent with his presentation? Is there something else you would check to assist you in your understanding?

He has a heart rate of 62 bpm (irregular with occasional PVCs). This is not consistent with his pain score of 10/10, anxiety and diaphoresis. It would be important to assess his 12 lead ECG findings to determine if he is in a dysrhythmia (i.e. heart block) or may be experiencing an acute coronary syndrome. The paramedic would also review his medication list to see if the patient is taking a betablocker for hypertension, as this would slow his heart rate and blunt a normal physiological response to pain and/or shock.

Case Progression

You have called the helicopter emergency medical service (HEMS) for transport and your partner is organising the stair chair to extricate the patient from the upstairs bedroom. You then insert an IV and, after clarifying that he has no allergies, you prepare to administer analgesia.

Patient assessment triangle

General appearance

The patient is alert, anxious and moaning in pain, continuing to shift position on the bed.

Circulation to the skin

Significantly pale, evidence of diaphoresis.

Work of breathing

No evidence of shortness of breath.

SYSTEMATIC APPROACH

Danger

Nil.

Response

Alert on the AVPU scale, but anxious.

Airway

Clear, but now complaining of nausea.

Breathing

Rate: 20 bpm. Effort: no increased effort. Accessory muscle use: no. Auscultation: clear air entry throughout on auscultation.

Circulation

Heart rate: 62 bpm. Heart regularity: irregular. Radial pulses strong bilaterally. Capillary refill time: 2 seconds.

Vital signs

RR: 20 bpm

HR: 62 bpm

BP: right arm 176/100 mmHg, left arm 180/99 mmHg

SpO$_2$: 95% on 2 L/min via nasal cannula

Blood sugar: 11.7 mmol/L
Temperature: 36.3 °C
Lead II ECG: sinus rhythm with occasional PVCs
12 Lead ECG: nil evidence of ST elevation or depression

Exposure
10/10 lower abdominal pain radiating to left flank described as 'tearing'. No obvious evidence of pulsatile mass. Patient unable to lie still for assessment. Strong radial pulses bilateral with equal capillary refill time (CRT) 2 seconds. Strong right pedal pulse, CRT 2 seconds; weak left pedal pulse, CRT 4 seconds. Left leg mottled and cool to touch.

What questions would you ask this patient specifically related to abdominal pain and possible complications associated with abdominal aortic aneurysm as part of the history-taking process?

See Table 4.6.

Table 4.6 History-taking questions

Aneurysm
When did the pain start and have you had this pain before?
Was it a sudden or gradual onset?
Can you specifically describe the nature of the pain?
Does it move anywhere else?
Is the pain constant or does it come and go?
Are you having any chest pain?
Did you 'pass out' or have a fainting episode?
Do you have any nausea or did you vomit with the pain?
Have you had normal bowel motion and normal urination?

Medication history
What was the change to your blood pressure medications?
Do you take any other medications?

F/SH (family and social history)
Do you drink alcohol? If so, how much and how often?
Do you use recreational substances?

Past medical history (PMH)
Do you have any past medical conditions?
Have you had any abdominal surgery?
Have you ever been assessed for an abdominal aneurysm? If yes, do you know the size?

Differential diagnosis (DDx) – what else could this be?
Thoracic aneurysm
Acute coronary syndrome (ACS)
Cholecystitis (gallstones)
Renal colic
Bowel obstruction

Case Progression

Your patient is in severe pain and you are suspicious that he may be experiencing complications associated with an abdominal aortic aneurysm, including possible dissection and/or extremity ischaemia secondary to an embolisation of a thrombus from within the aneurysm.

How would you manage his symptoms?

- Anxiety – provide reassurance, as this patient is potentially unstable. There is a very high mortality rate for patients who experience ruptured aneurysms in the out-of-hospital setting.
- Nausea – administer an anti-emetic (e.g. ondansetron 4 mg IV) to manage episodes of vomiting that might further aggravate a dissecting aneurysm.
- Pain – be aware of the haemodynamic effects of different analgesic options and administer them cautiously.
- Blood pressure – if in your scope of practice, consider the benefits of addressing the hypertension (e.g. GTN patch), but this needs to be balanced with the potential to lower it too fast or too much. If the patient was presenting with low to low normal blood pressure, then it would be reasonable to allow for permissive hypotension. Always follow your medical control guidelines.

There is a very high mortality rate for dissecting aneurysms that occur in the out-of-hospital setting. Knowing this, what would you communicate to either the patient and/or his wife?

It is not easy to acknowledge the seriousness of this situation and the potential of death if the aneurysm were to rupture. It would be important to broach the subject with the patient and his wife in some way to ensure that they are prepared for the seriousness of the situation. This may allow the wife to spend a few important minutes with her husband prior to transport. It may also facilitate a conversation around 'not for resuscitation', as the patient may have documented wishes in the event of a cardiac arrest.

LEVEL 3 CASE STUDY
Gallbladder and biliary obstruction

Information type	Data
Time of origin	02:06
Time of dispatch	02:10
On-scene time	02:22
Day of the week	Saturday
Nearest hospital	32 minutes
Nearest backup	Intensive care crew, 15 minutes
Patient details	Name: Davina Osborn DOB: 07/03/1977

CASE
You have been called to a wealthy residential address for a 43-year-old female who is restless with severe abdominal pains. She is forcefully vomiting and feels lightheaded.

Pre-arrival information
The patient is conscious and breathing.

Windscreen report
The upstairs lights are on at the address. An exterior light illuminates the driveway as the ambulance stops and you can see the front door has been left ajar.

Entering the location
The patient's husband welcomes you inside and shows you through to a small bathroom. He tells you that his wife often has short-duration abdominal pains after mealtimes, but never as severe as this.

On arrival with the patient
The female patient is changing her body position constantly, and she is clutching her upper abdomen. She is on her knees, leaning into a bathtub where there is a pool of green vomit.

Patient assessment triangle
General appearance
The patient is alert but restless.

Circulation to the skin
Moderately pale.

Work of breathing
Mildly increased respiratory rate.

SYSTEMATIC APPROACH
Danger
Bodily fluids splash risk.

Response
Alert on the AVPU scale.

Airway
Clear, violently vomiting.

Breathing
Rate: 24 bpm. Effort: no increased effort. Accessory muscle use: no. Auscultation: clear air entry throughout on auscultation.

Circulation
Heart rate: 138 bpm. Strength: weak. Heart regularity: regular. Capillary refill time: 4 seconds, pale.

Vital signs
RR: 24 bpm
HR: 138 bpm
BP: 74/48 mmHg
SpO$_2$: 95%
Blood sugar: 6.1 mmol/L
Temperature: 38.2 °C
Lead II ECG: sinus tachycardia

Exposure
9/10 right upper quadrant (RUQ) abdominal pain. The pain has been gradually increasing throughout the night from shortly after eating her evening meal. Pain is focused between the RUQ and epigastrium, radiating through to her back. The patient has a raised BMI.

TASK
Look through the information provided in this case study and highlight all of the information that might concern you as a paramedic.

Using what you currently know about the case at this point, including what you may have seen and how the patient is presenting to you, which vital signs and assessment should you undertake next?

The airway is clear and although the respiratory rate is raised, the patient's respiratory system is not unstable. The patient is pale, so it is important to assess circulation and then attempt to identify the cause of clinical shock. Checking the temperature will help to identify if an infection is the cause; however, it is important to remember that life-threatening sepsis can occur with unremarkable temperature readings. It will be difficult to gain the patient's cooperation to perform a thorough abdominal examination because of her persistent vomiting and constant pain. The increased respiratory and heart rate, low blood pressure and fever should help you recognise her septic shock.

Once you have undertaken the essential vital signs and performed a general and focused assessment, what would your next action be?

An IV opiate is likely to be required to control the pain; however, this is contraindicated due to hypotension. Medications administered orally are likely to be vomited back, or poorly absorbed due to reduced blood flow to the gastrointestinal system from shock. Paracetamol 1 g IV would be a good starting point and would also treat the patient's fever. Saline 0.9% IV administered in bolus doses could improve the hypotension, which would in turn allow an IV opiate to be given safely. Anti-emetic options can include ondansetron 4 mg IV/PO/SL or metoclopramide 10 mg IV/IM. Initial treatment should be aimed at improving hypotension, while reducing pain and vomiting so that the patient can be moved safely to the ambulance.

You now begin to relate this patient's presentation to your knowledge of biliary tract problems. What is the pathophysiology of this condition?

Bile is green and is produced by the liver. It then flows slowly along the hepatic ducts into the gallbladder, which stores bile, emptying it into the duodenum after eating. This flow of bile through the system prevents infection. Gallstones are common and occur 2–3 times more often in women than men. The prevalence increases with age, but then decreases after the sixth decade. 80% of stones are formed by cholesterol derived from diet but, paradoxically, they also occur after rapid weight loss. Short episodes (<2 hours) of RUQ pain after meals are classic of gallstones, which are usually treated conservatively. This is biliary colic, but the term is inaccurate as the pain is constant in nature, not colicky. Stones that obstruct the system (pain >2 hours) cause obstructive choledocholithiasis, or the infective conditions cholecystitis (inflamed gallbladder) and cholangitis (inflamed biliary tract). Obstructed bile flow ultimately leads to jaundice when hepatic duct flow ceases.

Case Progression

You have inserted an IV line and, after clarifying that the patient has no allergies, you administered paracetamol 1 g, sodium chloride 0.9% 500 mL, ondansetron 4 mg and morphine 5 mg.

Patient assessment triangle
General appearance
The patient is alert and calm.

Circulation to the skin
Slightly pale.

Work of breathing
No evidence of shortness of breath.

SYSTEMATIC APPROACH
Danger
Nil.

Response
Alert on the AVPU scale.

Airway
Clear, nausea has decreased.

Breathing

Rate: 20 bpm. Effort: no increased effort. Accessory muscle use: no. Auscultation: clear air entry throughout on auscultation.

Circulation

Heart rate: 110 bpm. Strength: weak. Heart regularity: regular. Capillary refill time: 3 seconds, pale.

Vital signs

RR: 20 bpm
HR: 110 bpm
BP: 102/60 mmHg
SpO$_2$: 94%
Blood sugar: 6.1 mmol/L
Temperature: 38.2 °C
Lead II ECG: sinus rhythm

Exposure

3/10 RUQ abdominal pain. There is RUQ tenderness. Murphy's sign positive: the RUQ is deeply palpated, but pain halts the patient from completing an inspiratory breath during RUQ palpation. There is no pain at the left upper quadrant (LUQ) when the test is repeated on the opposite side. No rebound tenderness or peritoneal irritation. No jaundice.

What questions would you ask this patient specifically related to biliary obstruction as part of the history-taking process?

See Table 4.7.

Table 4.7 History-taking questions

Gallbladder and biliary system

Does the pain radiate to the back or right shoulder?
Has the pain been prolonged in duration?
Have you experienced this type of pain previously after meals?
Have you had any recent rapid weight loss?
What colour is the vomit? (Patients often mistake stomach acid for bile)
Is the vomiting forceful?

Medication history

Have you tried any medications for this pain?

F/SH (family and social history)

What does your diet consist of?
Do you drink alcohol? If so, how much and how often?
Does the patient fit the demographic? 'Female, Forties, Fat, Fertile'

Past medical history (PMH)

Do you have any past medical conditions?
Do you know if you have gallstones?
Have you had an RUQ ultrasound scan?

Differential diagnosis (DDx) – what other conditions can cause RUQ pain?

Pancreatitis
Hepatitis
Cancer of the gallbladder
Pyelonephritis

What are the triad and pentad of symptoms closely linked to this condition?

- Charcot's triad: jaundice, fever and RUQ pain.
- Reynolds' pentad: Charcot's triad plus hypotension and altered mental status.

References and further reading

ACT Emergency Services Agency (2019) Clinical Management Guidelines 2019. https://esa.act.gov.au/emergency-services/ambulance/clinical-management-guidelines (accessed 2 July 2020).

Bickey, L. & Szilagyi, P. (2009) *Bates' Guide to Physical Examination and History Taking*. Philadelphia, PA: Wolters Kluwer.

Burroughs, A. & Westaby, D. (2009) Liver, biliary tract and pancreatic disease. In *Kumar and Clark's Clinical Medicine*, 7th edn (eds P. Kumar & M. Clark), Edinburgh: Saunders Elsevier, pp. 319–386.

Chen, Y., Liu, B. & Kirk, M. (2015) High incidence of hospitalisation due to infectious gastroenteritis in older people associated with poor self-rated health. *BMJ Open*, 5: e010161.

Curtis, K. & Ramsden, C. (2016) *Emergency and Trauma Care for Nurses and Paramedics, Australia and New Zealand Edition*, 2nd edn. Chatswood: Elsevier.

Fairclough, P. & Silk, D. (2009) Liver, biliary tract and pancreatic disease. In *Kumar and Clark's Clinical Medicine*, 7th edn (eds P. Kumar & M. Clark), Edinburgh: Saunders Elsevier, pp. 241–318.

Gralnek, I., Baskin, A. & Bardon, M. (2008) Management of acute bleeding from a peptic ulcer. *New England Journal of Medicine*, 359: 928–937.

Harty, J. (2014) Prevention and management of acute kidney injury. *Ulster Medical Journal*, 83(3): 149–157.

Johnson, M., Boyd, L., Grantham, H. & Eastwood, K. (2015) *Paramedic Principles and Practice ANZ: A Clinical Reasoning Approach*. Chatswood: Elsevier.

New South Wales Ambulance Service (2016) NSW Ambulance Protocols and Pharmacology. https://nswambulance.wordpress.com (accessed 2 July 2020).

Queensland Ambulance Service (2019) Clinical Practice Manual (CPM). https://www.ambulance.qld.gov.au/clinical.html (accessed 2 July 2020).

Simon, C., Everitt, H. & van Dorp, F. (2010) *Oxford Handbook of General Practice*. Oxford: Oxford University Press.

Summers, A. & Willis, S. (2010) Human factors within paramedic practice: The forgotten paradigm. *Journal of Paramedic Practice*, 2(9): 424–428.

Talley, N. & O'Connor, S. (2016) *Clinical Examination Essentials*, 4th edn. Chatswood: Elsevier.

Thomas, J. & Monaghan, T. (2010) *Oxford Handbook of Clinical Examination and Practical Skills*. Oxford: Oxford University Press.

Tintinalli, J., Stapczynski, B., Ma, O. et al. (2016) *Tintinalli's Emergency Medicine: A Comprehensive Study Guide*, 8th edn. Maidenhead: McGraw-Hill Education.

Wyatt, J., Taylor, R.G., de Wit, K. & Hotton, E.J. (2015) *Oxford Handbook of Emergency Medicine*. Oxford: Oxford University Press.

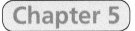

Chapter 5 Palliative and end-of-life care

Alisha Hensby and Samantha Sheridan
Charles Sturt University, Bathurst, NSW, Australia

CHAPTER CONTENTS

LEVEL 1 CASE STUDY
Exacerbation of illness in a patient with a cancer diagnosis

Information type	Data
Time of origin	17:40
Time of dispatch	18:01
On-scene time	18:10
Day of the week	Sunday
Nearest hospital	25 minutes
Nearest backup	Intensive care crew, 25 minutes
Patient details	Name: Jennifer Owens DOB: 16/04/1982

CASE
You have been called to a private address after a report of a 38-year-old female with abdominal pain and difficulty in breathing. The caller states the patient has a known diagnosis of liver cancer with multiple metastases and has become increasingly agitated and uncomfortable across the course of the weekend.

Pre-arrival information
The patient is conscious and breathing. She is currently receiving treatment from the local community and palliative care team. They are not in attendance at the scene.

Windscreen report
The area outside the house appears to be safe. No obvious activity outside. Lights are on inside the residence.

Clinical Cases in Paramedicine, First Edition. Edited by Sam Willis, Ian Peate, and Rod Hill.
© 2021 John Wiley & Sons Ltd. Published 2021 by John Wiley & Sons Ltd.

Entering the location

You are greeted by a male who appears distressed. He tells you that his wife has been diagnosed with liver cancer. He also tells you that the cancer has now metastasised and that she is receiving palliative care from the local community healthcare and cancer team. The husband states that his wife has had increasing pain and discomfort over the weekend with difficulty sleeping and a new onset of shortness of breath. He is concerned about her pain and wonders if her medications are effective. The palliative care team does not work on weekends.

On arrival with the patient

The female patient is in bed. She appears short of breath and in general discomfort. She is noted to be moving in an agitated fashion in an attempt to gain comfortable positioning.

Patient assessment triangle

General appearance

The patient is alert and she looks at you as you enter the room. She appears to be pale and sweaty and in moderate discomfort.

Circulation to the skin

Mildly pale. ?Jaundice.

Work of breathing

Tachypnoeic. Poor tidal volume.

SYSTEMATIC APPROACH

Danger

Nil.

Response

Alert on the AVPU scale.

Airway

Clear.

Breathing

Rate: 32 bpm. Effort: moderately increased. No accessory muscle use. On auscultation: crackling sound is heard. Poor tidal volume.

Circulation

Heart rate: 104 bpm. Effort: weak. Heart regularity: regular. Capillary refill time: 2 seconds.

Vital signs

RR: 32 bpm
HR: 104 bpm
BP: 150/95 mmHg
SpO_2: 92%
Blood sugar: 5.4 mmol/L
Lead II ECG: sinus tachycardia
Temperature: 36.1 °C (afebrile)
Pain: Patient reports abdominal pain of 8/10
Allergies: Latex

Exposure

Pale and sweaty. Short of breath.

> **TASK**
> Look through the information provided in this case study and highlight all of the information that might concern you as a paramedic.

Using what you currently know about the case, what are your treatment priorities for this patient?

Easing respiratory work and effort, making the patient as comfortable as possible by relieving pain if able.

What kinds of questions would you ask this patient specifically related to her medical diagnosis as part of the history-taking process?

See Table 5.1.

Table 5.1 History-taking questions

Cancer – palliative care
Do you think your pain and shortness of breath are related to your cancer diagnosis?
When did this episode start? (How long have you been like this today?)
What were you doing when this started?
When did you last see the palliative care team?
Have you ever been admitted to hospital before with similar symptoms? If so, when and what was the cause?
Have you been compliant in your treatment and medication regime?

Medication history
Do you take any regular pain medication?
If so, what and how frequently?
Are your medications relieving your pain and any other associated symptoms?
Have you suffered any side effects to your medication regime? If so, what and how have these been managed?
Has your prescription changed at all?
Do you take any medications for any other condition?
Do you have an escalation plan or breakthrough pain management strategy?

F/SH (family and social history)
Who do you live with and are they your primary carer?
What do you do for work?

Past medical history (PMH)
Apart from your cancer diagnosis, do you have any other medical conditions?

Differential diagnosis (DDx) – what else could this be?
Chest infection
Acute infection (of other origin)
Bowel obstruction

Given the patient's diagnosis, what might your considerations be in regard to your treatment plan?

- Provide basic airway management (suction and positioning if required).
- Breathing not within normal limits. On chest auscultation audible crackles at lung bases. Reduced SpO_2. Provide oxygen therapy to the patient.

- Refer to patient's care plan and contact the patient's palliative care team to receive further advice on how best to manage her.
- Provide breakthrough pain relief. This should be outlined on the patient's palliative care plan. If pain management details are not provided, refer to standard paramedic pain management protocols, with the knowledge that the patient may need an adjusted dose based on her current treatment regime and medications.
- Offer transport to a medical facility, be that an Emergency Department or identified palliative care facility if this is in line with the patient's wishes.
- Ensure both the patient and carer are given adequate information to allow for informed, patient-centred decisions.

From the following list of teams involved in patient care, which services may be able to assist you in your approach to patient care?
a. Palliative care team and services.
b. Community health team.
c. Intensive care/advanced care paramedic.
d. Local hospital.
e. Extended care paramedic/paramedic practitioner.
f. Family member on scene.
g. All of the above.

g. All of the above

Given the patient's condition, do you believe this patient can be managed at home or does she require transport to hospital? Explain your decision.

The patient may choose to be managed at home or within a healthcare facility. Ultimately the decision should be made by the patient if she has the capacity to do so at the time of assessment. Healthcare providers cover a wide range of professions, though all are limited by interventions able to take place within the home. Palliative care adopts a team-based approach to providing end-of-life care to a person and his or her primary carers. All efforts should be made to provide patient with their requests in the environment in which they are most comfortable. The patient in this case may therefore be treated at home or at hospital, though as mentioned there may be limitations in the home environment.

LEVEL 1 CASE STUDY
Shortness of breath in the patient with a life-limiting illness

Information type	Data
Time of origin	18:15
Time of dispatch	18:30
On-scene time	18:45
Day of the week	Monday
Nearest hospital	25 minutes
Nearest backup	Intensive care crew, 20 minutes
Patient details	Name: Sarah Shiners DOB: 03/04/1990

CASE

You have been called to a private address for reports of a 30-year-old female with difficulty breathing. The caller states the patient has a known diagnosis of multiple sclerosis (MS) and has been having problems with eating. The evening carers have called due to concerns about the patient's breathing and increased agitation.

Pre-arrival information

The patient is semi-conscious with rapid, noisy breathing. She is currently receiving treatment from local carers and a palliative care team.

Windscreen report

The area outside the house appears to be safe. No obvious activity outside. Lights are on inside the residence.

Entering the location

You are greeted by one of the carers who appears distressed. She states that they visit every evening to assist the patient with a night-time routine, as she has MS and is now unable to mobilise herself. The patient's husband states that his wife has had increasing difficulty breathing across the course of the weekend, and a few times he has had to assist her when choking. The patient's specialist MS nurse visited today and has referred the patient for a PEG tube due to increasing difficulty swallowing. He is concerned about her breathing as it is very noisy and she seems more agitated than usual. He tried to call the specialist nurse, but it is out of hours. On arrival the carer called the ambulance.

On arrival with the patient

The female patient is in bed. She appears cyanosed around the mouth, short of breath and in general discomfort. Her breathing is noisy.

Patient assessment triangle
General appearance

The patient looks at you as you speak to her. She appears to be pale and cyanosed and in a moderate level of discomfort.

Circulation to the skin

Mildly pale. Cyanosed around the mouth

Work of breathing

Tachypnoeic. Poor tidal volume. Audible rattling sound heard without auscultation.

SYSTEMATIC APPROACH

Danger

Nil.

Response

Verbal on the AVPU scale.

Airway

Secretions present.

Breathing

Rate: 32 bpm. Effort: moderately increased. No accessory muscle use. On auscultation: breath sounds are crackling at bases bilaterally. Poor tidal volume.

Circulation

Heart rate: 115 bpm. Effort: weak. Heart regularity: regular. Capillary refill time: 3 seconds.

Vital signs

RR: 32 bpm
HR: 115 bpm
BP: 110/82 mmHg
SpO_2: 89%

Blood sugar: 7.1 mmol/L
Lead II ECG: sinus tachycardia
Temperature: 36.4 °C (afebrile)
Patient unable to speak, speech has gone due to MS diagnosis.

Exposure
Exposed the chest to undertake a respiratory assessment: Central pallor and shortness of breath.

TASK
Look through the information provided in this case study and highlight all of the information that might concern you as a paramedic.

Using what you currently know about the case, what are your treatment priorities?

- Secretions in the airway – provide basic airway management (suction and positioning).
- Breathing not within normal limits. On chest auscultation audible crackles at lung bases. Reduced SpO$_2$ – oxygen therapy and consider more advanced treatment for fluid on lungs. Refer to patient's care plan.

What kinds of questions would you ask this patient and/or her carer specifically related to her medical diagnosis as part of the history-taking process?

See Table 5.2.

Table 5.2 History-taking questions

MS – palliative care
Do you think your shortness of breath is related to the MS diagnosis?
When did this episode start? (How long have you been like this today?)
What were you doing when this started?
When did you last see the palliative care team?
Have you ever been admitted to hospital before with similar symptoms? If so, when and what was the cause?
Have you been compliant in your treatment and medication regime?
Why was the MS nurse referring you for a PEG tube?
Do you have a referral pathway plan in case of emergency?

Medication history
Do you take regular medication?
If so, what medications do you take?
Are they working?
Has your prescription changed at all?
Do you take any medications for any other condition?
Do you have an escalation plan for medication?

F/SH (family and social history)
Who do you live with and are they your primary carer?
To what extent do they care for you? Are you able to mobilise, for example feed yourself?

Past medical history (PMH)
Apart from your MS diagnosis, do you have any other medical conditions?
At what stage is your MS currently, is it very active?

Differential diagnosis (DDx) – what else could this be?
Aspiration
Aspirated pneumonia
Acute infection (of other origin)

Given the patient's diagnosis, what might be your considerations in regard to your treatment plan?

The priority is to clear the airway and treat shortness of breath; oxygenation and suctioning where appropriate. Reassurance and communication are key in patient care and will assist in the overall management of the patient.

From the following list of teams involved in patient care, which services may be able to assist you in your approach to patient care?
a. Palliative care team and services.
b. Community health team.
c. Intensive care/advanced care paramedic.
d. Local hospital.
e. Extended care paramedic/paramedic practitioner.
f. Family member on scene.
g. All of the above.

g. All of the above.

Given the patient's condition and the differential diagnoses, what is your course of action?

It is unlikely that the shortness of breath is a symptom of MS progression, as it is unusual for it to affect the autonomic nervous system. Given the decline in the patient's condition, airway priority and assessment findings and recent history of dysphagia, the patient is likely to have aspirated and is at risk of contracting pneumonia. Follow the patient's care pathway if and where possible; however, the best course of action may be emergency transport for further assessment and ongoing care. Careful consideration must be taken of the patient's and carers' wishes if deciding to transport the patient.

LEVEL 2 CASE STUDY
Pain management during end-of-life care situations

Information type	Data
Time of origin	07:40
Time of dispatch	08:15
On-scene time	08:55
Day of the week	Sunday
Nearest hospital	45 minutes
Nearest backup	30 minutes
Patient details	Name: Paul Lord
	DOB: 08/01/1978

CASE
You have been called to a private address by a palliative care nurse who has arrived to find her 42-year-old male patient in bed and in extreme, uncontrolled pain. The nurse reports that the patient lives at home alone and requires daily visits to ensure his pain is well managed along with his current medications. The patient has a port-a-cath in situ and currently has a syringe driver attached to manage his ongoing pain. The syringe driver and associated medications are managed by the community health and palliative care teams.

Pre-arrival information
The patient is conscious and breathing. He has a history of metastatic cancer and has been well managed by the palliative care team at home to this point. The patient has an advance care directive in place.

Windscreen report

The area outside the house appears to be safe. No obvious activity outside. The front door is open.

Entering the location

You are greeted by a nurse, who briefly outlines the patient's medical history and informs you that he has a current advance care directive in place. The nurse also informs you that his pain has been increasing over the last few days and that his current pain management plan is no longer effective. The patient has no social support. He lives alone and does not want to go to hospital for any further treatment.

On arrival with the patient

The patient is supine on the bed. He appears distressed and in significant pain.

Patient assessment triangle

General appearance

The patient is agitated and distressed. He notes your presence, but is not too interested that you are there.

Circulation to the skin

Pallor and diaphoresis noted on the face.

Work of breathing

Tachypnoeic. Poor tidal volume.

SYSTEMATIC APPROACH

Danger

Nil.

Response

Alert on the AVPU scale.

Airway

Clear, pale, dry.

Breathing

Rate: 36 bpm. Increased effort, on auscultation the breath sounds are clear and equal in all fields. Poor tidal volume.

Circulation

Heart rate: 108 bpm. Effort: weak, regular. Capillary refill time: 3 seconds.

Vital signs

RR: 36 bpm
HR: 108 bpm
BP: 85/65 mmHg
SpO_2: 94%
Blood sugar: 4.1 mmol/L
Lead II ECG: tachycardic, regular
Temperature: 36.3 °C
Allergies: penicillin

Exposure

Pale and sweaty.

TASK

Look through the information provided in this case study and highlight all of the information that might concern you as a paramedic.

Using what you currently know about this case, what are your treatment priorities?

- Reassurance.
- Communication in regard to the patient's wishes and advance care directive.
- Pain management in consultation with the palliative care team.
- Discussing blood pressure management with the palliative care team.

What are your differential diagnoses for this patient?

- Exacerbation of cancer diagnosis.
- Bowel obstruction.
- Fracture (pathological).
- Sepsis/infection.
- Shock.

Given the patient's diagnosis and current condition, what might be your considerations in regard to your treatment plan?

- Access the advance care directive.
- Communicate with both the patient and the palliative care team to identify the patient's needs and expectations.
- Provide breakthrough pain management in consultation with the palliative care team.
- Offer transport to an appropriate facility.
- Ensure follow up with all healthcare providers to amend/adjust advance care directive and pain management plan.

What kinds of questions would you ask this patient and/or the palliative care team specifically related to his medical diagnosis as part of the history-taking process?

See Table 5.3.

Table 5.3 History-taking questions

General questions

Do you believe the pain and presenting condition are related to your cancer diagnosis?

If no, have you had this before?

If you have experienced this before, please tell me about it, including how similar this is to last time, how it was managed and who looked after you.

When did this episode start?

Has this happened before?

Are you in the care of a palliative care team?

Do you have an advance care directive?

What is your pain management plan?

Have you ever been admitted to hospital before with similar symptoms? If so, when and what was the cause?

Have you been compliant in your treatment and medication regime?

Medication history

Are you aware of all of your current medications and what they are taken for?

What is your current treatment regime inclusive of medication administered through the syringe driver?

Have there been any recent changes to your medication regime?

Do you take any medications for any other condition that is not directly associated with your cancer diagnosis?

Do you have medications listed on your advance care directive?

F/SH (family and social history)

Do you have any social support? If so, what?

What do you/did you do for work?

(Continued)

Table 5.3 (Continued)

Past medical history (PMH)
Apart from the cancer diagnosis, do you have any other medical conditions?

Differential diagnosis (DDx) – what else could this be?
Bowel obstruction
Exacerbation of condition
Fracture (pathological)
Infection/sepsis
Shock

Case Progression

This patient is able to produce an advance care directive. As part of the directive, the pain management component of the plan outlines that the patient is able to be administered 100 mg morphine/fentanyl for breakthrough pain relief. This dose is clearly outside your standard scope of practice.

Are you able to administer this? Why or why not?

- Yes. The paramedics in attendance are able to deliver these medications in order with the advance care directive provided they are authorised to do so by their ambulance service as part of their normal scope of practice. If the paramedics in attendance cannot normally utilise morphine or fentanyl as part of their clinical practice, then they should call for someone of an advanced clinical level with this training.
- The dose is likely to be more than the standard pain relief dose and therefore outside of the normal scope of practice. Paramedics are able to deliver this increased dose as part of the completed advance care directive.

The patient declines your offer of transport against your clinical recommendation. What risk-mitigation strategies can you employ to ensure patient safety?

- Thorough documentation that outlines all information that was given to the patient, inclusive of possible risks and adverse outcomes.
- Clear communication to ensure the patient is making an informed decision and is aware of all options, advice and risks.
- Explore alternative options for further care. For example, contact the local GP to book an appointment, or contact palliative care or home care services to ensure a timely follow-up occurs in the patient's home environment.
- With the patient's consent, attempt to make contact with family or friends to ensure general follow-up and support for the patient.
- Encourage the patient to revisit his advance care directive to ensure any changes that need to be made to better support him are made by the primary healthcare provider.

LEVEL 2 CASE STUDY
The unconscious patient

Information type	Data
Time of origin	06:45
Time of dispatch	07:00
On-scene time	07:15
Day of the week	Friday
Nearest hospital	90 minutes
Nearest backup	Intensive care crew, 20 minutes
Patient details	Name: Simon Swallow
	DOB: 19/02/1968

CASE

You have been called to a private rural address for reports of an unconscious 52-year-old male. The caller states the patient has a recent diagnosis of a brain tumour.

Pre-arrival information

The patient is unconscious and breathing. He has recently flown back from Sydney after an increase in headache frequency and severity. The caller is unsure of the results of the investigations, but states that he is aware the patient has commenced different medications for his new diagnosis.

Windscreen report

The area outside the house appears to be safe. No obvious activity outside.

Entering the location

You are greeted by a young male who appears distressed. He tells you that his father has been diagnosed with a brain tumour within the last month. His father has been complaining of headaches for approximately 3 months and had this investigated by his GP. He was then informed he had developed a brain tumour and was flown to Sydney for further investigation. The son tells you that his father returned from seeing the specialist in Sydney and hasn't been himself since. The son states that he has been home helping his dad with the farm since the diagnosis, but is not entirely sure of the specifics relating to his father's condition as his father has not wanted to talk about it. The son states they went to bed last night as usual, though his father was very quiet. He went to check on his father this morning as he is normally up before him and found his father unconscious on his bed.

On arrival with the patient

The patient is supine on the bed. He appears unresponsive. Audible gurgling can be heard. As you begin your assessment, two other siblings arrive on scene. You request immediate backup.

Patient assessment triangle

General appearance

The patient is unresponsive.

Circulation to the skin

Pale and sweaty.

Work of breathing

Bradypnoeic, irregular, poor tidal volume.

SYSTEMATIC APPROACH

Danger

Nil.

Response

P on the AVPU scale.

Airway

White, frothy sputum dried to corner of mouth.

Breathing

Rate: 8 bpm, laboured. On auscultation the breath sounds are clear and equal. Poor tidal volume.

Circulation

Heart rate: 64 bpm, weak, irregular. Capillary refill time: 3 seconds.

Vital signs

RR: 8 bpm
HR: 64 bpm
BP: unreadable, the patient's arm is stiff

SpO$_2$: 89%
Blood sugar: 3.4 mmol/L
Lead II ECG: bradycardic, irregular
Temperature: 36.1 °C
Allergies: paracetamol

Exposure
Pale and sweaty.

TASK
Look through the information provided in this case study and highlight all of the information that might concern you as a paramedic.

Using what you currently know about the case, what are your treatment priorities?

- Airway – improved positioning. Suctioning if required. Basic airway management techniques, with consideration given to airway adjuncts inclusive of OPA, NPA, LMA or ETT.
- Breathing – oxygenation to the patient. Given that the patient has poor tidal volume and is bradypnoeic, intermittent positive-pressure ventilation (IPPV) should be initiated.
- Circulation – priority given to airway and breathing. Continue to reassess and when possible complete 12 lead ECG and consider appropriate intervention.
- Disability – investigation into cause of reduced level of consciousness. Ensure all basic investigations are completed, including pupil assessment, temperature assessment and blood glucose assessment, before assuming it is resulting from the brain tumour.

What are your differential diagnoses for this patient?

- Seizure.
- Overdose.
- Hypoglycaemic episode.
- Stroke/TIA.
- Exacerbation of current condition – brain cancer/tumour.

Given the patient's diagnosis and current condition, what might be your considerations in regard to your treatment plan?

See the suggested history-taking questions in Table 5.4. In the first instance, it would be worthwhile asking what are the expectations of the patient and family in regard to the patient's condition and interventions, and in particular if the patient's wishes are known to the family given that the patient is unconscious.

Given that the patient has recently been to Sydney for further investigations, asking a family member to call the discharging hospital and specialist to gain clarification on the patient's condition may be beneficial if this information is freely available.

Consideration must be given to an advance care directive, though it appears in this instance that the patient does not have one.

If unable to ascertain any of the above information, paramedics should proceed with standard patient care until more information is able to be ascertained. Signs and symptoms should be treated in accordance with available guidelines.

Table 5.4 History-taking questions

General questions

Do you believe the patient's condition is related to his cancer diagnosis?

When did this episode start? (How long has he been like this today?)

Has this happened before?

What was his recent visit to the specialist for?

Is he in the care of a palliative care team?

Has he ever been admitted to hospital before with similar symptoms? If so, when and what was the cause?

Has the patient been compliant in his treatment and medication regime?

Does the patient have a current advance care directive or end-of-life care plan?

How do you think the patient is coping? Has he spoken to anyone about his condition and diagnosis?

Medication history

Do you know the patient's regular medication?

What is the patient's current treatment regime?

Have there been any changes to his treatment?

Does he take any medications for any other condition?

Does he have an escalation plan?

F/SH (family and social history)

Are you his primary carer?

What do you do for work?

Past medical history (PMH)

Apart from his cancer diagnosis, does he have any other medical conditions?

Differential diagnosis (DDx) – what else could this be?

Seizure due to condition

Overdose

Exacerbation of condition

Hypoglycaemia

Stroke/TIA

Case Progression

A backup crew arrives. No further information is able to be ascertained apart from what is already known. There is no advance care directive in place.

Based on the information provided in this case study, what would you do now?

Suction the airway, provide an OP tube, start bag-valve-mask (BVM) ventilation with 15 L of oxygen, warm the patient, administer glucose IV and remove him to hospital with a pre-alert.

While you are assessing the patient he begins to have a seizure. You are yet to perform any of the interventions listed for the previous question. What are your immediate actions?

- Ensure the patient is safe from harm from himself and others.
- Consider placing the patient in the lateral position to better manage his airway.
- Administer oxygen. Consider IPPV if required.
- Consider reversible causes and initiate treatment.

- Administer midazolam (or appropriate benzodiazepine) as outlined by the specific paramedic guideline. This may require more than the initial dose. Consider that if medication has been taken as overdose, pharmacological intervention may be ineffective. Consider transport.
- Once the seizure is controlled, support ABCs and consider advanced airway and IPPV if required.
- Treat associated conditions such as:
  - Hypovolaemia.
  - Trauma.
  - Hyperthermia.
- Transport to hospital and pre-notify hospital if possible.

Primary brain tumours are a diverse group of neoplasms, affecting approximately 7 persons per 100,000 population annually. Brain tumours have a high mortality rate and unpredictable disease trajectories.

List the common (and uncommon) presenting signs and symptoms you may encounter in someone with a brain tumour.

- Fatigue.
- Headaches.
- Blurred vision.
- Nausea and vomiting.
- Behavioural dysfunction.
- Cognitive decline, e.g. reduced capacity to make decisions.
- Ataxia.
- Speech difficulties.
- Reduced or altered vision.

Note that this is not a comprehensive list, but rather some suggestions of possible responses. It is important to note that not all signs and symptoms are physical in nature and that diagnosis and treatment of brain tumours should not rely solely on physical symptom presentation.

LEVEL 3 CASE STUDY
Interventions and end-of-life care in the aged population

Information type	Data
Time of origin	07:50
Time of dispatch	07:55
On-scene time	08:09
Day of the week	Thursday
Nearest hospital	35 minutes
Nearest backup	Unknown
Patient Details	Name: Betty Gable DOB: 12/12/1933

CASE
You have been called to an aged care facility where it is reported that an 87-year-old female has been found unresponsive in her bed. The patient was last seen 1 hour prior by staff who delivered her breakfast.

Pre-arrival information
The patient has been found unconscious. Staff are on scene with the patient, who is located in the dementia wing/high care unit of the aged care facility. The patient has a history of advanced dementia, hypertension, atrial fibrillation and

recurrent falls. She has had two previous strokes with mobility impairment. It is not known if there is an advance care directive in place.

Windscreen report
On your arrival there is no clear entry point to the aged care facility. You approach the administrative staff, who contact the registered nurse on duty. You are eventually met by staff with a total time delay to patient of approximately 10 minutes.

Entering the location
The care facility appears busy. Staff are rushing around and it appears to be short staffed.

On arrival with the patient
You are met by the enrolled nurse on duty who states that she found the patient as she is now while doing her medication rounds this morning. The patient is noted to be lying supine, with snoring, laboured respirations and audible gurgling on inspiration. She is unconscious and unresponsive, and appears pale and centrally cyanotic. No further assessment or treatment has been undertaken by the staff.

Patient assessment triangle
General appearance
The patient is pale and centrally cyanotic. She is unconscious and has laboured, irregular breathing.

Circulation to the skin
Pale. Capillary refill time >4 seconds.

Work of breathing
Bradypnoeic. Irregular. Poor tidal volume.

SYSTEMATIC APPROACH
Danger
Nil.

Response
Unresponsive on the AVPU scale.

Airway
Obstructed due to positioning of the patient.

Breathing
Rate: 8 bpm, poor effort. On auscultation: breath sounds bilaterally diminished. Poor tidal volume.

Circulation
Heart rate: 52 bpm, weak, irregular. Capillary refill time: >4 seconds.

Vital signs
RR: 8 bpm
HR: 52 bpm
BP: unable to obtain
SpO_2: 78%
Blood sugar: not taken
Lead II ECG: irregular
Temperature: 36.0 °C
Allergies: unknown

Exposure
Pale and centrally cyanosed.

> **TASK**
> Look through the information provided in this case study and highlight all of the information that might concern you as a paramedic.

Using what you currently know about the case, what are your treatment priorities?

- Establishing clear treatment goals and expectations.
- Clear communication in regard to patient's/family's wishes and advance care directive.
- Basic ABC interventions inclusive of oxygen and pain relief if required while further information is ascertained.
- If in doubt or in the case of dispute, treatment may be commenced.
  Refer to Chapter 11, Legal and ethical cases, for further information in regard to this question.

What are your differential diagnoses for this patient?

- Stroke/TIA.
- Infection/sepsis.
- Overdose.
- Choking/aspiration.

When a person resides in an aged care facility, advance care/health directives are routinely completed on admission. Explain who should ideally be involved in this process and the specifics that should be outlined in any advance care/health directive.

An advance care/health directive can only be completed by the person for whom the directive is intended. The person must display both competence and capacity at the time of completion. Ideally this directive should be completed by the person and:
- GP or primary health care provider.
- Any medical treatment decision maker identified by the person.
- Any family and/or friends of the person's choosing.

Specifics to be outlined in an advance care directive may vary slightly between countries and states. Paramedics and patients should refer directly to the relevant guidelines and directives. However, most advance care directives include:
- Personal details.
- Details of primary medical treatment decision maker.
- Current major health problems.
- Specific interventions involved in the patient's overall healthcare.
- People the patient would like involved in decision-making processes.
- Unacceptable outcomes.
- Organ and tissue donation.

What if there is a dispute in relation to treatment and care between family members and aged care providers? Who is able to make medical decisions for the patient?

Refer to Chapter 11, Legal and ethical cases, for further information in regard to this question.

LEVEL 3 CASE STUDY
Family conflict – the paediatric patient

Information type	Data
Time of origin	05:40
Time of dispatch	05:45
On-scene time	05:55

Information type	Data
Day of the week	Tuesday
Nearest hospital	55 minutes
Nearest backup	Unknown
Patient details	Name: Jade Faxter
	DOB: 29/04/2017

CASE

You have been called to a private address in a regional town. A father has called and reports that he requires assistance for his 3-year-old daughter who has severe congenital muscular dystrophy (CMD). The father states that she was found unresponsive in her bed this morning and has noted laboured breathing. The child is cared for at home by her parents and extended family and requires daily medication to manage her condition. Her parents have been advised that due to the severity of her illness, this is a life-limiting condition for the child.

Pre-arrival information

The patient is unconscious with laboured breathing. She has a history of CMD. More recently the patient has been managed in hospital for multiple episodes of aspiration pneumonia.

Windscreen report

On your arrival, there appear to be many people outside the house. It is assumed that these are extended family and friends of the patient.

Entering the location

You are greeted by the patient's father, who appears calm and sombre. He clearly explains the patient's chronic and declining medical history. He is able to produce an advance care plan that outlines comfort treatment and pain management only. It clearly states that no lifesaving or invasive interventions are to be performed. The father states that the family has extended family and friend support and that the decline of the patient is not unexpected. He further explains that his wife is not accepting of the imminent death of their daughter and that she was initially unaware that the ambulance had been called. The father would like to follow the end-of-life care plan to which both he and his wife agreed. His wife now wants all lifesaving treatment undertaken.

On arrival with the patient

The patient is lateral on the sofa with her head cradled by her mother. The mother is sobbing and appears extremely distressed. She asks you to treat her child.

Patient assessment triangle

General appearance

The patient is pale, unconscious and has laboured, irregular breathing.

Circulation to the skin

Pale. Capillary refill time >4 seconds.

Work of breathing

Bradypnoeic. Irregular. Poor tidal volume.

SYSTEMATIC APPROACH

Danger

Nil.

Response

Unresponsive on the AVPU scale.

Airway
Obstructed due to positioning of the patient.

Breathing
Rate: 10 bpm, increased effort. On auscultation breath sounds are bilaterally diminished. Poor tidal volume.

Circulation
Heart rate: 82 bpm. Effort: weak. Heart regularity: regular. Capillary refill time: >4 seconds.

Vital signs
RR: 10 bpm
HR: 82 bpm
BP: 55/40 mmHg
SpO_2: 82%
Blood sugar: 3.1 mmol/L
Temperature: 38.3 °C
Lead II ECG: regular

Exposure
Central cyanosis, mild subcoastal recession.

TASK
Look through the information provided in this case study and highlight all of the information that might concern you as a paramedic.

Using what you currently know about the case, what are your treatment priorities?

- Reassurance and empathy to the family.
- Establishing clear treatment goals and expectations.
- Clear and empathetic communication in regard to patient's/family's wishes and advance care directive. Is there legal documentation available?
- Basic ABC interventions inclusive of oxygen therapy.
- Consider pain relief if the patient regains consciousness in discussion with the family.
- If in doubt or in the case of a dispute, treatment may be commenced.
  Refer to Chapter 11, Legal and ethical cases, for further information in regard to this question.

List four differential diagnoses for this patient.

- Exacerbation of CMD.
- Infection/sepsis.
- Seizure.
- Aspiration pneumonia.

In the case of paediatric palliative care, collaborative communication is encouraged. Explain what you think this means and utilise the case as an example of how to undertake this process.

Collaborative communication is distinguished by the desire to accomplish five complex tasks:
- Establishing a common goal or set of goals that guide collaborative efforts.
- Exhibiting mutual respect and compassion for each other.
- Developing a sufficiently complete understanding of our differing perspectives.
- Assuring maximum clarity and correctness of what we communicate to each other.
- Managing intrapersonal and interpersonal processes that affect how we send, receive and process information.

Ensure you use examples relating to the case for each of these key points.

- The Australian Commission on Safety and Quality in Health Care published a national consensus statement in December 2016. It outlines 10 essential elements for safe and high-quality paediatric end-of-life care. Under the heading 'Processes of Care', the first five elements are specifically directed at clinicians who work within settings where acute care is provided to palliative care paediatric patients:Family-centred communication and shared decision making.
- Teamwork and coordination of care.
- Components of care.
- Use of triggers to recognise children approaching the end of life.
- Response to concerns.

References and further reading

ANZSPM (2020) Australian and New Zealand Society of Palliative Medicine. http://www.anzspm.org.au/c/anzspm (accessed 14 January 2020).

Australian Commission on Safety and Quality in Health Care (2016) *National Consensus Statement: Essential Elements for Safe and High Quality Paediatric End of Life Care.* Sydney: ACSQHC.

Better Health Channel (2020) Palliative care in a hospital or community residential home. https://www.betterhealth.vic.gov.au/health/servicesandsupport/palliative-care-in-a-hospital-or-community-residential-home?viewAsPdf=true (accessed 5 January 2020).

Cancer Council (2019) Brain and spinal cord tumours. https://www.cancercouncil.com.au/brain-cancer/

Feudtner, C. (2007) Collaborative communication in pediatric palliative care: A foundation for problem-solving and decision-making. *Pediatric Clinics of North America*, 54(5), 583607. doi: 10.1016/j.pcl.2007.07.008

MS (2019) Swallowing. https://www.ms.org.au/what-is-multiple-sclerosis/symptoms/common-symptoms/swallowing.aspx (accessed 10 December 2019).

National Cancer Institute (2019) Treatment option overview for adult primary CNS tumors. https://www.cancer.gov/types/brain/hp/adult-brain-treatment-pdq#_69 (accessed 13 December 2019).

National Multiple Sclerosis Society (2019) Breathing problems. http://www.nationalmssociety.org/Symptoms-Diagnosis/MS-Symptoms/Respiration-Breathing-Problems (accessed 10 December 2019).

NHS (2015) New guidelines on end of life care published by NICE. https://www.nhs.uk/news/medical-practice/new-guidelines-on-end-of-life-care-published-by-nice/ (accessed 10 December 2019).

Palliative Care Australia (2020). Palliative care. https://palliativecare.org.au (accessed 27 January 2020).

Queensland Ambulance Service (2016) Clinical practice guidelines: Neurological/seizures. https://www.ambulance.qld.gov.au/docs/clinical/cpg/CPG_Seizure.pdf (accessed 2 July 2020).

Queensland Government (2020) Advance health directive. https://www.qld.gov.au/law/legal-mediation-and-justice-of-the-peace/power-of-attorney-and-making-decisions-for-others/advance-health-directive (accessed 28 January 2020).

Song, K., Amatya, B. & Khan, F. (2015) Advance care planning in patients with brain tumours: A prospective cohort study. *Journal of Cancer Research and Therapy*, 3(7): 85–91. doi: 10.14312/2052-4994.2015-12

Townsend, R. & Luck, M. (2019) *Applied Paramedic Law, Ethics and Professionalism*, 2nd edn. Chatswood: Elsevier.

Victoria State Government (2018) Medical Treatment Planning and Decisions Act 2016. https://www2.health.vic.gov.au/hospitals-and-health-services/patient-care/end-of-life-care/advance-care-planning/medical-treatment-planning-and-decisions-act (accessed 2 July 2020).

Victoria State Government (2020) Advance care planning forms. https://www2.health.vic.gov.au/hospitals-and-health-services/patient-care/end-of-life-care/advance-care-planning/acp-forms (accessed 25 January 2020).

Chapter 6 — Medical emergencies

Tom E. Mallinson
BASICS Scotland, Auchterarder, UK

LEVEL 1 CASE STUDY
Hypoglycaemia

Information type	Data
Time of origin	02:58
Time of dispatch	03:08
On-scene time	03:34
Day of the week	Sunday
Nearest hospital	25 minutes
Nearest backup	Prehospital care doctor, 20 minutes
Patient details:	Name: Andrew May DOB: 12/09/1977

CASE
You have been called to a residential property for a 43-year-old male acting strangely. The call originated from the patient's flatmate.

Pre-arrival information
The patient is conscious and breathing, but acting strangely.

Windscreen report
The area outside the house appears to be safe; there are a number of people making their way out of the building. The house is well lit with lights on in all windows.

Clinical Cases in Paramedicine, First Edition. Edited by Sam Willis, Ian Peate, and Rod Hill.
© 2021 John Wiley & Sons Ltd. Published 2021 by John Wiley & Sons Ltd.

Entering the location

You are greeted by a middle-aged man who directs you upstairs. The house is in slight disarray: it appears a house party has just ended. He tells you that his flatmate was pacing back and forth upstairs, slurring his words and stumbling, and has now become quiet.

On arrival with the patient

The male patient is slumped on the floor in the corner of his room.

Patient assessment triangle:
General appearance

The patient is alert and he looks at you as you enter the room, although he doesn't acknowledge you.

Circulation to the skin

He appears pale and diaphoretic.

Work of breathing

Normal work of breathing.

SYSTEMATIC APPROACH

Danger

Nil.

Response

Alert on the AVPU scale.

Airway

Clear, patent and self-maintained.

Breathing

Rate: 16 bpm. Effort: normal. Accessory muscle use: no. Auscultation: bilateral equal air entry, vesicular breath sounds.

Circulation

Heart rate: 118 bpm. Effort: strong radial pulse. Heart regularity: regular. Capillary refill time: 3 seconds.

Vital signs

RR: 16 bpm
HR: 118 bpm
BP: 107/77 mmHg
SpO_2: 99%
Blood sugar: 2 mmol/L
GCS: E4, V4, M5 = 13/15
Lead II ECG: Sinus tachycardia

Exposure

No signs of traumatic injury. Noticeably diaphoretic.

TASK

Look through the information provided in this case study and highlight all of the information that might concern you as a paramedic.

Putting aside his low capillary blood glucose reading for a minute, what is your differential for this man's abnormal behaviour?

The differential for abnormal behaviour is vast, and a systematic primary and secondary survey is needed to narrow down the possible causes. Some important differentials are presented in Table 6.1.

Table 6.1 Differential diagnoses for abnormal behaviour

Hypoglycaemia	Ethanol intoxication
Overdose of prescription drugs	Recreational drug use
Head injury	Psychiatric emergency
Stroke	Delirium
Intracranial lesion	Infection
Hypoxia	Psychological distress

During the secondary survey for this case, what key findings might assist your diagnostic process?

Medical alert jewellery is a key source of information in an unwell patient. Such jewellery may take the form of a necklace or bracelet, or there may be data on the rear of a watch face. Further, more specific clues such as repeat prescriptions found in pockets or a continuous blood glucose monitor attached to the patient's skin may provide a wealth of information.

Case Progression

On further assessment the patient has confused conversation. His neurological examination reveals the following: pupils equal and receive size 4, symmetrical face; power and sensation assessment is limited due to patient's lack of cooperation. Plantars are downgoing with normal patella reflexes.

You have administered 1 mg IM glucagon 16 minutes ago. There has been no clear improvement. You have placed the patient on supplemental oxygen via a nasal cannula.

Patient assessment triangle
General appearance
The patient is rousable, but appears sleepy. When stimulated with a gentle squeeze to the shoulder, he looks in your direction but says nothing.

Circulation to the skin
Diaphoretic.

Work of breathing
Normal

SYSTEMATIC APPROACH
Danger
Nil.

Response
Responsive to pain on the AVPU scale.

Airway
Slight snoring when not stimulated.

Breathing
Rate: 20 bpm. Effort: normal. Accessory muscle use: no. Auscultation: clear, no added sounds.

Circulation
Heart rate: 122 bpm. Effort: strong. Heart regularity: regular. Capillary refill time: 2 seconds.

Vital signs
RR: 20 bpm

HR: 122 bpm

BP: 153/91 mmHg

SpO_2: 100% with FiO_2 of approx. 0.6

Blood sugar: 1.3 mmol/L

Lead II ECG: Sinus tachycardia

Temperature: 37.2 °C

Exposure

On exposure, the patient is systemically diaphoretic and pale. His breath smells of intoxicating liquor.

PRACTICAL TIP

Always ensure that drugs are checked with a colleague before administration. This is especially important in time-critical situations, where it is easier to become mentally overloaded and make cognitive errors.

Why do you think glucagon has been ineffective in this case? What other reasons could there be for treatment failure specific to this case?

In this case there appears to have been a party underway before your patient became unwell. This may provide a clue regarding the apparent ineffectiveness of the glucagon. Hypoglycaemia is associated with a number of recreational drugs, and commonly with alcohol. Alcohol stimulates an increase in the release of insulin from the pancreas, lowering circulating blood glucose levels. Ethanol metabolism also disrupts gluconeogenesis within the liver (further reducing the glucose available to circulate in the blood) and also leads to excess production of ketones and reactive Oxygen species.

Considering that this patient might be suffering hypoglycaemia secondary to alcohol intake, what would be the next appropriate treatment option and why?

An appropriate course of action here would be to initiate an IV infusion of glucose or to facilitate rapid transport to someone who can. An open mind should also be maintained for other potential causes of his low GCS and hypoglycaemia.

LEVEL 1 CASE STUDY
Convulsions

Information type	Data
Time of origin	08:40
Time of dispatch	08:44
On-scene time	09:02
Day of the week	Tuesday
Nearest hospital	11 minutes
Nearest backup	Critical care paramedic, 22 minutes
Patient Details	Name: Amy Witchell
	DOB: 12/09/2000

CASE

You are working on a double-crewed ambulance with an experienced colleague. You are dispatched to a 20-year-old female who is having a seizure in a shop.

Pre-arrival information

You are sent to a local food store you know well to attend a woman who is unresponsive and having a seizure. No further details are provided.

Windscreen report

On arrival, you are flagged down by a member of staff. You can see a small crowd of people in the front of the shop.

Entering the location

On entering the shop you approach the small crowd. They are surrounding a woman who appears to be in her mid-20s.

On arrival with the patient

You reach the side of the patient. A member of staff is supporting her head off the concrete floor. She appears to be experiencing a grand mal seizure.

Patient assessment triangle

General appearance

The patient is displaying disordered movement of her arms, legs and head. She appears to have been incontinent of urine. Her teeth are clenched and her eyes are open but not focusing.

Circulation to the skin

She has a good colour. Her capillary refill time is 2 seconds.

Work of breathing

It is almost impossible to accurately assess her work of breathing while she is still experiencing a seizure.

SYSTEMATIC APPROACH

Danger

There is no clear danger. The small crowd are cooperative and eager to help, and they are not crowding you.

Response

The patient in unresponsive to voice and painful stimuli. She is actively seizing.

Airway

It is difficult to assess the airway, there is trismus and on close examination a small amount of blood around the lips.

Breathing

Rate: approx. 26 bpm. Effort: difficult to assess while seizing, Accessory muscle use: difficult to assess. Auscultation: there is equal air entry, it is difficult to further assess while seizing.

Circulation

Heart rate: 122 bpm. Effort: weak. Heart regularity: regular. Capillary refill time: 2 seconds.

Vital signs

RR: Disordered
HR: 122 bpm
BP: Unrecordable
SpO$_2$: Unrecordable
Blood sugar: 5.5 mmol/L

Exposure

Systemic seizure activity, no injuries found.

TASK

In your working environment, where are the supplies needed to administer drugs to terminate a seizure? How quickly can you access these?

What is your initial treatment of this patient?

Patients experiencing seizures should be managed using the ABCDE approach. As soon as possible you need to secure their airway, administer oxygen at a high FiO_2, assess cardiac output and respiratory function and secure intravascular access. Terminating a seizure may accomplish many of these goals rapidly. The most common first-line treatment for seizures is a drug from the benzodiazepine family, such as diazepam or lorazepam (SIGN, 2018).

When considering using a benzodiazepine for this patient, what is the mechanism of action of this group of medications?

Benzodiazepines work through interaction with the benzodiazepine receptors that are present in the central nervous system. These receptors facilitate the activity of γ-aminobutyric acid (GABA) receptors, activation that leads to an influx of chloride ions and hyper-polarises the cell membrane, making it less likely to depolarise.

What are the main actions of benzodiazepine medications?

Benzodiazepines have a number of common effects, with some being more predominant for some drugs. Common effects include sedation and anxiolysis, hypnosis, amnesia and muscle relaxation, in addition to their anticonvulsive action. Bradypnoea or apnoea are also signifcant side effects of benzodiazepines, which may present after administration.

Case Progression

You have administered your first-line treatment for prolonged seizures, which was a benzodiazepine via the IV route. The patient has stopped convulsing, but has a decreased level of consciousness.

Patient assessment triangle
General appearance
The patient appears pale.

Circulation to the skin
Capillary refill time is around 3 seconds centrally on the sternum.

Work of breathing
There is no increased work of breathing, although the respiratory rate is low.

SYSTEMATIC APPROACH
Danger
Nil.

Response
Pain on the AVPU scale, and localises to pain.

Airway
Clear with simple manoeuvres (head tilt, chin lift).

Breathing
Rate: 4 bpm. Effort: reduced. Accessory muscle use: no. Auscultation: slight crackles to the right upper zones.

Circulation
Heart rate: 110 bpm. Effort: strong. Heart regularity: regular. Capillary refill time: 3 seconds.

Vital signs
RR: 4 bpm
HR: 110 bpm
BP: 98/63 mmHg
SpO_2: 89%
Blood sugar: 5.2 mmol/L
Temperature: 36.4 °C
Lead II ECG: sinus tachycardia

Exposure
Slow deep respirations, equal chest rise and fall.

PRACTICAL TIP

Patients with prolonged tonic-clonic seizures lasting more than 5 minutes require drug therapy to terminate the seizure. It is likely that any patient who is still convulsing on your arrival will have been seizing for over 5 minutes.

How would you manage a benzodiazepine-induced respiratory depression?

While it is tempting to reach for the reversal agent (flumazenil), this is unlikely to be the best option. Respiratory depression, or arrest, is a condition that can be appropriately managed with a combination of basic airway adjuncts and a bag-valve-mask or breathing circuit. Introducing a benzodiazepine antagonist at this juncture may result in refractory seizures that will be unresponsive to further benzodiazepine therapy.

What factors would you need to take into account before safety discharging a patient at scene who has had a seizure?

In general, it is unlikely that it would be safe to discharge a patient who has had a seizure, if any of the following conditions are met:

- Benzodiazepine administration.
- First seizure.
- GCS <15.
- Unexplained hypoglycaemia.
- Evidence of drug overdose as a cause.
- Head injury.

LEVEL 2 CASE STUDY
Cardiac arrest

Information type	Data
Time of origin	12:08
Time of dispatch	12:10
On-scene time	12:21
Day of the week	Thursday
Nearest hospital	30 mins
Nearest backup	30 mins
Patient details	Name: Alice Lewis
	DOB: 10/09/1985

CASE

You are called to a private address to a 20-year-old female complaining of difficulty in breathing.

Pre-arrival information
The patient appears unwell and is complaining of chest pain.

Windscreen report
On arrival there is another ambulance already in attendance, the crew have propped the door open to a residential property.

Entering the location
On entering the property you hear the sounds of an ongoing resuscitation coming from the front room. A paramedic crew you know well are already in attendance and undertaking good-quality cardiopulmonary resuscitation.

On arrival with the patient
The patient is a female in her early 20s. She is lying on her back in the middle of the living room. Resuscitation is ongoing.

Patient assessment triangle
General appearance
Apnoeic, cyanotic with ongoing cardiopulmonary resuscitation.

Circulation to the skin
Cyanosis with apparent venous congestion to the upper chest, neck and head.

SYSTEMATIC APPROACH
Danger
No concerns.

Response
Unresponsive.

Airway
Intubated with a cuffed size 8 ET tube, 22 cm at the teeth, pilot balloon filled.

Breathing
Being ventilated using a bag valve at a rate of 10/min, with equal chest rise and fall.

Circulation
No palpable pulses.

Vital signs
RR: end-tidal CO_2 (ETCO$_2$) 10 mmHg/1.5 KPa, your colleagues report it was initially higher
HR: no palpable pulse
BP: unrecordable
SpO$_2$: unrecordable
Blood sugar: 9.4 mmol/L
Lead II ECG: irregular narrow complex rhythm with ventricular rate of approx. 140/min (see Figure 6.1)

Exposure
As appropriate for the situation.

Collateral history
Fit and well. According to family she smokes 5–10 cigarettes a day. Recently returned from a vacation abroad. Takes a regular contraceptive pill and a multivitamin.

> **TASK**
>
> Look through the information provided in this case study and highlight all of the information that might concern you as a paramedic.

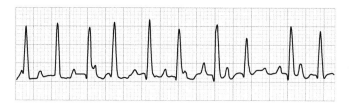

Figure 6.1   Multifocal atrial tachycardia. Reproduced with permission from Morris, F., Brady, W.J. & Camm, A.J. (2009) *ABC of Clinical Electrocardiography*, 2nd edn. Chichester: Wiley-Blackwell.

What do you consider is the most likely cause of this patient's cardiac arrest? Do you have a mnemonic to remind you to consider all the causes?

A review of reversible causes of cardiac arrest using the 4Hs and 4Ts is a useful place to start (Table 6.2).

In this case there is no evidence of trauma, toxin ingestion, hypovolaemia or hypothermia. There is also not enough history for an acute electrolyte disturbance to be a high probability. Thromboembolic disease is the most likely cause of the cardiac arrest here.

Table 6.2   Reversible causes of cardiac arrest (4Hs and 4Ts)

Hs	Ts
Hypovolaemia	Tamponade (cardiac)
Hypothermia	Tension pneumothorax
Hypo- or hyper-electrolyte disturbance	Thromboembolic
Hypoxia	Toxins

As an advanced practitioner, what key intervention could you undertake to maximise this patient's chance of survival?

Good-quality chest compressions with effective ventilation will maximise the efficacy of your resuscitation. However, thinking beyond the basics, this patient is likely to have a catastrophic thromboembolism. Treatment for this is either clot evacuation or thrombolysis. Pre-hospital thrombolysis could lead to return of spontaneous circulation in this case, and immediate thrombolysis is indicated where a cardiac arrest may be due to a PE (Resuscitation Council UK, 2015; Australian Resuscitation Council, 2016).

If you opt to thrombolyse a patient in cardiac arrest, you then need to commit to continuing resuscitation for between 60 and 90 minutes. Why do you think this is?

In cardiac arrest, intrinsic blood flow is interrupted and drugs administered into the venous circulation will not circulate without effective chest compressions. In the case of thrombolysing a pulmonary embolism, enough time is required for the drug to reach the suspected clot in the pulmonary vasculature and then to have a significant fibrinolytic effect to reduce the size of the thrombus and lessen the obstruction to blood flow it is causing.

Case Progression

You have administered IV thrombolysis after discussing this through your services clinical support pathway with a senior colleague. After 30 minutes of ongoing resuscitation, you notice a rise in ETCO$_2$ and respiratory effort. You reassess the patient.

Patient assessment triangle
General appearance
Unresponsive.

Circulation to the skin
Less cyanosis and venous congestion than when previously assessed.

Work of breathing
Respiratory effort is being made at a rate of around 4 bpm. Insufficient ventilation is being achieved.

SYSTEMATIC APPROACH

Danger
Nil.

Response
Unresponsive on the AVPU scale.

Airway
Intubated with a cuffed ET tube, 23 cm at the teeth, pilot balloon inflated.

Breathing
Rate: 4 bpm. Effort: abdominal muscle use noted, poor ventilation. Auscultation: poor air entry, some right-sided crackles.

Circulation
Heart rate: 105 bpm. Effort: weak radial pulse. Heart regularity: regular. Capillary refill time: 2 seconds.

Vital signs
RR: 4 bpm
HR: 105 bpm
BP: 85/30 mmHg
SpO$_2$: 97% when ventilated with FiO$_2$ of 1.0
Blood sugar: 10 mmol/L
Temperature: 35.8 °C
Lead II ECG: sinus tachycardia

Exposure
Full exposure achieved during ongoing resuscitation. No injuries found.

PRACTICAL TIP

It is worthwhile having a pre-prepared checklist (Table 6.3) for action after achieving a return of spontaneous circulation (ROSC). This will reduce cognitive burden and enable effective steps to be taken to optimise post-resuscitation care.

Table 6.3 Checklist for use in cases of return of spontaneous circulation

AIRWAY

   Reassess airway, consider need to change adjunct

   Consider inserting a orogastric or nasogastric tube (to allow gastric decompression)

BREATHING

   Ventilate to achieve $ETCO_2$ of 35 mmHg (30–40) or 4.5 KPa (4–5)

   Monitor waveform $ETCO_2$

   Adjust FiO_2 and positive end-expiratory pressure (PEEP) to achieve SpO_2 of 94–98%

   Ventilate with 6–8 mL/kg

CIRCULATION

   Aim for systolic blood pressure of >90 mmHg

   Aim for mean arterial pressure (MAP) of >65 mmHg

   Consider inotropic support

   Consider limited fluid resuscitation (if hypovolaemia suspected)

   Obtain a 12 lead ECG

   Secure intravascular access (IO or IV)

   Consider inserting a urinary catheter

DISABILITY

   Consider point-of-care ultrasound (PoCUS; if results will alter management)

   Consider sedation and paralysis strategy

   Tape patient's eyes closed (to protect cornea)

PRE-ALERT

   Chosen destination

Source: Adapted from Deakin et al. (2015)

In terms of a patient's history, what are the red flags for pulmonary embolism (PE)?

Some common red flags for pulmonary embolism are presented in Table 6.4.

Table 6.4 Red flags for pulmonary embolism

Lifestyle

Recent travel of >4 hours

Smoking

Medication

Endogenous oestrogen (HRT or combined contraceptive)

Comorbidities

Previous DVT or PE

Surgery in last 3 months

Lower limb cast in last 3 months

Pregnancy

Malignancy

Obesity

COPD

Heart failure

Thrombophilia

While considering red flags can be useful, another way of considering causes for an unwanted thrombus or embolus is Virchow's triad. Can you outline the components of Virchow's triad and how the red flags fit under its three components?

Figure 6.2 demonstrates the components of Virchow's triad. Disruption to any of the three components can lead to the formation of a thrombus and subsequent embolisation. All of the risk factors for a pulmonary embolus with affect one or more of the components of the triad (Table 6.5).

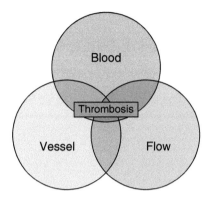

Figure 6.2   Virchow's triad. Reproduced with permission from Paramothayan, S. (2018) *Essential Respiratory Medicine*, Chichester: Wiley-Blackwell.

Table 6.5 Risk factors for pulmonary embolism categorised by components of Virchow's triad

Hypercoagulable state	Stasis of flow	Vessel/endothelial disruption
Malignancy	Immobility	Previous DVT/PE
Thrombophilia	Pregnancy	Thrombophlebitis
Pregnancy	Heart failure	Vessel trauma

LEVEL 2 CASE STUDY
Hypothermia

Information type	Data
Time of origin	04:40
Time of dispatch	04:50
On-scene time	05:02
Day of the week	Monday
Nearest hospital	55 minutes
Nearest backup	30 minutes
Patient details	Name: Jeanette Wallis DOB: 27/01/1961

CASE
You have been tasked with assisting your local mountain rescue team with a patient they have retrieved from the hills. The patient is a 59-year-old female who became disorientated and lost last night and has been outside unaccompanied since then. The mountain rescue team do not believe she is injured, but they are concerned about hypothermia.

Pre-arrival information
The patient is conscious and breathing. No further vital signs are available.

Windscreen report
You arrive at the road head just as the mountain rescue team approach carrying a stretcher.

On arrival with the patient
The mountain rescue team have wrapped the patient in a blanket with a foil blanket over the top. The mountain rescue medic tells you they found the patient around 30 minutes ago, but it is likely she has been outside since around midday yesterday, and she was not equipped for a night on the hill. She has been very confused with them and was cold to the touch.

Patient assessment triangle
General appearance
The patient is alert and is looking around. However, when you try to engage her in conversation she appears distracted and starts tugging at her blankets.

Circulation to the skin
She appears very pale.

Work of breathing
Normal work of breathing, slightly tachypnoeic.

SYSTEMATIC APPROACH
Danger
There is no immediate danger.

Response
Alert on the AVPU scale.

Airway
Clear.

Breathing
Rate: 28 bpm. Effort: normal. Accessory muscle use: no. Auscultation: mild crackles across all zones.

Circulation
Heart rate: 54 bpm. Effort: weak. Heart regularity: irregular. Capillary refill time: unrecordable on peripheries.

Vital signs
RR: 28 bpm
HR: 54 bpm
BP: initially unrecordable
SpO_2: unrecordable
Blood sugar: unable to gain enough blood from a fingertip
Lead II ECG: sinus tachycardia, abnormal QRS complex

Exposure
The weather is cool, and you move into the ambulance to provide some shelter.

TASK
Look through the information provided in this case study and highlight all of the information that might concern you as a paramedic.

You suspect hypothermia may be contributing to this patient's condition. What is the best way of measuring core temperature in the pre-hospital environment?

There are multiple modalities available to measure core body temperature. However, core temperature measurement is sometimes impossible or impractical in the pre-hospital phase (Strapazzon et al., 2014; Zafren et al., 2014). The four main options are oesophageal, rectal, tympanic and dermal, with the first two being preferred (in terms of gaining an accurate result). Table 6.6 provides an overview of the staging of accidental hypothermia.

You are eager to rewarm this patient. Which options are available in a pre-hospital setting?

There are a number of options available internationally, and some are summarised in Table 6.7. What is available in your service?

Table 6.6 Staging of accidental hypothermia

Degree	Swiss stage	Clinical condition	Core temperature C
Mild	1	Conscious and Shivering	32–35°C
Moderate	2	Impaired consciousness with an absence of shivering	28–32°C
Severe	3	Unconscious without shivering but maintaining a cardiovascular output	24–28°C
Profound	4	Cardiac Arrest or Extreme Low Flow Stage	<24°C
	5	Death due to irreversible hypothermia	<13.7°C

Table 6.7 Rewarming strategies

Rewarming type		Techniques	Rationale
Passive		Shivering	Shivering increases thermogeneration to five times the resting metabolic rate, resulting in a core temperature increase of 3 °C per hour
		Insulation	Insulation from further heat loss, ideally in the form of a blanket or bag structure that is insulating, reflective and also acts as a vapour barrier
		Activity	For mild hypothermia, physical activity may generate enough heat to regain normothermia; however, exertion may also precipitate afterdrop
		Calorie supplementation	Providing warmed calorific drinks will provide additional energy to fuel shivering
Active	Non-invasive	Heat pads or packs applied to the torso	In a shivering patient, shivering will decrease the patient's energy consumption and decrease the discomfort that shivering causes
		Body-to-body rewarming	Likely reduces thermal discomfort and minimises shivering, but is unlikely to cause significant core temperature rise
		Forced air warming	Rarely available in the pre-hospital setting; initially only the trunk is warmed to avoid afterdrop
	Invasive	Heated and humidified oxygen	Reduces insensible heat loss, but is unlikely to lead to a significant rise in core temperature
		Heated IV fluids	Isotonic crystalloid fluids warmed to around 40 °C and administered IV may support blood pressure and contribute to rewarming
		Lavage	Peritoneal or pleural lavage/irrigation with warmed fluids can increase core temperature; gastric or colonic lavage can cause unwanted electrolyte shifts and should be avoided
		Extracorporeal blood rewarming	Various techniques can be used to facilitate heating a patient's blood outside his or her body

This patient's electrocardiogram is described as having abnormal QRS complexes. What changes in an ECG would you anticipate in a patient with hypothermia?

Presence of an Osborne or J-wave is the typical finding of a hypothermic patient's ECG (see Figure 6.3). However, there are a number of other common changes, including atrial fibrillation with a slow ventricular response, sinus bradycardia, prolongation of the QRS, and various ST segment and T-wave abnormalities. Such changes are more marked once the core temperature drops below 30 °C.

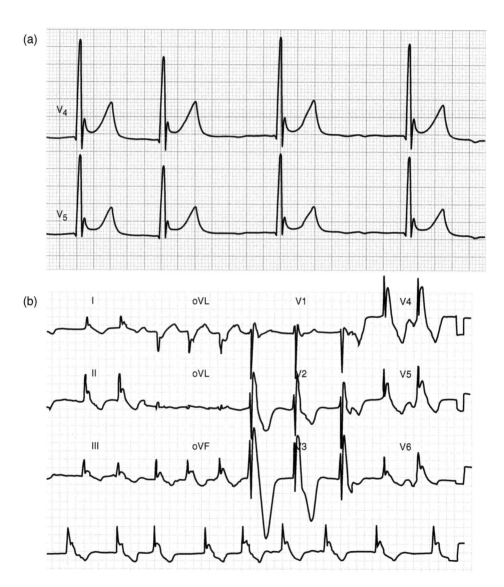

Figure 6.3 Hypothermia ECG – the J-wave. (a) J-waves in moderate hypothermia (temp. 30 °C). (b) Marked J-waves in severe hypothermia (temp. <27 °C). Reproduced with permission from Morris, F., Brady, W.J. & Camm, A.J. (2009) *ABC of Clinical Electrocardiography*, 2nd edn. Chichester: Wiley-Blackwell.

Case Progression

You have the patient wrapped in three layers (wool blanket, foil blanket, wool blanket) and have ambulance heaters on.

Patient assessment triangle
General appearance
She is looking much brighter and is now engaging with you.

Circulation to the skin
Good colour with a capillary refill time of 4 seconds.

Work of breathing
Normal work of breathing.

SYSTEMATIC APPROACH
Danger
Nil.

Response
Alert on the AVPU scale.

Airway
Clear.

Breathing
Rate: 17 bpm. Effort: normal. Accessory muscle use: no. Auscultation: mild crackles in all zones.

Circulation
Heart rate: 66 bpm. Effort: strong. Heart regularity: regular. Capillary refill time: 4 seconds.

Vital signs
RR: 17 bpm
HR: 66 bpm
BP: 111/64 mmHg
SpO_2: 96%
Blood sugar: 3.2 mmol/L
Temperature: 37 °C
Lead II ECG: sinus rhythm

Exposure
On exposure, no injuries found. Fingers and toes appear hyperaemic.

PRACTICAL TIP

Ambulances are very poorly insulated, and aircraft far worse! Whenever possible, heaters in ambulances should be running automatically to pre-warm the passenger compartment. This will benefit any trauma patients, children, the elderly and of course hypothermic patients.

Hypothermic patients should be handled gently, which may be challenging during rescue operations. Why is this?

Rough handling of this patient may irritate the hypothermic myocardium and stimulate ventricular dysrhythmias. Below around 28 °C such a rhythm may be ventricular fibrillation, which may be precipitated by a developing acidosis, hypocarbia, hypoxia or by sudden movement or injudicious patient handling (Zafren et al., 2014). A balance must be struck between avoiding unnecessary movement and undertaking life-saving interventions.

If this patient were in cardiac arrest, how might you modify your resuscitation?

If cardiopulmonary resuscitation is required, appropriate modifications may include limiting adrenaline to three standard doses and after three unsuccessful defibrillation attempts withholding further defibrillation until core temperature is above 30 °C. Consideration could also be given to withholding chest compressions if required to facilitate a faster evacuation.

When would you recognise death in a hypothermic patient?

This is a challenging decision to make, as recognition of death in those with hypothermia is difficult. The saying 'no one is dead until they are warm and dead' exists to remind us of this point. If in doubt, commence resuscitation efforts. However, there are some situations where we can confidently say that death has occurred (Zafren et al., 2014):

- Avalanche victims buried for >35 mins in whom the airway is obstructed by snow or ice.
- Chest wall too stiff to undertake chest compressions.
- Other fatal injuries are present.

LEVEL 3 CASE STUDY
Anaphylaxis

Information type	Data
Time of origin	11:40
Time of dispatch	11:45
On-scene time	12:02
Day of the week	Wednesday
Nearest hospital	1 hour
Nearest backup	22 minutes
Patient details	Name: Jack Harper DOB: 12/09/1958

CASE
You have been called to a car on the outskirts of town for a 62-year-old male with breathing difficulties.

Pre-arrival information
Patient is conscious with difficulty in breathing.

Windscreen report
You drive along the road you have been sent to, which is bordered by fields on both sides. After about a mile you come across a car at the side of the road, with a man dressed in white slumped in the driver's seat.

Entering the location
The man does not acknowledge you when you bang on the car window, but the car is unlocked. As you open the car door, around 40 honey bees fly out of the car and disappear into the field behind you.

On arrival with the patient
The gentleman is sitting slumped sideways in the car. He is wearing white overalls with a veil and hat attached (unzipped and hanging over his shoulder). He is breathing in rapid, shallow breaths and is covered in a red raised rash.

Patient assessment triangle
General appearance
The patient is not alert. He appears to be *in extremis*.

Circulation to the skin
Widespread blotchy, raised red rash to his hands, face and neck.

Work of breathing
Significant tachypnoea with upper airway noises.

SYSTEMATIC APPROACH

Danger
A few dead bees are clinging to the patient's suit and you try to brush these off him. You ask your cremate if they're allergic and fortunately neither of you are.

Response
Unresponsive on the AVPU scale.

Airway
Stridor is evident, with accompanying tracheal tug.

Breathing
Rate: 40 bpm. Effort: markedly increased. Accessory muscle use: yes. Auscultation: wheeze bilaterally and upper airway noises.

Circulation
Heart rate: 132 bpm. Effort: weak central pulse. Heart regularity: regular. Capillary refill time: 2 seconds.

Vital signs
RR: 40 bpm
HR: 132 bpm
BP: unrecordable
SpO_2: 88%
Lead II ECG: sinus tachycardia

Exposure
When you have removed the patient from his vehicle and laid him supine, he moans and tries to open his eyes, which appear swollen. His chest and back are covered with raised erythematous weals. He is displaying tracheal tug, and intercostal and subcostal recession.

TASK
Looking at the information provided here, explain the patient's loss of consciousness in relation to the suspected pathology.

From the information presented, what immediate intervention does this patient require?

This patient is presenting with the signs and symptoms of anaphylaxis. The initial treatment is IM adrenaline, which should be administered immediately (Deakin et al., 2015). The appropriate doses are presented in Table 6.8.

Table 6.8 Intramuscular adrenaline doses in anaphylaxis

Age	Dose for IM administration	Volume of 1:1000 preparation	
Adult	500 µg	0.5 mL	
Child aged >12 years	500 µg	0.5 mL	Repeated after 5 minutes if no
Child aged 6–12 years	300 µg	0.3 mL	clinical improvement seen
Child aged <6 years	150 µg	0.15 mL	

Source: Adapted from Resuscitation Council UK (2012)

Once this first drug has been administered, what are the next pharmacological interventions this patient needs?

While adrenaline is the mainstay of treatment, this patient will require a number of other medications. Most pressingly, a fluid challenge of intravascular crystalloid is needed (500–1000 mL for an adult), followed by an antihistamine and a steroid.

If you were to use a patient's own adrenaline auto injector (AAI), which of the following statements are _false_?

a. An AAI can only be administered in the thigh.
b. All AAIs administer the same dose of adrenaline.
c. You need to 'press and hold; an AAI against the patient's muscle, to give time for it to deliver the drug.
d. AAIs contain a mixture of adrenaline and noradrenaline.
e. AAIs can be administered by paramedics.

a, b and d are _false_. An AAI can be administered into any large muscle group. Doses vary by brand and age group. AAIs only contain adrenaline.

Case Progression

You have administered 500 µg IM adrenaline, 10 mg IV chlorphenamine and 200 mg of IV hydrocortisone. 1 L crystalloid has also been infused, and a second 1 L is running in now, through a large-bore cannula. The patient is receiving high-flow oxygen.

Patient assessment triangle
General appearance
The patient is responsive to pain. The angioedema to his face is worsening.

Circulation to the skin
Generalised urticaria has developed across his whole body.

Work of breathing
Persistently high, but improving.

SYSTEMATIC APPROACH
Danger
Nil, you have moved the patient into your ambulance.

Response
Pain on the AVPU scale.

Airway
Stridor is improving.

Breathing
Rate: 28 bpm. Effort: increased. Accessory muscle use: yes. Auscultation: widespread polyphonic wheeze.

Circulation

Heart rate: 131 bpm. Effort: weak. Heart regularity: regular. Capillary refill time: <1 second.

Vital signs

RR: 28 bpm

HR: 131 bpm

BP: 81/33 mmHg

SpO_2: 97%

Blood sugar: 7 mmol/L

Temperature: 36.5 °C

Lead II ECG: sinus tachycardia

Exposure

Ventilation has improved, but generalised rash and oedema continue to worsen.

This patient has had an incomplete response to first line therapies for anaphylaxis. The degree of respiratory compromise appears to be improving, however they have ongoing significant cardiovascular compromise. They are likely to require further pharmacological support, possibly in the form of an inotrope infusion (RCUK, 2012). This may be an intervention available to all paramedics in your area, or may require early activation of an enhanced care team or specialist.

PRACTICAL TIP

In anaphylaxis, adrenaline is the key lifesaving intervention. Antihistamines and steroids are beneficial, but are not going to benefit your patient immediately. If in doubt, administer IM adrenaline as soon as possible.

What drug options do you carry to provide further cardiovascular support to this patient?

Repeated doses of IM adrenaline can be undertaken if no response is seen. However, it may be that IV adrenaline is required (Resuscitation Council UK, 2012). IV adrenaline must be carefully titrated and ideally administered as an infusion; Tables 6.9 and 6.10 give further details of this. Glucagon is also an option for anaphylaxis refractory to adrenaline, but this is unlikely to be required in a standard pre-hospital setting.

Table 6.9 Intravenous adrenaline dosages

Drug	Dosage (titrated to effect)	Preparation
Adrenaline infusion	0.1 µg/kg/min	10 mL 1:10,000 in 1 L 0.9% saline
Adrenaline as a push-dose vasopressor	50 µg boluses	0.5 mL 1:10,000

Table 6.10 Infusion table for adrenaline 1 µg/mL (1 mg adrenaline in 1 L 0.9% saline)

Weight (kg)	Micrograms per minute (µg/min)	Millilitres per minute (mL/min)	Millilitres per hour (mL/hr)
10	1	1	60
20	2	2	120
30	3	3	180
40	4	4	240
50	5	5	300
60	6	6	360
70	7	7	420
80	8	8	480
90	9	9	540
100	10	10	600
110	In obese patients, consider commencing infusion as per a 100 kg patient		

In patients with ongoing cardiovascular instability from anaphylaxis, intravenous adrenaline may be lifesaving. However its use is complicated by the risk of significant unwanted effects including acute hypertension, cardiac dysrhythmias and cardiac ischaemia, these can be life threatening. Intravenous adrenaline should only be undertaken by clinicians experienced in the titration of intravenous inotropes.

What safety netting would your ongoing management plan involve for any patient who has received IM adrenaline for suspected anaphylaxis?

All patients presenting with suspected anaphylactic reaction should be observed for at least 6 hours from point of exposure in a healthcare setting able to treat life-threatening developments. Furthermore, this patient group should be warned about the risk of a biphasic reaction occurring within the next 24 hours (Resuscitation Council UK, 2012).

LEVEL 3 CASE STUDY
Seizure

Information type	Data
Time of origin	16:28
Time of dispatch	16:32
On-scene time	16:40
Day of the week	Thursday
Nearest hospital	80 minutes
Nearest backup	22 minutes
Patient details	Name: Paul Boates
	DOB: 06/09/1970

CHAPTER 6: MEDICAL EMERGENCIES

CASE
You are dispatched to the local shopping centre for reports of a 50-year-old male having a seizure.

Pre-arrival information
The man is not conscious and breathing is unknown

Windscreen report
You are directed to a side entrance of the shopping centre by employees in hi-vis jackets.

Entering the location
On entering the shopping centre, you see a crowd of people surrounding your patient, who is experiencing a tonic-clonic seizure. A first aider is supporting his head and attempting to keep the onlookers at bay.

On arrival with the patient
The patient is a male who appears to be around 50 years old. There is a shopping bag lying next to him from the grocery store. He is actively seizing.

Patient assessment triangle
General appearance
Active tonic-clonic seizure activity.

Circulation to the skin
Slight cyanosis to lips.

Work of breathing
Disordered breathing.

SYSTEMATIC APPROACH
Danger
Nil, crowds are calm and disperse somewhat on your arrival.

Response
Unresponsive on the AVPU scale.

Airway
Some upper airway noises with air movement. Small amount of blood in mouth.

Breathing
Rate: difficult to assess. Effort: disordered muscle contractions. Auscultation: equal air entry, minimal air movement.

Circulation
Heart rate: rapid at approx. 120 bpm. Effort: weak radially. Heart regularity: appears regular. Capillary refill time: 2 seconds.

Vital signs
RR: difficult to assess
HR: 120 bpm
BP: unrecordable
SpO_2: unrecordable
Blood sugar: 6.8 mmol/L
Lead II ECG: unreadable due to artefact

Exposure
Generalised tonic-clonic seizure activity, incontinent of urine.

TASK
In relation to this case, list as many possible sources of collateral history or medical information that may be available to you as you can.

This patient requires early benzodiazepines to stop the seizure. For a patient who does not respond to initial benzodiazepine therapy, what are your next actions?

Such a case requires significant bandwidth to enable two lines of management concurrently: first, direct care of the patient: ensuring the medication was delivered, considering a second dose, optimising oxygenation and ventilation; second and concurrently, formulating an onward plan of care. This plan may involve requesting further help or rapid conveyance to hospital. Further management may involve the preparation and administration of further medications to curtail the seizure.

What are some potential strategies to optimise oxygenation while a patient is seizing?

High-flow oxygen via a nasal cannula can provide significant oxygenation, even for the apnoeic patient. Equally it may be possible to ventilate with some success used a bag-valve mask. Other simple manoeuvres should not be overlooked: for instance, it may be necessary to suction a patient's airway while they are seizing, especially if significant blood has soiled the airway from tongue biting.

What would be the properties of an *ideal* medication to terminate a seizure?

In the case of an anticonvulsant medication for use for patients experiencing a seizure, an *ideal* medication probably has multiple properties:

- Can be administered quickly and easily without requiring significant preparation.
- Administration does not require the use of needles, or gaining intravascular access.
- Wide therapeutic range to avoid overdosing or underdosing – theophylline is an example of a medication with a very narrow therapeutic range, requiring significant monitoring.

- Absence of side effect such as apnoea or confusion.
- Rapid predictable onset and offset (e.g. thiopentone).
- Long shelf life, with no specific storage requirements.

Case Progression

Despite administration of the full dose of benzodiazepine, the patient is still displaying generalised tonic-clonic seizure activity. You have applied a high-flow nasal cannula and placed two nasopharyngeal airways and a non-rebreather mask with 15 L/min oxygen.

Patient assessment triangle
General appearance
Actively seizing.

Circulation to the skin
In general skin colour is normal, perhaps with a touch of cyanosis to the lips.

Work of breathing
Difficult to assess while the patient is seizing.

SYSTEMATIC APPROACH
Danger
Nil.

Response
Unresponsive on the AVPU scale.

Airway
Appears clear.

Breathing
Rate: unclear. Effort: unable to assess. Accessory muscle use: seizure activity obscures accessory muscles. Auscultation: unable to hear any crackles or wheeze, but with the patient seizing it is difficult to discern breath sounds.

Circulation
Heart rate: 125 bpm. Effort: weak. Heart regularity: regular. Capillary refill time: 1 second.

Vital signs
RR: unclear
HR: 125 bpm
BP: unobtainable
SpO_2: unobtainable
Blood sugar: 5.7 mmol/L
Temperature: 37 °C
Lead II ECG: significant movement artefact

Exposure
On exposure a small haematoma is found on the patient's occiput and he has been incontinent of urine.

PRACTICAL TIP

Non-convulsive status epilepticus is problematic to diagnose and an EEG is usually required (SIGN, 2018). If in doubt, treat the patient as being in status epilepticus.

In a situation where you have requested additional assistance from an advanced care team for a patient in status epileptics, what steps can you undertake before their arrival?

As far as possible, secure the airway and deliver supplemental oxygen, while ensuring monitoring is in place for vital signs (including $ETCO_2$). Establish two secure points of large-bore intravascular access. Ensure the full dose of first-line medications has been given. If there is any suggestion of hypoglycaemia, administer IV glucose, and if there is any chance of alcohol abuse or nutritional deficiency, administer IV thiamine (vitamin B_1) if available.

What would be your anaesthetic strategy for this patient?

The key priority for induction of anaesthesia here is to minimise further hypoxia and secure an airway as quickly as possible to allow positive pressure ventilation to be administered. Ideally such an induction of anaesthesia would also terminate the seizure activity in the cerebrum.

In practice, such an anaesthetic would be a modified rapid sequence induction. This should be undertaken with propofol, thiopentone, ketamine or midazolam as the induction agent with an appropriate paralytic agent.

References and further reading

Australian Resuscitation Council (2016) Medications in adult cardiac arrest. https://resus.org.au/guidelines/ (accessed 30 October 2019).

Brown, D.J., Brugger, H., Boyd, J. & Paal, P. (2012) Accidental hypothermia. *New England Journal of Medicine*, 367(20): 1930–1938.

Deakin, C., Brown, S., Jewkes, F. et al. (2015) Prehospital resuscitation – Resuscitation Council. https://www.resus.org.uk/resuscitation-guidelines/prehospital-resuscitation/ (accessed 1 December 2019).

McIntosh, S., Opacic, M., Freer, L. et al. (2014) Wilderness Medical Society practice guidelines for the prevention and treatment of frostbite: 2014 update. *Wilderness & Environmental Medicine*, 25(4 suppl): S43–S54.

Reid, C., Brindley, P., Hicks, C. et al. (2018) Zero point survey: A multidisciplinary idea to STEP UP resuscitation effectiveness. *Clinical and Experimental Emergency Medicine*, 5(3): 139–143.

Resuscitation Council UK (2012) *Emergency Treatment of Anaphylactic Reactions: Guidelines for Healthcare Providers*. London: Resuscitation Council UK.

Resuscitation Council UK (2015) Advanced life support: Treat reversible causes. https://www.resus.org.uk/resuscitation-guidelines/adult-advanced-life-support/#reversible (accessed 30 October 2019).

SIGN (2018) *Diagnosis and Management of Epilepsy in Adults: A National Clinical Guideline*. Edinburgh: Scottish Intercollegiate Guidelines Network.

Strapazzon, G., Procter, E., Paal, P. & Brugger, H. (2014) Pre-hospital core temperature measurement in accidental and therapeutic hypothermia. *High Altitude Medicine and Biology*, 15: 104–111.

Zafren, K., Giesbrecht, G.G., Danzl, D.F. et al. (2014) Wilderness Medical Society practice guidelines for the out-of-hospital evaluation and treatment of accidental hypothermia. *Wilderness and Environmental Medicine*, 25: 425–445.

CHAPTER 6: MEDICAL EMERGENCIES

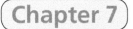
Non-technical skills

Georgette Eaton
Clinical Practice Development Manager, Advanced Paramedic Practitioner Urgent Care,
London Ambulance Service, NHS Trust, London, UK

> **CHAPTER CONTENTS**
> Level 1: Situational awareness
> Level 1: Communication
> Level 2: Egoism
> Level 2: Team working
> Level 3: Decision making
> Level 3: Flexibility

In addition to the technical knowledge and skills that will have been interwoven throughout the chapters so far, paramedic practice is also dependent on the ability to practice the cognitive and social skills that complement these technical skills. These 'non-technical' skills are *"not new or mysterious but are what the best practitioners do in order to achieve consistently high performance and what the rest of us do on a good day"* (Flin & O'Connor, 2017, p. 1). Awareness of these skills, which are just as cognitively technical as the ability to undertake a physical examination, are elements of practise that we all must strive to master.

LEVEL 1 CASE STUDY
Situational awareness

Information type	Data
Time of origin	04:30
Time of dispatch	06:30
On-scene time	07:15
Day of the week	Friday
Nearest hospital	40 minutes
Nearest backup	Advanced paramedic, 30 minutes
Patient details	Name: Sarah Shiner
	DOB: 05/07/1978

> **CASE**
> You have been called to a female patient who has fallen.
>
> **Pre-arrival information**
> The patient is conscious and breathing.
>
> **Windscreen report**
> The large garden surrounding the house is well-established and overgrown. There is evidence of previous well-kept borders and a vegetable garden, both of which are scattered with leaves and frost. The door to the house is open.

Clinical Cases in Paramedicine, First Edition. Edited by Sam Willis, Ian Peate, and Rod Hill.
© 2021 John Wiley & Sons Ltd. Published 2021 by John Wiley & Sons Ltd.

Entering the location
Your breath hangs in the air as you loudly announce your arrival in the house and are greeted by a middle-aged female who is wrapped in many coats. She tells you that she found her aunt on the floor this morning and she's struggling to talk to her.

On arrival with the patient
The female patient is lying prone in a narrow utility room. There is evidence of blankets around her, but none actually covering the patient, who is wearing outer clothes and wellington boots. The utility room is long and narrow, flanked by a washing machine and cupboard on one side, and a wall with an open window on the other. There is only space for the patient on the floor and you at her head.

Patient assessment triangle
General appearance
You cannot see the patient's face, but she quietly responds to your voice and touch.

Circulation to the skin
Capillary refill time >2 seconds.

Work of breathing
Normal, quiet breathing.

TASK
Look through the information provided in this case study and highlight all of the information that might concern you as a paramedic.

Using what you currently know about the case at this point, including what you may have seen and how the patient is presenting to you, what are your first actions?

Due to the patient's positioning, you cannot undertake a full primary survey, and so the initial action needs simply to be considering moving the patient onto her back or side.

Once you have moved the patient to see her face, what are your next actions?

You need to complete the primary survey, including determining the correct level of consciousness.

SYSTEMATIC APPROACH
Response
Verbal.

Airway
Patent.

Breathing
Rate 14 bpm. No accessory muscle use. Shallow effort.

Circulation
Heart rate 40 bpm. Capillary refill time >2 seconds

Vital signs
RR: 14 bpm
HR: 40 bpm
BP: 82/40 mmHg
SpO$_2$%: 91%
Blood sugar: 4.2 mmol/L

Once you have undertaken the essential vital signs, what would your next action be?

This patient is primary survey positive, with more than one deranged vital sign. Oxygen would be indicated by the British Thoracic Society (BTS) (2016) and the Thoracic Society of Australia and New Zealand (2015). The next action you need to consider is whether you move the patient before undertaking the secondary survey (Case Progression A) or undertake the secondary survey with the patient in situ (Case Progression B).

Case Progression A

The patient is primary survey positive. You have chosen to administer 6 L oxygen via a partial rebreather mask and move the patient to a more accessible environment before undertaking any further observations.

Patient assessment triangle
General appearance
The patient has her eyes closed, but responds verbally to your voice. She cries out as you attempt to move her.

Circulation to the skin
Capillary refill time >2 seconds.

Work of breathing
Normal, quiet breathing.

Which of the following are your differential diagnoses?
a. Sepsis.
b. Not enough information collected to form a differential diagnosis.
c. Fall, unknown cause.

You don't yet have enough information to make a differential diagnosis. However, you have recognised that there is at least one deranged vital sign, and you cannot exclude trauma, sepsis or specific system failure. You have become focused on the patient and may cause harm by moving her without undertaking a more thorough assessment.

Case Progression B

The patient is primary survey positive. You have chosen to administer 6 L oxygen via a partial rebreather mask and complete a secondary survey with the patient in situ.

Patient assessment triangle
General appearance
The patient has her eyes closed, but responds verbally to your voice and does not move as you obtain undertake your secondary survey.

Circulation to the skin
Capillary refill time >2 seconds.

Work of breathing
Normal, quiet breathing.

SYSTEMATIC APPROACH
Danger
Nil.

Response
Voice on the AVPU scale.

Airway
Clear.

Breathing

Rate 14 bpm. Shallow effort.

Circulation

Heart rate 40 bpm. Capillary refill time >2 seconds.

Vital Signs

RR: 14 bpm

HR: 40 bpm

BP: 82/40 mmHg

SpO_2 (on oxygen): 94%

Temperature: 32 °C

Lead II ECG: sinus bradycardia

Exposure

Obvious shortening and external rotation to the left leg.

Which of the following are your differential diagnoses?

a. Neck-of-femur fracture.

b. Sepsis.

c. Hypothermia.

On recognising there is more than one deranged vital sign, you have undertaken a secondary examination. This has shown that the patient likely has a traumatic injury (such as a fracture to the left neck of femur) and is symptomatic for hypothermia. With this additional information, you are now able to focus your differential diagnoses and begin to formulate an action plan, considering any appropriate treatment prior to moving the patient. You have balanced the information obtained from the environment with the physiological presentation of the patient in order to make a decision.

Discussion

Endsley's 3-level theory of situational awareness holds that there are three stages to situational awareness formation (Hunter et al., 2020):

Perception – The first step in achieving situational awareness is to perceive the relevant dynamics of the environment. This involves the process of recognition, cue detection or monitoring which enable the clinician to build a picture of the current state of the environment based on multiple situational elements.

Review the narrative at the start of this case study. What objects, events, people, systems, environmental factors and their current states (locations, conditions, modes, actions) did you pick up on initially? Is there anything you notice now that you did not before?

You may have considered the following:

- The patient was found by her niece.
- The garden is well-established and overgrown.
- There are leaves and frost.
- The door to the house is open.
- Your breath hangs in the air.
- A middle-aged female relative is wrapped in many coats.
- The narrow utility room is flanked by a washing machine and cupboard on one side, and a wall with an open window on the other.
- Evidence of blankets around the patient, but none actually covering her.
- The patient is wearing outer clothes and wellington boots.

Comprehension – The next step in achieving situational awareness is the synthesis of the disjointed elements perceived. This is likely to be achieved through all forms of decision making, including pattern recognition, interpretation and evaluation (Collen, 2017).

How does the previous information influence your approach to this patient?

This scenario is clearly set in the colder months of the year, with leaf fall and frost present. There is evidence that the occupant of the house is starting to struggle with independence, with the overgrown garden. Your breath hangs in the air as you enter the house, meaning it is no warmer inside than outside. The relative is 'wrapped in many coats'. They have likely been in the house for some time, so their multiple layers tell you both that it is cold, but also that they have not been able to move much – thus the patient is likely immobile. The room the patient is in is unlikely to have heating, but in any case, with an open window, it is likely to be a heat inefficient room and thus generally colder. The fact that the patient is on the floor means that heat will have been lost through conduction - a patient who has fallen will lose significantly more heat to being in contact with the ground than they will to the air (Du Point & Dickinson, 2017). The patient is wearing outdoor clothing, meaning she either fell very early this morning, or last night. The blankets around the patient indicate three things: Firstly, that the patient was, at some point, cold. Secondly, that someone was able to put the blankets around the patient, likely the female relative. Thirdly, that the patient has removed them from herself, which is likely to be paradoxical undressing as part of the cognitive response to hypothermia (Mizukami et al., 1999).

Projection – The third stage of situational awareness involves the ability to project the current situation in an attempt to predict the evolution of the situation. This is achieved through knowledge particular to the situation (such as that which is necessary to be a paramedic) and comprehension of the situation achieved through the first two stages. This supports short-term planning and leads to decision making and subsequent action.

What were your predictions based on the case progression you chose?

If you opted to move the patient (Case progression A), you may have done so because you predicted that she would continue to deteriorate. If you opted to undertake a thorough assessment (Case progression B), you may have done so to gain more information to determine the presence of injury and severity of the condition, to better help you inform the treatment required prior to movement and transfer. There is no 'right' answer for this case example, but the ability to perceive, comprehend and then consider the outcome is an important element for this case.

PRACTICAL TIP

Every incident requires the paramedic to be situationally aware. This is important from the initial assessment all the way through to examination. It is particularly important to consider when preparing to undertake, or performing, a technical task. Situational awareness is lost when we become too focused on the task, or undertake a task without due attention to the environment.

LEVEL 1 CASE STUDY
Communication

Information type	Data
Time of origin	22:21
Time of dispatch	22:25
On-scene time	22:35
Day of the week	Saturday
Nearest hospital	90 minutes by road, 20 minutes by air
Patient details	Name: Adam Dimmond DOB: 29/06/1986

The ability to effectively communicate is outlined in regulatory guidance for paramedics (Health and Care Professions Council, 2016; Paramedicine Board of Australia, 2018), where the focus is on the clinician-patient partnership and the ability to act in the best interests of the patient. Poor communication in healthcare leads to various negative outcomes, including the compromise of patient safety, discontinuity of patient care and patient dissatisfaction (Vermeir et al. 2015).

CASE

You have been called to a 34-year-old male who has been stabbed.

Pre-arrival information

Helicopter Emergency Services (HEMS) are enroute.

Windscreen report

The stabbing has taken place on the sidewalk of a busy road. Whilst there is street lighting, the Police are standing and kneeling around a young person on the floor are using torches to light the scene.

Approaching the scene

A Police Officer approaches you advises that the scene is safe, and this was an isolated stabbing. They are concerned there is a lot of blood loss, and the knife is still in situ.

On arrival with the patient

The patient is lying supine on the floor and is conscious. He is shouting verbal abuse to the bystanders and police officers, and it is obvious that there is a knife protruding from the left side of his upper thorax (chest) and evidence of blood loss on his clothing as well as on the floor. A police officer is trying to reassure the patient and deescalate the rising tension. You hear that HEMS has landed.

Patient assessment triangle

General appearance

The patient is conscious and pale.

Circulation to the skin

Capillary refill time <2 seconds.

Work of breathing

Normal breathing, shouting in full sentences.

TASK

What organs may have been injured by the stab wound?

Using what you currently know about the case at this point, including what you may have seen and how the patient is presenting to you, what are your first actions?

The patient's airway is clear and the patient is breathing and managing to raise his voice. The knife is obviously protruding from the chest and there is significant blood loss. Your initial actions should follow the CABC primary survey approach, considering that additional expertise in the form of HEMS is imminently available.

Case Progression

As you complete your primary survey, the HEMS crew approach you. The physician introduces themselves to the patient and asks you to get the trolley bed from the ambulance, before beginning their assessment. They have taken control of the scene and care of the patient.

TASK

Reflect on how you feel having been interrupted during your primary survey and asked to get the trolley bed.

> **Case Progression**
>
> The physician eventually decides to anaesthetise the patient and asks your crewmate to assist, alongside the HEMS paramedic. They are completely focussed on the task. You place the trolley bed at the foot of the patient and return to the ambulance to retrieve the scoop stretcher. When you return, you see the physician directing the Police and your crewmate to pick up the patient, now sedated and intubated, and place them on the trolley bed, rather than waiting for the scoop stretcher. The HEMs physician tells you sharply, 'too late'. However, you realise that they have placed the patient the wrong way around on the trolley bed – the head being at the foot end of the trolley bed.

What are your next actions?

In the majority of emergency ambulances, the trolley bed will only lock into position when placed headfirst into the ambulance. The error must be corrected before the trolley bed is loaded onto the ambulance, otherwise the bed will not lock into position.

> **Case Progression**
>
> You tell the HEMS physician that the patient is on the trolley bed the wrong way around. You explain that if they continue, the bed will not lock into position. Despite this, they ignore you and proceed to load the trolley bed into the ambulance, it does not lock into position and the HEMS physician becomes agitated and realises the error.

What factors contributed to the trolley bed being loaded incorrectly into the ambulance?

There are several factors that could have contributed to this error. The trolley bed could have initially been positioned it in a way that would have reduced the chance of error. The physician, who was dominating the control of the scene, was also task-focussed. In dynamic, high-stress, environments, adhering to the instructions from more dominant personalities is a human response to authority (Preuschoft & Schaik, 2000), and such a response often results in the loss of original thought.

> **Case Progression**
>
> The HEMS physician acknowledges that the trolley bed does not lock into the ambulance, and orders that the patient is turned round. You, your cremate and the HEMS paramedic duly comply and the patient is repositioned on the trolley bed and secured for transport to hospital.

Discussion

The use of assertive communication is important to challenge any action or behaviour that is inappropriate or unsafe. The 'probe, alert, challenge and escalate' (PACE) tool is particularly useful to empower any healthcare professional of any type or seniority to use graded assertiveness.

Probe – Gain attention or raise a concern using a question. This may be in the form of a pre-emption, and can be a powerful way to inform others within the team when they are at risk of violating safe practice, and function to sensitise them to the need to alter their behaviour (Tarrant et al. 2017).

How could you have probed or raised concerns using a question in this incident?

Simply asking 'Is the patient the correct way round on the trolley bed?' may have been enough of a probe to prompt the other clinicians to consider the position.

Alert – Repeat this concern or increase your volume to be heard. Repetition and consistency have long been held as important components of health communication (Schiavo, 2013).

How could you have alerted the others to the problem in this incident?

This would have been about speaking more loudly, addressing the physician and stating the problem: 'Doctor, the patient is the wrong way round on the trolley bed.'

Challenge – Formally state your concern and challenge the decision. This requires a high level of assertation, but challenges can be a powerful tool to ensure everyone in the team listens (Tarrant et al., 2017). Unlike probing and alerting, challenges demand an answer.

Who would you challenge in this incident?

It is obvious that the physician has taken control of this incident, so the challenge should be directed at her: 'Doctor, the patient is the wrong way round on the trolley bed and it will not load correctly in the ambulance for you to be able to continue to manage his airway. Can I take over?'

Escalate – Gain eye contact and prepare to take over the task. This requires assertion and confidence. It includes an element of repetition and challenge but you also suggest the potential outcome to ensure risk is adverted.

How do you escalate in this incident?

If the other aspects of assertive communication have failed, it would be appropriate to address your crewmate, the HEMS paramedic and other bystanders: 'The patient is the wrong way round on the trolley bed and it will not load correctly. We need to turn the patient round so that he can continue to be managed.'

PRACTICAL TIP

Effective communication is the cornerstone of healthcare delivery and working together within a team. However, it is not always easy! Graded assertiveness is a useful tool for communicating within the team to avoid error, especially if there are opposing views or you have spotted a problem no one else has.

LEVEL 2 CASE STUDY
Egoism

Information type	Data
Time of origin	11:59
Time of dispatch	12:01
On-scene time	12:07
Day of the week	Monday
Nearest hospital	25 minutes (traffic)
Patient details	Name: Phillip Beer
	DOB: 01/01/1983

Grounded in several ethical doctrines, egoism describes relationships between self-interest, morality and behaviour. Egoism is held within a branch of ethics called consequentialism, in which the main theme is that an action is considered 'good' if the outcome or result is good (Eaton, 2019). With its belief that one's primary obligation is to ourselves, and self-interest is a virtue, Egoism is completely disconnected from beneficence, which has been widely regarded as the common morality of healthcare. Paramedicine is typically a career choice for those who wish to help people (Ross et al., 2016) and work has been done to frame anti-egoism within the profession: Not only being selfless, but actively working in the interests of others, even if it costs you something (Townsend, 2017).

CASE

You have been called to a private address for a 37-year-old male in cardiac arrest.

Pre-arrival information

This was a witnessed cardiac arrest, with cardiopulmonary resuscitation being performed by bystanders.

Windscreen report

The area outside the house appears to be safe, despite rubbish piled up the front wall and the garden littered with children's toys.

Entering the location

You are greeted by two adult males who appear distressed. They inform you that their friend collapsed while watching the football on TV and their other friend has been performing cardiopulmonary resuscitation since then.

On arrival with the patient

The patient is lying supine on the floor and is unconscious. Chest compressions are being performed.

Patient assessment triangle
General appearance
The patient is unconscious and pale.

Circulation to the skin
Capillary refill time <2 seconds.

Work of breathing
No breathing

After starting CPR you attach the automatic external defibrillator and administer one shock, before continuing chest compressions and moving through the arrest algorithm under guidance from your mentor. Despite opening the airway (Australian and New Zealand Committee on Resuscitataion, 2016; Deakin et al., 2015), there is minimal chest rise noted during ventilation.

Before thinking through this case study, reflect on how you would define egoism.

Grounded in several ethical doctrines, egoism describes relationships between self-interest, morality and behaviour. Egoism is held within a branch of ethics called consequentialism, in which the main theme is that an action is considered 'good' if, all things considered, the outcome or result is good (Eaton, 2019).

What may be causing minimal chest rise?

Poor chest rise during ventilation can be caused by several factors, such as airway blockage, lung injury (such as tension pneumothorax), chest wall trauma, or aspiration of regurgitated gastric contents into the lungs. The latter is common in patients who received CPR prior to arrival of the ambulance service, and is exacerbated by stomach inflation during rescue breaths (Simons et al., 2007). Aggressive ventilation increases airway pressure and increases gastric inflation, therefore increasing the chance of regurgitation (Simons et al., 2007).

Case Progression

A second crew arrives on scene to assist you, whereby one person undertakes the role of clinical team leader and oversees the incident. Your mentor assigns you to manage the airway. You have been signed off as competent in the full range of airway skills, but have not yet performed an endotracheal intubation on a patient.

What would be the most appropriate way to manage the airway in this case?

With gastric regurgitation, the airway needs more definitive management. Simple airway adjuncts will not reduce aspiration of gastric contents. Supraglottic airways reduce gastric inflation compared with the use of a bag-valve mask, whereas correct tracheal intubation abolishes this risk completely (Deakin et al., 2015). While tracheal intubation has long been considered the gold standard in pre-hospital airway management, the difficulties associated with successful intubation and outcome data have challenged this concept (Soar & Nolan, 2013). Ultimately, the optimal airway technique for cardiac arrest is dependent on the skills of the operator, the anticipated pre-hospital time and individual patient-dependent factors (Benger et al., 2018).

> **TASK**
> Consider the ethical arguments presented in this case.

Discussion

This case would require you to balance the patients need (to secure their airway), alongside the most contemporaneous evidence (such as the AIRWAYS-2 trial by Benger et al., 2018). You could argue that endotracheal intubation fulfils both points – the airway would be secured, and it is a sanctioned skill within the evidence-base. However, egoists will always rank the most important duties as those that bring them the greatest reward. Airway management in cardiac arrest requires no more than necessary to enable adequate oxygenation and ventilation (Deakin et al., 2015). Therefore, whilst endotracheal intubation would not be an incorrect choice, it is the choice that would benefit you more, when the patient may benefit just as well from a supraglottic airway device.

> **PRACTICAL TIP**
>
> Without awareness, egoistic actions may prevail over the altruistic intentions in treatment. Awareness is the key point, and adopting an anti-egoist mindset is important in working in a culture where putting the interests of others ahead of the self is considered part of the regulatory framework within the profession (Health and Care Professions Council, 2016; Paramedicine Board of Australia, 2018; Townsend, 2017).

LEVEL 2 CASE STUDY
Team working

Information type	Data
Time of origin	09:05
Time of dispatch	09:06
On-scene time	10:35
Day of the week	Tuesday
Nearest hospital	40 minutes
Patient details	Name: Jessica Brearsley
	DOB: 12/08/1982

Key components of teamwork include communication, sharing the same goal or vision and mutual trust and understanding (Salas et al., 2005). Regardless of the profession, when teamwork in healthcare fails, negative patient outcomes occur (Chapman et al., 2017; Francis, 2013; Patterson et al., 2012).

> **CASE**
> You have been called to a multiple vehicle road traffic collision on a busy major route.
>
> **Pre-arrival information**
> You are the third ambulance on scene, with police and fire services already in attendance.
>
> **Windscreen report**
> You arrive on scene to see six vehicles rear-ended into each other, each with significant damage. The scene is safe. Police have cordoned off the carriageway and the ambulance incident commander is approaching you.

Entering the location

You are directed to assist with extrication of an obese patient from one of the vehicles in the middle of the accident. The patient, a 38-year-old female, has been assessed and triaged, but they have been unable to clear her cervical spine of a fracture, and so the decision has been made to extricate the patient and you and your crewmate will provide the clinical oversight for extrication.

Patient assessment triangle

General appearance

The patient is conscious, appears well and is talking to the firefighters who are with her.

Circulation to the skin

The patient is well perfused. IV access was previously obtained, and the cannula is in situ but without any drug administration.

Work of breathing

The patient is talking in full sentences. A 28% rebreather mask supplying oxygen has been applied to her.

TASK

Consider the best, evidence-based method of extrication for a patient with isolated central neck pain who is sat in a vehicle.

Case Progression

Firefighters have been maintaining manual in-line stabilisation. Their longboard is on the ground next to the patient. The crew commander approaches you and discusses their plans with you. They would like to remove the roof of the car, which would enable them to slide the longboard down the back of the patient then tilt the chair back to then slide the patient out on the longboard.

What are your initial thoughts regarding this plan?

The crew commander is taking charge of this situation and plans for extrication are very much the responsibility of the fire and rescue services. The proposed plan is a standard method of extrication (Dunbar, 2012) and would be an appropriate method given the clinical condition of this patient. However, while the crew commander may be leading on the extrication, you still have clinical primacy of care for the patient, and so you will need to ensure you work together to facilitate the best outcome.

Case Progression

You agree to the plan and your crewmate swaps with one of the firefighters who has been maintaining manual in-line stabilisation. You explain the plan to the patient, and she sits and talks happily to you while the firefighters prepare the vehicle. Preparation finished, the crew commander asks if you have an update for them and enquires after the clinical condition of the patient.

Is there anything you need to inform the crew commander of?

As previously outlined, good communication is a cornerstone of successful healthcare delivery. The crew commander is ensuring that you are still involved in the extrication, and this would be a good opportunity to update on the clinical progression of the patient. This would also be a good opportunity to check the progression of their extrication plan, and whether there have been any changes to what was originally discussed.

PRACTICAL TIP

If you are not asked for an update, give one and ask for one too! Good teamwork relies on good communication, especially when different professional groups are contributing to reach the same goal. The best decisions can only be made with the most up-to-date information.

> **Case Progression**
>
> You undertake the secondary assessment, administer analgesia and remove the oxygen as per the patient's physiological parameters. The crew commander informs you that they are ready to start the extrication process and outlines in what order they will be cutting the vehicle in order to remove the roof. They have asked you and your crewmate to step away from the vehicle and the patient to allow them to do this, and one of the firefighters will stay with the patient to maintain manual inline stabilisation.

Is it appropriate for you to step away from the patient at this point?

In this case, without appropriate PPE, you cannot safely stay with the patient. However, it is important that the firefighters are made aware of anything to watch for while they take primacy of this element of the incident. For example, if opiate-based analgesia was given, the firefighters should be alert to any decrease in the patient's consciousness.

Discussion

Multi-professional teamwork represents collaboration between health professionals and sometimes other emergency services. Whilst teambuilding is considered a non-technical skill in itself, successful teamwork relies on situational awareness and good communication between relevant professionals involved in order to make, and follow, a plan. Appreciating the different knowledge and skills other professionals bring to the team is important, as it is the mix of these skills, when communicated and planned in the right way, that ensure effective and safe care is given to the patient.

LEVEL 3 CASE STUDY
Decision making

Information type	Data
Time of origin	15:33
Time of dispatch	19:27
On-scene time	19:50
Day of the Week	Thursday
Nearest hospital	15 minutes
Nearest backup	Advanced paramedic, 25 minutes
Patient details	Name: Amy Smythe
	DOB: 12/09/2015

Whilst decision making is a fundamental component of paramedic practice, it is incredibly complex. The dual-process theory of Epstein and Hammond (Epstein, 1994) outlines two 'systems' which control our cognitive operations: System 1 (the intuitive system) and System 2 (the analytical system).

In system 1 thinking, the available information is channelled through a subconscious pattern recognition based on similar past situations. This system is responsible for 'gut feeling' (Hogarth, 2001). System 2 is the more analytical side to the thinking process and conclusions are made through logical judgment, and a mental search for additional information acquired through past learning and experience. It is a much slower mechanism for thinking, requiring significant cognitive effort, but more likely to lead to better decisions (Hogarth, 2005). This analytical system is usually engaged when there is uncertainty or complexity, and when there is time to think.

Although System 2 (analytical) thinking is more deliberate than System 1, the latter is still very important for paramedics. System 1 thinking is required for those emergency situations, where rapid decisions must be made using pre-existing knowledge – essential for time critical situations. Complex, cognitive, operations eventually migrate from System 2 to System 1 as proficiency and skill are acquired, and pattern recognition replaces cognitive processing (Croskerry, 2009).

CASE

You have been called to a 5-year-old child with a high temperature.

Pre-arrival information

The parents have reported a high temperature for four days, and the child is crying and inconsolable.

Windscreen report

The front door is ajar to the large, detached property.

Entering the location

You are greeted by one adult female, who informs you that her child has had a temperature and today has begun to develop a rash.

On arrival with the patient

The patient is wrapped in a blanket on the sofa in the living room, watching a children's television programme.

Patient assessment triangle
General appearance

The patient is conscious and appears flushed, with an obvious blotchy redness to her face.

Circulation to the skin

Capillary refill time <2 seconds.

Work of breathing

Breathing at 28 bpm. No use of accessory muscles.

TASK

Look through the information provided in this case study and highlight all of the information that might concern you as a paramedic.

Which of the following are your first actions?

a. Expose the patient to review the rash.
b. Obtain a history of the presenting complaint.
c. Remove the blanket and turn off the television.
d. Obtain the patient's vital signs.

It is very tempting to get drawn into what you can see when faced with a patient where there a physical symptom. Whilst noticing this is part of your situational awareness, pattern recognition can be a really poor clinical decision-making technique when used in isolation (Banning, 2007). Therefore, you will need to focus on obtaining a thorough history of presenting complaint.

Using what you currently know about this case, what questions will you ask the mother to ascertain the history of the presenting complaint?

See Table 7.1.

These questions are not only related to what you already know (such as the fever) and what you can see (such as a skin compliant), but they also are looking to find out if there are any associated, severe symptoms. Once these are safely ruled out, you can continue gathering more information as part of your decision-making process.

Are there any other important questions you need to ask at the moment?

See Table 7.2.

The second set of questions should consider past medical history, medications, allergies and family history. Immunisation history should also be explored. This patient is 5 years old and so it is reasonable to enquire about her vaccination status according to national vaccination schedules (Australian Government Department

Table 7.1 Obtaining the history of the presenting complaint

History-taking question	Answer
When did the fever develop?	After school on Monday evening
How have you measured the child's fever?	With the back of my hand on her head
What have you tried to reduce the fever?	I have given regular paracetamol and plenty of water
Has she had any other symptoms?	She's had the usual cough/cold symptoms – with a runny nose and cough
Has she had any breathing difficulties?	No
Has she complained of any pain?	No, not really, just a generalised aching
Has she been eating and drinking as normal?	She's been happy to drink, but has had a loss of appetite over the week – eating a small amount each mealtime
Has she been toileting as normal?	Yes – she's been pooing and weeing every day as normal
Has she reported any abdominal pain?	No
Has she reported any headache?	No
Has anything made her any better?	No – I've tried wrapping her up in blankets, I've tried cooling her with the window open, I've tried difficult herbal drinks, but none of it is working
Has anything made her any worse?	No
When did the rash develop?	I noticed it this morning, it wasn't there yesterday
Has it spread since you noticed it?	I think it's spread downwards, from her face to her chest
Have you noticed any other symptoms?	She has grey spots inside her mouth, I didn't think anything of them as she hasn't complained of a sore throat or anything

Table 7.2 Further history taking

History-taking question	Answer
Does the patient have any past medical history?	No
Is the patient prescribed any medications?	No
Is the patient allergic to anything?	No
Who lives with the patient – has anyone else in the household been unwell?	It's just me, my partner and my child, we've both been fine
Does she attend school?	Yes, she started school this year
Has she had all her vaccinations?	She had her vaccinations up to the age of 1 year, and then we stopped
When did you last give paracetamol?	2 hours ago

of Health, 2019b; Ministry of Health NZ, 2020b; NHS, 2019). In this case, the parents stopped the vaccination regime, so the patient is likely not immunised against conditions such as measles, mumps, rubella, meningitis, whooping cough and others.

Case Progression

As you ascertain the history of the presenting complaint, you undertake your secondary survey with the consent of the mother and compliance of the patient.

SYSTEMATIC APPROACH

Response
Alert.

Airway
Patent.

Breathing
Rate 26 bpm. Dry cough present. No accessory muscle use. Talks full sentences and replies to you. SpO$_2$: 100%. Auscultation – bilateral air entry, chest clear.

Circulation
Heart rate 125 bpm. Capillary refill time <2 seconds. Hot to touch.

Vital signs
RR: 26 bpm
HR: 125 bpm
Blood sugar: 4.2 mmol/L
Temperature: 39.8 °C

Exposure
A blotchy, flat rash spread over the face, neck and torso.

Which of the following are your differential diagnoses?
a. Pyrexia of unknown origin.
b. Meningitis.
c. Viral illness.
d. Infectious disease.

You have all the information here to follow an analytical decision-making process. The patient has been experiencing a fever for 4 days, with coryzal symptoms as well as some grey spots in the mouth. The rash, flat and red, started 3 days after the temperature began and is moving from the head downwards. The child has a high-grade pyrexia, and her other physiological signs are towards the upper end of normal parameters. The child has not received her childhood vaccinations and, with the current rise in measles within countries that claimed previous elimination (Australian Government Department of Health, 2019a, 2019c; Public Health England, 2019), this infectious disease should be top of your differential list. The pyrexia is likely caused as part of the body's response to the virus. While measles is a viral illness, it is reportable under various public health legislation (Australian Government Department of Health, 2019c; Ministry of Health New Zealand, 2020a; Public Health England, 2019) and so a firm diagnosis is required to be made by a physician. However, you can be reasonably clear in your decision making to ensure that this notification is made to the relevant public health body, and the patient is reviewed.

Discussion

When caring for paediatric patients, 75% of diagnostic failures can be attributed to clinical decision making failure (Thammasitboon & Cutrer, 2013). Clinical judgements are based on sound decision making, and the ability to form a correct clinical impression is central to ongoing patient care (Collen, 2017). It is tempting to make a decision intuitively, based on what is seen – rather than considering why the presentation has occurred. Undertaking an analytical process in decision making allows the paramedic to piece all relevant information together, especially in new clinical situations with different presentations compared to those seen before (Tay et al., 2016). Thus, the paramedic's ability to provide safe, high-quality care is dependent upon their ability to reason, think, and judge.

LEVEL 3 CASE STUDY
Flexibility

Information type	Data
Time of origin	23:59
Time of dispatch	00:19
On-scene time	00:43
Day of the week	Wednesday
Nearest hospital	47 minutes
Nearest backup	Clinical team leader, 11 minutes
Patient details	Name: Jasmine Willis
	DOB: 31/08/1998

Cognitive flexibility is the ability to adjust one's thinking from old situations to new situations, by overcoming habitual thinking or responses and adapt to new situations (Scott, 1962). In paramedicine, it is the ability to have an awareness and understand all the possible options and alternatives simultaneously within any given situation. Flexible thinking is a key element of the critical thinking process and avoids tunnel vision by ensuring the clinicians' mind is open to all possible causes of the patient's current condition.

CASE

You have been called to a 22-year-old female with difficult breathing.

Pre-arrival information

The patient has also been drinking alcohol.

Windscreen report

You approach a bar in the centre of a town, with loud music blaring from the inside. The patient is sat outside against the wall.

On arrival with the patient

The patient has her eyes closed and is crying, breathing heavily between sobs.

Patient assessment triangle
General appearance

The patient is conscious and is clearly crying.

Circulation of the skin

Capillary refill time <2 seconds.

Work of breathing

Breathing at 30 bpm. Accessory muscle use is noted and the patient cannot talk in full sentences.

TASK

Reviewing this information, what could be causing this patient's dyspnoea?

Case Progression

You are informed by one of the patient's friends that the patient had been dancing with her friends when she suddenly became short of breath, dizzy and unable to breathe. She wanted some fresh air and collapsed outside on the floor, crying and breathing heavily.

Which of the following questions do you need to ask first?
a. The amount of alcohol consumed.
b. The use of any illicit drugs.
c. Whether the patient has any respiratory conditions.
d. Whether anything has upset the patient.
e. All of the above.

These are all important questions to start the consultation. At this point there could be a variety of causes for this patient's dyspnoea, including an anxiety attack, cardiac event, exacerbation of asthma, pulmonary embolism or use of synthetic illicit drugs (such as LSD or ecstasy). Asking a variety of initial, early questions will ensure you do not have tunnel vision in your approach and can consider a range of diagnoses.

Case Progression

A friend with the patient denies the group was using any illicit drugs and outlines they have had a range of cocktails, alcoholic shots and vodka in the last 4–6 hours. The patient had seen her recent Tinder date with another girl earlier this evening and that had upset her, but she's 'totally over it now'. You move on to your secondary survey.

SYSTEMATIC APPROACH

Danger
Nil.

Response
Alert on the AVPU scale.

Airway
Clear, able to talk in incomplete sentences.

Breathing
Rate 30 bpm. Increased work of breathing, use of accessory muscles. Respiratory auscultation: bilateral air entry, chest clear.

Circulation
Heart rate 138 bpm. Capillary refill time <2 seconds.

Vital signs
RR: 30 bpm
HR: 138 bpm
BP: 118/62 mmHg
SpO_2: (on oxygen): 92%
Temperature: 36.3 °C
Lead II ECG: sinus tachycardia

Exposure
No swelling or lower leg pain.

Of the possible causes of dyspnoea considered earlier, which is now the most likely?
a. Anxiety attack, pulmonary embolism.
b. Anxiety attack, cardiac event.
c. Illicit drug use, exacerbation of asthma.
d. Anxiety attack, illicit drug use.

There is no obvious cause of distress and the report of a collapse and the physiological symptoms of dyspnoea, tachypnoea, tachycardiac and low saturations also indicate there could be an underlying physical cause.

Case Progression

You administered supplemental oxygen therapy as per local guidelines (British Thoracic Society, 2016; Thoracic Society of Australia and New Zealand, 2015) and, as a pulmonary embolism (PE) is the mostly likely diagnosis with these symptoms, consider undertaking a Wells score to determine the probability of PE. Based on the information obtained so far, this scores PE as unlikely (Torbicki et al., 2008).

Are there any other questions you could consider now?

See Table 7.3.

Table 7.3 History-taking questions

History-taking question	Answer
Does you have any past medical history?	Thrombophilia
Any recent surgery?	No
Do you take any medications?	Only the oral contraceptive pill
Are you allergic to anything?	No
Does anyone in your family suffer with any medical problems?	Mother has thrombophilia

These answers demonstrate that the patient may actually be a higher risk for a PE than determined by the Wells' score. A past medical and family history of thrombophilia, as well as the oral contraceptive pill, increase the likelihood that this patient is experiencing a PE (Doherty, 2017).

Discussion

Flexibility ensures that paramedics have the capability to adapt to new, different, or changing presentations. Considering the varying causes of the presentation and avoiding cognitive rigidity (tunnel vision) is an exceptionally useful non-technical skill that is honed and developed during the formulative years in undergraduate education, and built on whilst working in clinical practice (Loving, 1993).

References and further reading

Australian and New Zealand Committee on Resuscitation (2016) Guideline 8 Cardiopulmonary Resuscitation (CPR). https://www.hpw.qld.gov.au/__data/assets/pdf_file/0010/5203/anzcorguideline8cprjan16.pdf (accessed 3 July 2020).

Australian Government Department of Health (2019a) Measles outbreaks 2019. https://www1.health.gov.au/internet/main/publishing.nsf/Content/ohp-measles-outbreaks-2019.htm (accessed 3 July 2020).

Australian Government Department of Health (2019b) National Immunisation Program Schedule. https://www.health.gov.au/health-topics/immunisation/immunisation-throughout-life/national-immunisation-program-schedule (accessed 1 December 2019).

Australian Government Department of Health (2019c) National Notifiable Diseases Surveillance System. http://www9.health.gov.au/cda/source/cda-index.cfm (accessed 3 July 2020).

Banning, M. (2007) A review of clinical decision making: Models and current research. *Journal of Clinical Nursing*, 17(2): 187–195. doi: 10.1111/j.1365-2702.2006.01791.x

British Thoracic Society (2017) Guidelines for oxygen use in healthcare and emergency settings. https://www.brit-thoracic.org.uk/quality-improvement/guidelines/emergency-oxygen/ (accessed 3 July 2020).

Collen, A. (2017) *Decision Making in Paramedic Practice*. Bridgwater: Class Professional Publishing.

Doherty, S. (2017) Pulmonary embolism: An update. *Australian Family Physician*, 46(11), 816–820.

Dunbar, I. (2012) *Vehicle Extrication Techniques*. Nottingham: Holmatro.

Du Point, D. & Dickinson, E. (2017) Identifying and managing accidental hypothermia. *Journal of Emergency Medical Services*, 11(42).

Eaton, G. (2019) *Law and Ethics for Paramedics: An Essential Guide*. Bridgwater: Class Professional Publishing.

Endsley, M.R. (1995) Toward a theory of situation awareness in dynamic systems. *Human Factors*, 37(1): 32–64. doi: 10.1518/001872095779049543

Epstein, S. (1994) Integration of the cognitive and the psychodynamic unconscious. *American Psychologist*, 49(8), 709–724. doi: 10.1037/0003-066X.49.8.709

Flin, R. & O'Connor, P. (2017) *Safety at the Sharp End: A Guide to Non-technical Skills*. Boca Raton, FL: CRC Press.

Health and Care Professions Council (2014) Standards of proficiency – paramedics. https://www.hcpc-uk.org/resources/standards/standards-of-proficiency-paramedics/ (accessed 3 July 2020).

Health and Care Professions Council (2016) *Standards of Conduct, Performance and Ethics*. London: HCPC.

Ministry of Health New Zealand (2020a) List of diseases notifiable by health practitioners and laboratories to the Medical Officer of Health. https://www.health.govt.nz/our-work/diseases-and-conditions/notifiable-diseases (accessed 3 July 2020).

Ministry of Health New Zealand (2020b). New Zealand Immunisation Schedule. https://www.health.govt.nz/our-work/preventative-health-wellness/immunisation/new-zealand-immunisation-schedule (accessed 3 July 2020).

Mizukami, H., Shimizu, K., Shiono, H. et al. (1999) Forensic diagnosis of death from cold. *Legal Medicine*, 1(4): 204–209. doi: 10.1016/s1344-6223(99)80039-x

NHS (2019) Vaccinations. https://www.nhs.uk/conditions/vaccinations/ (accessed 1 December 2019).

Paramedicine Board of Australia (2018) Professional capabilities for registered paramedics. https://www.paramedicineboard.gov.au/Professional-standards/Professional-capabilities-for-registered-paramedics.aspx (accessed 3 July 2020).

Patterson, P., Weaver, M.D., Weaver, S.J. et al. (2012) Measuring teamwork and conflict among emergency medical technician personnel. *Prehospital Emergency Care*, 16(1): 98–108. doi: 10.3109/10903127.2011.616260

Preuschoft, S. & Schaik, C. (2000) Dominance and communication: Conflict management in various social settings. In *Natural Conflict Resolution* (eds F. Aureli & F. Waal), Berkeley, CA: University of California Press, pp. 77–105.

Public Health England (2019) Measles notifications and confirmed cases by oral fluid testing 2013 to 2019. https://www.gov.uk/government/publications/measles-confirmed-cases/measles-notifications-and-confirmed-cases-by-quarter-in-england-2013-to-2015 (accessed 1 December 2019).

Scott, W.A. (1962) Cognitive complexity and cognitive flexibility. *Sociometry*, 25(4): 414. doi: 10.2307/2785779

Simons, R.W., Rea, T.D., Becker, L.J. & Eisenberg, M.S. (2007) The incidence and significance of emesis associated with out-of-hospital cardiac arrest. *Resuscitation*, 74(3): 427–431. doi: 10.1016/j.resuscitation.2007.01.038

Soar, J. & Nolan, J.P. (2013) Airway management in cardiopulmonary resuscitation. *Current Opinion in Critical Care*, 19(3): 181–187. doi: 10.1097/MCC.0b013e328360ac5e

Thammasitboon, S. & Cutrer, W.B. (2013) Diagnostic decision-making and strategies to improve diagnosis. *Current Problems in Pediatric and Adolescent Health Care*, 43(9): 232–241. doi: 10.1016/j.cppeds.2013.07.003

Thoracic Society of Australia and New Zealand (2015) Oxygen guidelines for acute oxygen use in adults. https://www.thoracic.org.au/journal-publishing/command/download_file/id/34/filename/TSANZ-AcuteOxygen-Guidelines-2016-web.pdf (accessed 3 July 2020).

Torbicki, A., Perrier, A., Konstantinides, S. et al. (2008) Guidelines on the diagnosis and management of acute pulmonary embolism: The Task Force for the Diagnosis and Management of Acute Pulmonary Embolism of the European Society of Cardiology (ESC). *European Heart Journal*, 29(18): 2276–2315. doi: 10.1093/eurheartj/ehn310

Chapter 8

Trauma cases

Tom E. Mallinson[1] and Fenella Corrick[2]
[1] BASICS Scotland, Auchterarder, UK
[2] Western Isles, Scotland, UK

CHAPTER CONTENTS

LEVEL 1 CASE STUDY
Burns

Information type	Data
Time of origin	12:10
Time of dispatch	12:22
On-scene time	12:34
Day of the week	Thursday
Nearest hospital	40 minutes by road
Nearest burns unit	2 hours by road
Nearest backup	Helicopter-based critical care paramedic, 23 minutes
Patient details	Name: Stacey Ridcliffe
	DOB: 12/03/1996

CASE
A 24-year-old non-binary patient has called an ambulance after knocking over a pan of boiling water.

Pre-arrival information
The patient is conscious and breathing. They have burns to their right arm.

Windscreen report
You arrive in a residential area. It appears safe and unremarkable.

Entering the location
The front door of the house is open and you venture inside, following calls for help from a downstairs bathroom.

Clinical Cases in Paramedicine, First Edition. Edited by Sam Willis, Ian Peate, and Rod Hill.
© 2021 John Wiley & Sons Ltd. Published 2021 by John Wiley & Sons Ltd.

On arrival with the patient

The patient is standing with their right arm under the shower, they're tearful and clearly in significant pain. They tell you it was a pan of boiling oil, rather than water, and that they rushed to the shower as soon as it happened.

Patient assessment triangle
General appearance
Alert and orientated.

Circulation to the skin

Good colour to skin, no pallor or cyanosis. Their right arm is highly erythematous, with some areas of blistering and sloughing skin already apparent.

Work of breathing

They are tachypnoeic, but do not appear to have increased work of breathing.

SYSTEMATIC APPROACH

Danger

Your crewmate enters the kitchen to ensure there is no ongoing risk from the stove or oil. They report they have turned off the gas hob and the kitchen is safe.

Response

The patient is alert and responding normally to you.

Airway

Airway is clear and self-maintaining. There is no evidence of burns or inhalation injury.

Breathing

Respiratory rate is elevated, on auscultation normal air entry is heard in all lung fields.

Circulation

Radial pulse is strong with a rapid rate, capillary refill time is 2 seconds centrally.

Vital signs
RR: 20 bpm
HR: 110 bpm
BP: 144/85 mmHg
SoO_2: 99%
Lead II ECG: sinus tachycardia

Exposure

The right arm has widespread erythema on the anterior of the arm and circumferentially to the forearm and hand. The erythema to the arm is mild, while on the forearm and hand there is significant blistering and desquamation of skin.

TASK

Looking at the information in the case, which elements of this history and assessment make you most concerned and why?

What is your cooling strategy for this patient?

Tepid running water should be used to cool burns for 20 minutes within the first 3 hours post-burn (Stiles & Goodwin, 2018). Cooling beyond this time with cold water may result in unwanted hypothermia. Ice or iced water should not be used (Stiles & Goodwin, 2018).

This patient has burns to a *special area*, what are the areas considered special areas in relation to a burns injury?

The *special areas* in terms of a burns injury are those that pose the risk of a worse outcome or progression to further significant complications. They usually require discussion with a specialist burns unit. The following are considered special areas in relation to burns injuries:

- Face
- Hands
- Feet
- Joints
- Neck
- Perineum or genital area

What other aspect of this patient's burn makes you especially concerned?

This patient has circumferential burns to their forearm and hand. This alone makes this injury a serious burn requiring hospital assessment and possibly admission.

Case Progression

You have cooled the burn for 20 minutes under a tap, and the patient has been moved to the ambulance and wrapped in a blanket to maintain normothermia. You have gained IV access and given 1 g paracetamol. The burn has been covered with a sterile burns dressing.

Patient assessment triangle
General appearance
The patient was shivering slightly before being wrapped in blankets, and they still appear to be in pain.

Circulation to the skin
Normal colour of skin.

Work of breathing
Normal work of breathing.

SYSTEMATIC APPROACH
Danger
There is no danger.

Response
The patient is alert and orientated.

Airway
Patent, no compromise.

Breathing
Rate: 22 bpm. Effort: normal. Accessory muscle use: no. Auscultation: equal bilateral vehicular breath sounds.

Circulation
Heart rate: 122 bpm. Effort: strong. Heart regularity: regular. Capillary refill time: 2 seconds.

Vital signs
RR: 22 bpm
HR: 102 bpm

BP: 137/89 mmHg
SpO$_2$: 99% on air
Blood sugar: 8.2 mmol/L
Lead II ECG: sinus tachycardia
Temperature: 35.5 °C – tympanic

Exposure
No changes.

If you administer morphine to this patient, what other type of drug would it be useful to also administer?

The management plan for this patient will include a journey to hospital by road or air. As opioids are emetogenic, it would be sensible to administer an antiemetic early. Ondansetron would be a good choice.

This patient is still in pain despite cooling, paracetamol and morphine. What is your approach to providing adequate analgesia to this patient?

In general a multimodal approach to analgesia provision is warranted. In this case you have already utilised two different pharmacological interventions and the physical intervention of cooling and applying a dressing.

When considering analgesia provision, it is worth first considering non-pharmacological options such as reassurance, distraction, splinting and applying dressings. Then when thinking about pharmacological interventions, one useful approach is to consider the classes of the medications involved and if there is scope to add an agent from a different class. In this case paracetamol and an opioid have been used. To create a truly multimodal approach, consideration could be given to non-steroidal anti-inflammatories (NSAIDs), inhaled agents, ketamine and techniques such as regional anaesthesia (Porter et al., 2018; Smith et al., 2011).

LEVEL 1 CASE STUDY
Limb injury following a fall from height

Information type	Data
Time of origin	11:10
Time of dispatch	11:22
On-scene time	12:34
Day of the week	Thursday
Nearest hospital	40 minutes by road
Nearest burns unit	2 hours by road
Nearest backup	Helicopter-based critical care paramedic, 23 minutes
Patient details	Name: Charlotte Ballard DOB: 25/04/2000

CASE
You have been called to a 20-year-old female rock climber who has fallen approximately 3 metres while climbing.

Pre-arrival information
The casualty is conscious and breathing. She is unable to walk from the scene.

Windscreen report
On arrival in a car park, you see a young woman sitting at the base of a rocky wall, with a man crouching beside her.

Entering the location
A rope is secured up to a height of approximately 3 metres to bolts in the wall. Both the woman and the man are wearing helmets and climbing harnesses.

On arrival with the patient
The young woman is sitting with her right leg stretched out in front of her with deformity at the ankle.

Patient assessment triangle
General appearance
The patient is alert and orientated.

Circulation to the skin
Normal.

Work of breathing
Tachypnoeic, speaking in full sentences. No added sounds.

SYSTEMATIC APPROACH
Danger
There are no other climbers using the wall or at the top of the wall. It is safe to approach.

Response
Alert on the AVPU scale.

Catastrophic haemorrhage
There is no evidence of catastrophic external haemorrhage.

C-spine
No evidence of injury.

Airway
Clear.

Breathing
Rate: 18 bpm. Effort: normal. Accessory muscle use: no. Auscultation: good air entry throughout the chest, no added sounds.

Circulation
Heart rate: 112 bpm. Effort: normal. Heart regularity: regular. Capillary refill time: 2 seconds.

Vital signs
RR: 18 bpm
HR: 18 bpm
BP: 130/85 mmHg
SpO$_2$: 98%
Blood sugar: 5 mmol/L

TASK
Look through the information provided in this case study and highlight all of the information that might concern you as a paramedic.

What assessment must be included in the examination of a suspected limb injury?

As for all musculoskeletal examinations, the approach should be 'look, feel, move'.

If significant injury is suspected, it is essential to assess the neurovascular status of the limb distal to the injury. If there is evidence of neurovascular compromise distal to the wound, this must be documented and would warrant escalation of urgency in treatment. If there is no neurovascular compromise on initial assessment, this must be regularly reviewed and documented until handover to definitive care.

What is involved in assessment of neurovascular status?

For neurological assessment, both motor and sensory components of nerve function should be assessed. In the case described, movements distal to the ankle should be assessed such as toe plantar and dorsiflexion. Sensation should be assessed by testing both presence and subjective normality of light touch sensation.

Vascular status should be assessed by testing capillary refill time distal to the injury, for example in the great toe. Pulses distal to the injury should also be assessed and specifically documented as present or absent. In the case of suspected ankle injury, both dorsalis pedis and posterior tibialis pulses should be assessed.

What volume of blood might be lost in a closed fracture of the ankle? What is the most volume that might be lost in a fracture?

In a closed ankle fracture, estimated blood volume loss could be 500–1000 mL. The volume is limited by the relatively small calibre of vessels in the area and the tamponade (compressive) effect of the limited space available in the surrounding soft tissues. In contrast, in an open fracture there is potentially unlimited blood volume loss to exsanguination unless haemorrhage control is achieved.

What analgesia options would you consider for this patient?

For pain caused by fractures, splinting is a highly effective intervention for pain control.

In terms of pharmacological pain management, a multimodal approach to analgesia is often more effective than use of a single mode, due to acting at different sites and effectively 'diluting' side effects.

Simple analgesia such as IV paracetamol may be effective alone for mild to moderate pain or act synergistically with other analgesics in severe pain.

Opiates, which have already been administered to this patient, can be highly effective. There are multiple rapid and effective delivery modalities, including oral, intranasal, intravenous and intraosseous.

Inhalation agents can also be used. Due to their relatively short action, these may be particularly beneficial as adjuncts during interventions or moving the patient.

What is the purpose of splinting in long bone fracture management?

The goal of splinting is to reduce the abnormal position of fractured bones in order to reduce damage to surrounding tissues and to lessen associated pain and haemorrhage.

LEVEL 2 CASE STUDY
Car versus pedestrian

Information type	Data
Time of origin	16:58
Time of dispatch	17:00
On-scene time	17:22
Day of the week	Monday
Nearest hospital	40 minutes
Nearest backup	30 minutes
Patient details	Name: John Lonogan DOB: 30/09/1975

CASE

You are called to support an ambulance staffed by emergency care assistants who are attending a road traffic collision reported as 'car versus pedestrian'.

Pre-arrival information

A male in his 40s has been struck by a car. He is conscious and breathing.

Windscreen report

The road has been closed by the local police. The first ambulance on scene is parked in the fend- off position with its emergency warning lights cycling. No patient is visible on scene; you suspect he has been transferred to the ambulance already.

Entering the location

You are greeted by a colleague you know well, who is a fairly new ambulance attendant. She tells you the patient is a 45-year-old man who was crossing the road when he was struck by a car travelling at approximately 35 miles per hour (56 kilometres per hour). He has told your colleague he is a smoker, but is otherwise fairly healthy, taking no medications and with no allergies.

On arrival with the patient

The male patient is supine on the ambulance trolley, he has been immobilised and is receiving high-flow oxygen (15 Lpm) via a non-rebreather mask. He appears breathless.

Patient assessment triangle

General appearance

The patient is alert and looks at you as you reach his side. He is breathing quickly.

Circulation to the skin

He is diaphoretic and slightly pale.

Work of breathing

You note tachypnoea and dyspnoea with mild tracheal tug.

SYSTEMATIC APPROACH

Danger

Nil, the scene has been made safe.

Response

Alert on the AVPU scale.

Airway

Clear and self-maintaining.

Breathing

Rate: 40 bpm. Effort: marked increased effort. Accessory muscle use: yes. Auscultation: normal air entry on the right, 'echoing' breath sounds on the left.

Circulation

Heart rate: 140 bpm. Effort: strong radial pulse. Heart regularity: regular. Capillary refill time: 3 seconds centrally

Vital signs

RR: 40 bpm
HR: 140 bpm
BP: 110/52 mmHg
SpO$_2$: 91%
Blood sugar: 7.3 mmol/L
GCS 15/15
Lead II ECG: sinus tachycardia

Exposure

Mild bruising to the left side of his chest.

> **TASK**
>
> Look through the information provided in this case study and highlight all of the information that might concern you as a paramedic.

What are the clinical findings you would expect to present in a patient with a tension pneumothorax?

Tracheal deviation is often the first clinical sign students and clinicians describe when asked this question; however, tracheal deviation is a very late sign in cases of tension pneumothorax. Common signs and symptoms are listed in Table 8.1. The diagnosis is a clinical one and this is an emergency needing immediate intervention. Tension haemo- or pneumo-thorax should be suspected in patients with significant thoracic trauma (such as flail segments) or a mechanism suggestive of significant energy transfer.

Table 8.1 Signs and symptoms suggestive of a tension pneumothorax

Dyspnoea
Reduced breath sounds
Hypoxaemia
Tachypnoea
Tachycardia
Hypotension
Hyperresonance to percussion
Subcutaneous emphysema
Narrowing pulse pressure
Reduced chest expansion
Distended neck veins (unless also hypovolaemic)
Loss of consciousness
Tracheal deviation (rarely clinically apparent)
Cardiac arrest
Increased airway pressures in ventilated patients

You suspect a tension pneumothorax and plan to treat this with needle chest decompression. Outline the anatomical site you would select to insert the needle.

A frequently chosen first site for needle decompression is between the second and third ribs in the mid-clavicular line (Figure 8.1). This location benefits from being easily accessible; however, in patients with significant anterior chest musculature or large body habitus, the needle may not reach the thoracic cavity and the technique has a high failure rate (Laan et al., 2016). A lateral approach may be a more appropriate first-line choice. A lateral approach should be undertaken in the fourth or fifth intercostal space in the anterior axillary or mid-axillary line (Figure 8.2). Furthermore, specifically designed slightly longer catheters may be more appropriate for this intervention compared to standard IV cannulae. The triangle of safety is widely considered the 'safe zone' for lateral needle decompression and chest drain insertion (Faculty of Prehospital Care, 2016).

What is the optimal position in which to manage this patient?

In a patient with a significant thoracic injury, the supine position may not be the preferred position in terms of facilitating optimum ventilation. A semi-recumbent or upright position on the trolley may be preferred if other injuries allow, and many patients with thoracic injuries will find a more upright posture more comfortable (Dünser et al., 2018).

Needle Decompression	
Decompression Technique	**Decompression Landmarks**

1. Prepare equipment
   • Skin prep
   • Decompression needle or wide-bore cannula
   • Syringe
2. Identify landmarks
   • Fifth Intercostal Space, Mid-Axillary Line
   • Second Intercostal Space, Mid-Clavicular Line
3. Clean the skin
4. Insert the needle above the lower rib
5. Aspirate during insertion with syringe
6. When air is aspirated advance cannula
7. Withdraw needle (® hiss of air)
8. Stabilize cannula
9. Observe patient
	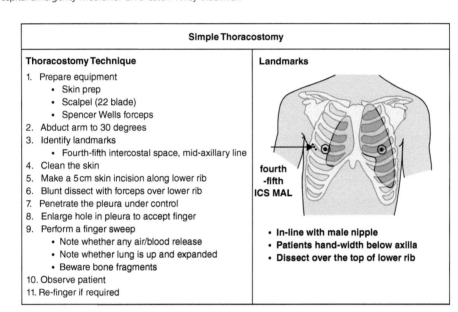
	second ICS MCL
	
	fifth ICS MAL
	
	· **Neurovascular bundle runs below rib**

Figure 8.1   Needle decompression landmarks. Reproduced by permission from Nutbeam, T. & Boylan, M. (eds) (2013) *ABC of Prehospital Emergency Medicine*. Chichester: Wiley-Blackwell.

Simple Thoracostomy	
Thoracostomy Technique	**Landmarks**

1. Prepare equipment
   • Skin prep
   • Scalpel (22 blade)
   • Spencer Wells forceps
2. Abduct arm to 30 degrees
3. Identify landmarks
   • Fourth-fifth intercostal space, mid-axillary line
4. Clean the skin
5. Make a 5 cm skin incision along lower rib
6. Blunt dissect with forceps over lower rib
7. Penetrate the pleura under control
8. Enlarge hole in pleura to accept finger
9. Perform a finger sweep
   • Note whether any air/blood release
   • Note whether lung is up and expanded
   • Beware bone fragments
10. Observe patient
11. Re-finger if required
	fourth -fifth ICS MAL
	
	• **In-line with male nipple**
	• **Patients hand-width below axilla**
	• **Dissect over the top of lower rib**

Figure 8.2   Simple thoracostomy. Reproduced by permission from Nutbeam, T. & Boylan, M. (eds) (2013) *ABC of Prehospital Emergency Medicine*. Chichester: Wiley-Blackwell.

Case Progression

A needle decompression has been undertaken on the left lateral side with a 5 cm 14-gauge cannula. Despite initial improvement in vital signs, the patient has now become unresponsive.

Patient assessment triangle
General appearance
The patient is pale and peripherally cyanotic.

Circulation to the skin
Capillary refill time is delayed at 4 seconds on the sternum.

Work of breathing
Accessory muscles are being used and the patient is demonstrating significant air hunger.

SYSTEMATIC APPROACH
Danger
Nil.

Response
Pain on the AVPU scale.

Airway
Clear and self-maintaining.

Breathing
Rate: 46 bpm. Effort: significant effort is being exerted. Accessory muscle use: yes. Auscultation: no breath sounds on the left, normal vesicular breath sounds on the right.

Circulation
Heart rate: 135 bpm. Effort: palpable carotid, but weak radial. Heart regularity: regular. Capillary refill time: 4 seconds.

Vital signs
RR: 46 bpm
HR: 135 bpm
BP: 90/77 mmHg
SpO_2: 82%
Lead II ECG: sinus tachycardia

Exposure
Notable asymmetry of the chest, the left side appears hyper-expanded with reduced ventilatory movements.

What is your next intervention for this patient?

This patient required rapid decompression of his tension pneumothorax, which can be attempted through repeating the needle decompression already performed. It is likely that the cannula you have already inserted has become blocked, kinked or dislodged. A more reliable technique can be through the surgical method of finger thoracotomy with subsequent chest drain insertion. It is important to note that if finger thoracotomy alone is undertaken, the patient cannot be left to breathe spontaneously and positive pressure ventilation must be instigated.

PRACTICAL TIP

In the majority of patients a needle decompression will either be ineffective or only a temporary measure.

If this patient experienced a cardiac arrest, how would you modify your standard resuscitation approach?

The standard ALS algorithm is designed for patents who have experienced a cardiac arrest from a medical cause. In traumatic cardiac arrest, your approach needs to be heavily modified. The HOTT acronym is a useful guide to this and is presented in Table 8.2.

Table 8.2 HOTT

H	Hypovolaemia	Hypovolaemia should be suspected and corrected. This involves stopping catastrophic or ongoing haemorrhage and replacing lost circulating volume with either blood (preferably) or crystalloid. Applying tourniquets, dressings or pelvic binders may be required.
O	Oxygenation	Oxygenation and ventilation should be optimised. This is likely to be via a cuffed tube in the trachea and intermittent positive pressure ventilation with 100% oxygen.
T	Tension pneumothorax	Tension pneumothorax and cardiac tamponade should be suspected and corrected when possible. This is likely to be by bilateral finger thoracotomies as a first intervention, followed up by formal
T	Tamponade	chest drain insertion or progression to clamshell thoracotomy where indicated.

PRACTICAL TIP

In a HOTT resuscitation, access is required to both axillae, which often requires the patient to be in a position with their arms spread away from the thorax. This position limits the utility of the humeral head as an option for intraosseous access. Furthermore, having another clinician at the head end managing a humeral IO may reduce the working space for thoracostomies or thoracotomy if these are required. Consider the proximal tibia as an alternative for IO access in such cases.

If this patient were to be transferred to hospital by air (rotary or fixed-wing aircraft), what specific interventions might you want to undertake prior to departure?

Patients need to be stabilised as well as possible before commencing an aeromedical transfer. This is especially important when the transfer will occur in an aircraft with limited in-flight access to the patient.

In cases where a pneumothorax is known or suspected, chest drains should be inserted prior to aeromedical transportation and should have their patency checked (Whiteley et al., 2011). Patients who have been intubated should ideally have the air in the cuff of the endotracheal tube replaced with water (not saline), to reduce the potential for tracheal pressure damage due to atmospheric pressure reduction with altitude causing expansion of the tracheal tube cuff. Air present in fluid-giving sets and fluid bags under pressure should also be evacuated, as this too will be affected by the pressure and temperature changes.

LEVEL 2 CASE STUDY
Motorcyclist

Information type	Data
Time of origin	16:58
Time of dispatch	17:00
On-scene time	17:22
Day of the week	Monday
Nearest hospital	40 minutes
Nearest backup	30 minutes
Patient details	Name: Jaime Lamire DOB: 20/01/1970

CASE

You have been called to a road junction for reports of a road traffic collision involving a male motorcyclist.

Pre-arrival information

The motorcyclist is conscious and breathing, but is distressed.

Windscreen report
You arrive at a traffic light–controlled three-way junction. Police officers are on scene and controlling traffic. You are directed to park by police officers, who tell you the patient is lying on the grass verge just beyond a fallen motorcycle.

Entering the location
There are skid marks several metres back from the motorcycle, which is lying on its side in the road with no visible damage. You hear a police officer reassuring the patient.

On arrival with the patient
The patient, a male of around 50 years old, is lying on his back with a motorcycle helmet on the ground beside him. He is dressed in casual clothing. His right leg is angulated laterally at mid-thigh and his left leg is twisted above the knee. A police officer is crouching at his side, keeping him calm.

Patient assessment triangle
General appearance
The patient is alert and groaning, trying to reach towards his legs with both arms.

Circulation to the skin
Appears pale.

Work of breathing
Tachypnoeic, speaking in full sentences. No added sounds.

SYSTEMATIC APPROACH
Danger
Environmental dangers are being managed by the police. Safe to approach.

Response
Alert on the AVPU scale.

Catastrophic haemorrhage
There is no evidence of catastrophic external haemorrhage.

C-spine
No evidence of injury. The police officer is able to provide manual in-line stabilisation when asked.

Airway
Clear.

Breathing
Rate: 24 bpm. Effort: normal. Accessory muscle use: no. Auscultation: good air entry throughout the chest, no added sounds.

Circulation
Heart rate: 122 bpm. Effort: normal. Heart regularity: regular. Capillary refill time: 4 seconds.

Vital signs
RR: 24 bpm
HR: 122 bpm
BP: 100/60 mmHg
SpO_2: 96%
Blood sugar: 5 mmol/L

> **TASK**
> Reading through the case information, identify what modifications of the primary survey have been made for this patient with trauma compared to a medically unwell patient.

What is the most likely explanation of the abnormal observations described in the case information?

The patient has bilateral femoral fractures with a raised respiratory rate, raised heart rate, low blood pressure and prolonged capillary refill time. Oxygen saturations are just below normal. Although pain associated with injuries will cause an increased heart rate, it is likely to increase rather than lower blood pressure and will not affect capillary refill time. The likeliest explanation for these findings is haemorrhagic shock.

What key interventions could be used to directly address the injuries you have identified?

On primary ABCDE assessment, this patient's first life-threatening issue is haemorrhagic shock secondary to bilateral femoral fractures. In addition, the significant mechanism of injury should raise a suspicion of pelvic injury, which may not be readily detected on examination and can cause unseen catastrophic haemorrhage. In motorcyclists, the commonest cause of pelvic fractures is impact with the fuel tank of their own vehicle (Meredith et al., 2016).

Like all unwell patients with significant traumatic injury, he should receive high-flow oxygen via a non-rebreather mask.

The mainstay of haemorrhage control in closed limb fractures is splinting. Splinting also reduces pain and can prevent further injury. By improving alignment of bone, splinting can mitigate blood loss from exposed and traumatised blood vessels. In addition, realignment and stabilisation reduce ongoing injury related to misaligned and sometimes sharp bone fragments, including nerve injury and laceration of blood vessels and highly vascular muscle. Common splints in pre-hospital use include box splints, vacuum splints and traction splints (Lee & Porter, 2005).

Suspected pelvic fracture should be managed through the application of a pelvic binder. These work through similar principles to limb splints, by reducing displacement caused by fracture and thereby reducing active blood loss.

What should be considered prior to applying these key interventions?

Although splinting ultimately reduces pain, application of splints is painful. Not only is this a humanitarian concern, pain may increase muscle tension and decrease the effectiveness of the intervention. Effective pain control prior to and during splinting is essential.

It is also important to assess and document the neurovascular status of the limb distal to the injury prior to applying splinting or traction. This should then be reassessed at regular intervals.

Some splints may be inappropriate depending on the presence of comorbid injuries. In this case, it would be important to ensure that any splint used is safe to apply in association with a possible pelvic fracture, as some traction devices rely on stabilisation against the pelvis.

Case Progression

The patient has been given high-flow oxygen. Bilateral IV cannulae have been inserted and opiate analgesia given IV, titrated to pain. A pelvic binder and traction splints have been applied.

Patient assessment triangle
General appearance
The patient is alert and speaking in full sentences.

Circulation to the skin
Normal colour. Warm.

Work of breathing
There is no increased work of breathing.

SYSTEMATIC APPROACH

Danger
Scene safety is being maintained by ancillary services.

Response
Alert on the AVPU scale.

Catastrophic haemorrhage
There is no evidence of catastrophic external haemorrhage.

C-spine
Manual in-line stabilisation is being maintained by a colleague.

Airway
Clear.

Breathing
Rate: 18 bpm. Effort: normal. Accessory muscle use: no. Auscultation: good air entry throughout the chest, no added sounds.

Circulation
Heart rate: 110 bpm. Effort: normal. Heart regularity: regular. Capillary refill time: 2 seconds.

Vital signs
RR: 18 bpm
HR: 110 bpm
BP: 96/58 mmHg
SpO_2: 100%
Blood sugar: 5 mmol/L
Temperature: 36.5 °C

Exposure
On exposure, no additional injuries are found. The patient is then covered by blankets.

What risks or contraindications to analgesia options would you consider in this patient?

Opiates can be an effective initial strategy for analgesia, but should be applied cautiously due to the risks of hypotension and respiratory depression. Dose should be titrated to pain, with the speed of administration depending on the specific opiate agent.

Inhalation agents such as methoxyflurane (e.g. Penthrox) and nitrous oxide (e.g. Entonox) are widely used both as first-line agents and as adjuncts (Porter et al., 2018). See Table 8.3 for contraindications to each.

What additional analgesia options might critical care teams be able to provide?

In addition to the analgesia already discussed, critical care teams may be able to provide additional or alternative analgesia. Ketamine is widely used in trauma management and has some advantages over opioid analgesia, as it is not associated with the same risks of hypotension and respiratory depression (Smith et al., 2011). In some cases, rapid sequence induction anaesthesia may be necessary for pain control, for instance where doses of other analgesia risk compromising airway management, or if severe pain is causing extreme patient distress and agitation.

Table 8.3 Cautions and contraindications of methoxyflurane and nitrous oxide

Inhalation analgesic	Contraindications and cautions	Reason
Methoxyflurane	History of malignant hyperthermia	Can be a causative agent
	Reduced level of consciousness	May be exacerbated by agent, and normal voluntary respiratory pattern required for safe delivery
	Pre-eclampsia or eclampsia	Risk of renal injury
	Untreated renal failure	Risk of renal injury
	Patients under 18 years of age	Check local guidelines; may be unlicensed use
	Acute behavioural disturbance	May exacerbate confused states and may not be able to comply with delivery
	Current tetracycline use	Increased effects on the kidneys when take together
Nitrous oxide	Severe head injury	Possible diffusion into and expansion of intracranial air
	Diving within the prior 24 hours	May cause expansion of nitrogen bubbles within the bloodstream ('the bends')
	Suspected pneumothorax, pneumomediastinum or pneumoperitoneum	Possible diffusion into and expansion of intrathoracic air
	Acute behavioural disturbance	May exacerbate confused states and the patient may not be able to comply with delivery instructions
	Intraocular injection of gas within the last 4 weeks	Possible diffusion into gas causing raised intraocular pressure
	Suspected intestinal obstruction	Possible expansion of bowel gas increasing risk of perforation

Source: Adapted from Porter et al. (2018) and Smith et al. (2011).

LEVEL 3 CASE STUDY
Severe burns

Information type	Data
Time of origin	14:55
Time of dispatch	14:56
On-scene time	15:08
Day of the week	Thursday
Nearest hospital	15 minutes
Nearest burns/trauma unit	40 minutes (by road) or 12 minutes (flight time)
Nearest backup	Intensive care crew, 15 minutes
Patient details	Name: Dean Gimble DOB: 16/06/1985

CASE
You are called to a house fire.

Pre-arrival information
35-year-old male. Clothing on fire. Conscious and breathing.

Windscreen report
On arrival at the residential property, there is a group of people in the front garden surrounding a person lying supine. There is a small fire of garden waste burning to the side of the house.

Entering the location

The small fire is being extinguished by two adults with a hosepipe. Your patient is lying supine on the floor, members of the surrounding group are patting at his clothing with a thick blanket, his clothing is still smoking and smouldering. Members of the crowd tell you they saw the patient pour accelerant of some kind onto the fire and described a fireball engulfing him.

On arrival with the patient

The male patient in his mid-30s is alert and clearly in pain. His upper body is burnt and remnants of his T-shirt are melted to his skin. Both his arms are severely burnt and have a blistered and leathery appearance.

Patient assessment triangle

General appearance

Acutely distressed and panicking.

Circulation to the skin

In areas, the skin on his arms is leathery and insensate with no capillary refill.

Work of breathing

Normal, with a rapid rate.

SYSTEMATIC APPROACH

Danger

The garden fire is being extinguished.

Response

Responsive and orientated to place and events.

Airway

Patent and self-maintaining.

Breathing

Rate: 32 bpm. Effort: normal. Accessory muscle use: some accessory muscle use to maintain the rapid rate. Auscultation: equal bilateral air entry with some mild scattered crackles.

Circulation

Heart rate: 140 bpm. Heart regularity: regular pulse. Capillary refill time: 3 seconds on forehead.

Vital signs

RR: 32 bpm

HR: 140 bpm

BP: the patient will not tolerate a cuff on his arm

SpO$_2$: 96% on air

Blood sugar: not obtained at this point

Lead II ECG: not obtained at this point, significant burnt skin over shoulders and arms hampers electrode placement

Exposure

You cut away the patient's tattered and charred clothing to reveal a large area of burnt skin across his thorax, neck and arms.

TASK

Now the patient's clothing has been extinguished, what are your priorities of care for this man?

How would you approach the decision making around requesting further support to the scene and rapid conveyance to hospital?

Transport time to the nearest hospital is the same as travel time for an intensive care ambulance to reach your location. Furthermore, travel time to a specialist burns and trauma unit is significant by road. While there is the temptation to 'scoop and run', it may be a better alternative to await the arrival of critical care colleagues and if possible facilitate primary transfer to a burns unit.

This patient is in significant pain from the burns to his arms. What is your analgesic and route of administration of choice?

You would want a fast-acting and effective analgesia for this patient's severe pain. Options such as paracetamol, ketorolac or ibuprofen are not appropriate as sole agents for this patient's pain due to their slow onset and low potency. Entonox or Penthrox may be an appropriate temporising option, but this too is unlikely to provide sufficient sole analgesia in this case (Porter et al., 2018).

Ketamine and fentanyl both have a rapid onset of action and are potent analgesics (Smith et al., 2011). They also both have the benefit that they may be administered via the intranasal route. Furthermore, fentanyl is fairly cardio-stable and unlikely to cause significant hypotension, while ketamine is positively inotropic and also a bronchodilator, which may be beneficial in this case.

Case Progression

You have requested attendance of the intensive care ambulance and moved the patient onto the stretcher in your vehicle. You have gained IV access at the patient's ankle and administered 7.5 mg morphine sulfate.

Patient assessment triangle
General appearance
The patient is complaining of severe pain in his hands, and is unable to bend his arms.

Circulation to the skin
Circulation to unaffected limbs is normal, but assessing the patient's arms is challenging, a number of large blisters have developed, and there are extensive patches of leathery skin.

Work of breathing
The patient is breathing very rapidly, but with coaching can slow this down.

SYSTEMATIC APPROACH
Danger
The patient has been removed to the safety of the ambulance and all his clothing has been extinguished and removed where possible.

Response
Alert and orientated.

Airway
Patent.

Breathing
Rate: 20 bpm. Effort: normal. Accessory muscle use: no. Auscultation: equal bilateral normal vesicular breath sounds.

Circulation
Heart rate:133 bpm. Effort: strong. Heart regularity: regular. Capillary refill time: 3 seconds on feet, no capillary refill on some areas of his arms.

Vital signs
RR: 20 bpm
HR: 133 bpm
BP: unable to acquire
SpO_2: 98%
Blood sugar: 7.2 mmol/L
Lead II ECG: significant artefact is present, but there appears to be a sinus tachycardia underlying this
Temperature: 36.7 °C

Exposure
Anterior chest is erythematous with two areas of blistering, where clothing is adhered. Both arms are extensively burnt with multiple large blisters and patches of leathering insensate skin. His neck and face are unaffected.

If this patient's thoracic burns were restricting ventilation, what intervention should you consider?

Escharotomy should be considered for patients with full-thickness circumferential burns, including burns to limbs, but especially when encircling the thorax (Chesters, 2017; Kupas & Miller, 2010). Escharotomy is a technically simple surgical skill, certainly when compared to interventions like surgical front of neck access (Kupas & Miller, 2010). However, that should not underestimate the challenges involved in a case requiring this intervention in terms of clinical judgement, decision making and onward care.

PRACTICAL TIP

When performing an escharotomy, the incisions should be deep enough for you to see fat (not muscle). They will bleed profusely, so have dressings to hand. Where the incision extends proximal/distal into unburnt skin, local anaesthetic will be needed. A finger sweep along the incision will identify any areas of constriction that have been missed.

If this patient required emergency anaesthesia, how would you modify your approach in light of his burn injuries?

It is often said that suxamethonium is contraindicated in cases of significant burns due to intracellular potassium release, causing hyperkalaemia, being increased to a dangerous level by the suxamethonium. Fortunately, this is not the case until around 24 hours post-burn, and is unlikely to be an issue during the pre-hospital phase. That being said, rocuronium would be the author's paralytic of choice for this patient. Choice of induction agent would depend on local policy, however in cases of burns ketamine provides many advantages, among them its positive inotropic action and bronchodilation.

LEVEL 3 CASE STUDY
Hanging

Information type	Data
Time of origin	10:46
Time of dispatch	11:04
On-scene time	11:09
Day of the week	Wednesday
Nearest hospital	22 minutes
Nearest backup	Critical care paramedic, 5 minutes
Patient details	Name: Tina Schiny DOB: 12/02/2003

CASE

You have been called to the local secondary school for a 17-year-old female. She had been noted as absent from a morning lesson and had been found hanging in the girls' toilets. Resuscitation attempts are underway by school staff.

Pre-arrival information

The patient is not conscious and is not breathing normally. CPR is underway.

Windscreen report

You are met by a member of staff at the school entrance, they tell you the school is in lockdown and police have also been called.

Entering the location

On entering the school it is eerily quiet and you notice all classrooms have the blinds drawn and doors closed. You are guided to a ground-floor toilet near the front of the building.

On arrival with the patient

The female patient is half in a toilet cubicle in the school toilets. Effective chest compressions are being delivered by a teacher. An automated external defibrillator is turned on and the pads are being applied in the correct positions to the patient's chest. A school tie remains attached to the toilet cubicle wall, and it appears to have been cut.

Patient assessment triangle
General appearance

The patient appears plethoric, and you note disordered abdominal movements. There is a ligature mark present high on the patient's neck, around the level of the hyoid bone.

Circulation to the skin

Plethoric appearance of the head and face with discolouration to the tongue.

Work of breathing

There is evidence of ventilatory effort, in that the abdomen is rising and falling paradoxically to the thorax. The teacher in attendance is undertaking continuous chest compressions.

SYSTEMATIC APPROACH

Danger

There is a multitool knife in the corner of the room, which you suspect was used to cut the patient down. There are no other dangers.

Response

Unresponsive.

Airway

On inspection of the mouth and oropharynx, there is no visible obstruction to the airway.

Breathing

There is active ventilatory effort, which is erratic. No air is being moved on a 'look, listen and feel' check. Attempted ventilation with the bag-valve mask using a jaw thrust is unsuccessful, with no air entry and no chest rise despite a good seal with the mask.

Circulation

Heart rate: difficult to count, intermittent impulses are felt, the rate is approximately 40–50 bpm. Effort: very weak at the carotids. Heart regularity: irregular. Capillary refill time: 4 seconds on sternum.

Vital signs

N/A

Exposure

Nothing untoward noted when placing the AED pads.

> **TASK**
> Looking at the information provided in this scenario, what aspects of this case might lead to an increased psychological impact on you or other clinicians in attendance?

You believe this patient has an obstructed airway. What are the signs and symptoms of a partial or complete obstruction to the airway?

The signs and symptoms of partial and complete airway obstruction include added audible noises when breathing, such as stridor or bubbling. Tracheal tug, paradoxical abdominal movements and cyanosis are all signs of airway compromise. Conscious patients may also reach for, or claw at, their neck/throat.

How will you approach the management of this patient's airway?

Two clear problems have been detected on primary survey: airway compromise and circulatory compromise.

It is likely that the cause of unconsciousness was compression of the blood vessels in the neck and that airway compromise occurred after this. While a standard approach to airway management could be utilised here, it may be appropriate in this case to rapidly escalate your interventions to the higher end of the airway ladder (Table 8.4). This is due to the anticipated airway trauma sustained and the likelihood of subsequent airway swelling. This may be orotracheal intubation, or surgical airway if intubation fails. See also Figures 8.3–8.6.

Table 8.4 Airway ladder

Simple manoeuvres	Jaw thrust
	Head tilt chin lift
	Triple manoeuvre
Simple adjuncts	Nasopharyngeal
	Oropharyngeal
Supraglottic airways	Laryngeal mask airway
	iGel airway
Intubation	Oral or nasal endotracheal intubation
Front of neck access	Needle cricothyroidotomy
	Surgical cricothyroidotomy

What are the likely causes of the complete airway obstruction in this case?

There are multiple factors that may contribute to airway obstruction that persists after removal of the ligature in a case such as this. These may include:

- Fracture of the hyoid bone and resultant oedema to the area.
- 'Fracture' of the lateral components of the larynx, leading to collapse of the glottic opening.
- Soft tissue oedema to the neck secondary to compression trauma from the ligature.
- Significant trauma to the cervical spine, resulting in anatomical disruption and compromise to the tracheal path.

Such injuries are far more likely to occur in 'long-drop' or judicial hangings. The cause of death in most domestic hangings is obstruction of blood flow through the vasculature of the neck, rather than spinal cord disruption or airway compromise. In this respect the case presented here is a statistical anomaly.

Based on the details presented so far, would you be requesting further support? What specific skills would you like such support to bring to the scene?

A case such as this would benefit from the attendance of a pre-hospital clinician with an armamentarium including advanced airway management and the ability to provide inotrope support as well as competencies in sedation or anaesthesia. This may be a physician, a critical care paramedic or an enhanced care team.

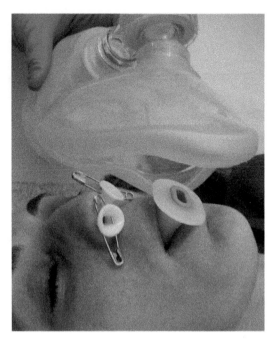

Figure 8.3   Multiple airway technique. Reproduced by permission from Nutbeam, T. & Boylan, M. (eds) (2013) *ABC of Prehospital Emergency Medicine.* Chichester: Wiley-Blackwell.

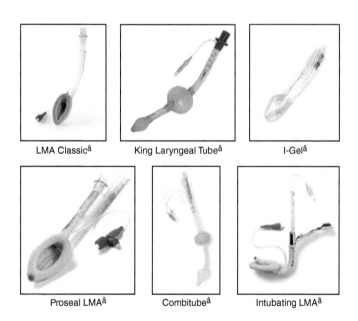

Figure 8.4   Supraglottic airways. Reproduced by permission from Nutbeam, T. & Boylan, M. (eds) (2013) *ABC of Prehospital Emergency Medicine.* Chichester: Wiley-Blackwell.

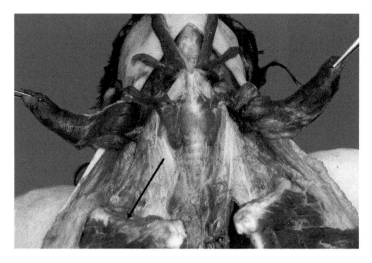

Figure 8.5   Layer-by-layer dissection of the anterior soft tissues of the neck (incomplete hanging). Arrow: haemorrhage on the clavicular origin of the right sternocleidomastoid muscle. Reproduced by permission from Madea, B. (ed.) (2014) *Handbook of Forensic Medicine*. Chichester: Wiley-Blackwell.

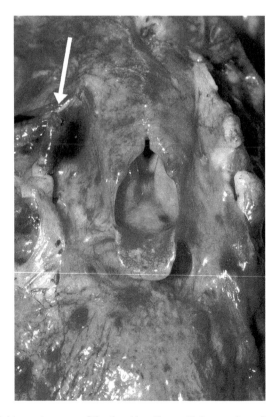

Figure 8.6   Fracture of the right superior cornu of the thyroid cartilage with haemorrhage (incomplete hanging). Reproduced by permission from Madea, B. (ed.) (2014) *Handbook of Forensic Medicine*. Chichester: Wiley-Blackwell.

Does this patient require spinal immobilisation and, if so, what form should this take?

Surprisingly, few hangings in domestic situations result in disruption to the cervical spine. However, in a patient who is unconscious with a history of significant trauma to the neck, it is appropriate to provide a degree of immobilisation (Quinn et al., 2014; NICE, 2016).

Pre-hospital care guidelines are moving away from the injudicious application of rigid collars to protect the cervical spine as further data is accumulated providing evidence that they can cause problems (Connor et al., 2013). These may include issues such as raising intracranial pressure, hampering airway management and causing pressure necrosis to the skin, while not limiting unwanted neck movements to any useful degree.

Case Progression

You are achieving good air entry via a surgical cricothyroidotomy.

Patient assessment triangle
General appearance
The patient has a good colour, cyanosis is no longer present. Tardieu spots are present on the patient's face, as is bilateral subconjunctival haemorrhage.

Circulation to the skin
Appears normal, with a capillary refill time of 2 seconds on the chest.

Work of breathing
Ventilated at 16 bpm with a 400 mL tidal volume.

SYSTEMATIC APPROACH
Danger
Nil.

Response
Unresponsive, intubated and sedated.

Airway
Surgical airway with inflated cuff.

Breathing
The patient is being ventilated at a rate of 16 bpm, with an inspiratory volume of 400 mL using a volume-controlled ventilator setting with a positive end-expiratory pressure (PEEP) of 8 cmH$_2$O. ETCO$_2$ is 32 mmHg with a good waveform. Oxygen delivery is being titrated to obtain an SpO$_2$ reading above 97%.

Circulation
Heart rate: varying between 60 and 90 bpm with frequent ectopy. Pulse character: strong carotid pulse. Heart regularity: irregularly irregular. Capillary refill time: 2 seconds.

Vital signs
RR: 16 bpm
HR: 60–90 bpm
BP: 90/68 mmHg
SpO$_2$: 97%
Blood sugar: 5 mmol/l
Lead II ECG: irregular narrow complex rhythm with frequent ectopy
Temperature: 35.8 °C on tympanic

Exposure
As above.

PRACTICAL TIP

Patients who have experienced a hanging injury may present with a presumed cardiac arrest or low output state prior to cessation of cardiac function. These patients have a fairly high chance of a positive outcome. Initial GCS is not useful in determining chance of survival.

What is your sedation and paralysis strategy for this patient?

This patient will require appropriate sedation and paralysis to facilitate safe and effective ventilation and onward transfer to definitive care. While approaches vary by region, an appropriate strategy would be to use a long-acting paralysis agent such as rocuronium, administered at a rapid sequence intubation (RSI) dose (1.2 mg/kg) alongside anaesthesia with an appropriate agent. The sedation agent will again vary with local guidelines, but an appropriate choice may be the judicial use of titrated midazolam or ketamine. It is important to remember that awareness is far more likely in those patients receiving paralytic agents (AAGBI, 2017).

While ventilating this patient you notice that her SpO$_2$ is dropping, despite ruling out mechanical dysfunction, tube malposition or a fault with the finger probe. On inspection of the ET tube you notice pink frothy secretions in the lumen. What is the most likely cause of these secretions?

This is most likely a result of negative pressure (post-obstructive) pulmonary oedema. In cases of hanging there may also be a neurogenic component to the development of pulmonary oedema due to a centrally mediated sympathetic storm. Such pulmonary oedema can be managed by increasing PEEP or with larger tidal volumes.

References and further reading

AAGBI (2017) Safer prehospital anaesthesia. *Anaesthesia*, 72: 379–390.

Araujo, M., Illanes, E., Chapman, E. & Rodrigues, E. (2017) Effectiveness of interventions to prevent motorcycle injuries: Systematic review of the literature. *International Journal of Injury Control and Safety Promotion*, 24(3): 406–422.

Baker, S.P., O'Neill, B., Haddon, W. & Long, W.B. (1974) The Injury Severity Score: A method for describing patients with multiple injuries and evaluating emergency care. *Journal of Trauma*, 14(3): 187–196.

Battalogu, E., Greasley, L., Leon-Villapalos, J. et al. (2019) *Management of Burns in Pre-hospital Trauma Care*. Edinburgh: Faculty of Prehospital Care, Royal College of Surgeons of Edinburgh.

Chesters, A. (2017) Medical emergencies in pre-hospital care. Crash cards: Drills for use in the emergency setting. Version 2. UK HEMS. https://associationoffairambulances.co.uk/wp-content/uploads/2017/11/UK-HEMS-Medical-Crash-Cards-v2.1.pdf (Accessed 27 April 2019).

Connor, D., Porter, K., Bloch, M. & Greaves, I. (2013) *Pre-Hospital Spinal Immobilisation*. Edinburgh: Faculty of Prehospital Care, Royal College of Surgeons of Edinburgh.

Davis, C., Engeln, A., Johnson, E. et al. (2014) Wilderness Medical Society practice guidelines for the prevention and treatment of lightning injuries: 2014 update. *Wilderness and Environmental Medicine*, 25(4): S86–S95.

de Rome, L., Ivers, R., Firzharris, M. et al. (2011) Motorcycle protective clothing: Protection from injury or just the weather? *Accident Analysis and Prevention*, 43(6): 1893–1900.

Dünser, M.W., Dankl, D., Petro, S. & Mer, M. (2018) The airway and lungs. In *Clinical Examination Skills in the Adult Critically Ill Patient* (eds M.W. Dünser & D. Dankl), Chaim: Springer, pp. 21–49.

Faculty of Prehospital Care (2016) *Manual of Core Material: Version* 3. Edinburgh: Royal College of Surgeons of Edinburgh.

Granhed, H., Altgarde, E., Akyurek, L.M. & David, P. (2017) Injuries sustained by falls: A review. *Trauma Acute Care*, 2: 38.

Kent, A. & Pearce. A. (2006) Review of morbidity and mortality associated with falls from heights among patients presenting to a major trauma centre. *Emergency Medicine Australasia*, 18(1): 23–30.

Kupas, D.F. & Miller, D.D. (2010) Out-of-hospital chest escharotomy: A case series and procedure review. *Prehospital Emergency Care*, 14(3): 349–354.

Laan, D.V., Vu, T.D.N., Thiels, C.A. et al. (2016) Chest wall thickness and decompression failure: A systematic review and meta-analysis comparing anatomic locations in needle thoracostomy. *Injury*, 47(4): 797–804.

Lapostolle, F., Gere, C., Borron, S.W. et al. (2005) Prognostic factors in victims of falls from height. *Critical Care Medicine*, 33(6): 1239–1242.

Lee, C. & Porter, K.M. (2005) Prehospital management of lower limb fractures. *Emergency Medicine Journal*, 22(9): 660–663.

McIntosh, S, Opacic, M., Freer, L. et al. (2014) Wilderness Medical Society practice guidelines for the prevention and treatment of frostbite: 2014 update. *Wilderness and Environmental Medicine*, 25(4): S43–S54.

Meredith, L., Baldock, M., Fitzharris, M. et al. (2016) Motorcycle fuel tanks and pelvic fractures: A motorcycle fuel tank syndrome. *Traffic Injury Prevention*, 17(6): 644–649.

NICE (2016) *Spinal Injury: Assessment and Initial Management*. London: National Institute for Health and Clinical Excellence.

Pointer, S. (2015) *Trends in Hospitalised Injury, Australia 1999–00 to 2012–13*. Canberra: Australian Institute of Health and Welfare.

Porter, K.M., Siddiqui, M.K., Sharma, I. et al. (2018) Management of trauma pain in the emergency setting: Low-dose methoxyflurane or nitrous oxide? A systematic review and indirect treatment comparison. *Journal of Pain Research*, 11, 11.

Quinn, R.H., Williams, J., Bennett, B.L. et al. (2014) Wilderness Medical Society practice guidelines for spine immobilisation in the austere environment: 2014 update. *Wilderness and Environmental Medicine*, 25(4): S105–S117.

Sauvageau, A. (2014) Death by hanging. In *Essentials of Autopsy Practice* (ed. G.N. Rutty), London: Springer, pp. 23–38.

Sauvageau, A., Laharpe, R., King, D. et al.; Working Group on Human Asphyxia (2011) Agonal sequences in 14 filmed hangings with comments on the role of the type of suspension, ischemic habituation, and ethanol intoxication on the timing of agonal responses. *American Journal of Forensic Pathology*, 32(2): 104–107.

Smith, S., Scarth, E. & Sasada, M. (2011) *Drugs in Anaesthesia and Intensive Care*, 4th ed. Oxford: Oxford University Press.

Stiles, K. & Goodwin, N. (2018) *British Burn Association: First aid clinical practice guidelines*. London: British Burn Association. https://www.britishburnassociation.org/wp-content/uploads/2017/06/BBA-First-Aid-Guideline-24.9.18.pdf (Accessed 5 May 2019).

Szostakowski, B., Smitham, P. & Khan, W.S. (2017) Plaster of Paris: Short history of casting and injured limb immobilization. *Open Orthopaedics Journal*, 11: 291.

Truhlář, A., Deakin, C.D., Soar, J. et al. (2015) European Resuscitation Council guidelines for resuscitation 2015: Section 4. Cardiac arrest in special circumstances. *Resuscitation*, 95: 148–201.

Whiteley, S., Macartney, I., Mark, J. et al. (2011) *Guidelines for the Transport of the Critically Ill Adult*, 3rd ed. London: Intensive Care Society.

World Health Organization (2015) *Global status report on road safety 2015*. Geneva: WHO. https://www.who.int/violence_injury_prevention/road_safety_status/2015/en/ (Accessed 1 December 2019).

World Health Organization (2018) *Fact sheet: Falls*. Geneva: WHO. https://www.who.int/news-room/fact-sheets/detail/falls (Accessed 1 December 2019).

Chapter 9 **Paediatric cases**

Erica Ley

Lincolnshire and Nottinghamshire Air Ambulance, Lincoln, and University of East Anglia, Norwich, UK

CHAPTER CONTENTS

LEVEL 1 CASE STUDY
Pyrexia of unknown origin (PUO)

Information type	Data
Time of origin	09:10
Time of dispatch	09:40
On-scene time	09:58
Day of the week	Wednesday
Nearest hospital	24 minutes
Nearest backup	EMT crew, 15 minutes
Patient details	Name: John Peterson
	DOB: 05/08/2008

CASE

You have been called to a residential address for reports of a 12-year-old child with a knee injury. The caller states the child has been unwell for 2 weeks with increasing knee pain and an intermittent temperature. The child has previously been seen by the GP, who advised the mother it was a viral illness and for the child to return home and keep up his fluid intake.

Pre-arrival information

He is conscious and breathing.

Windscreen report

Quiet street in a poorer area of town. The house is well kept from the outside and the front door is open. No obvious activity outside.

Clinical Cases in Paramedicine, First Edition. Edited by Sam Willis, Ian Peate, and Rod Hill.
© 2021 John Wiley & Sons Ltd. Published 2021 by John Wiley & Sons Ltd.

Entering the location

You are greeted by a female who shows you into the ground-floor living area. She tells you that her son has had a temperature for a few days. He came home early from school today due to knee pain.

On arrival with the patient

The child is sat on the sofa with his legs extended outwards.

Patient assessment triangle:

General appearance

The patient is alert and looks at you as you enter the room.

Circulation to the skin

Pink cheeks, good peripheral colour.

Work of breathing

Adequate, no accessory muscle use, effort appears normal.

SYSTEMATIC APPROACH

Danger

Nil.

Response

Alert on the AVPU scale.

Airway

Clear, pale.

Breathing

Rate: 16 bpm. Effort: normal. Accessory muscle use: no. Auscultation: good air entry to all lung fields.

Circulation

Heart rate: 108 bpm. Effort: strong. Heart regularity: regular. Capillary refill time: <2 seconds.

Vital signs

RR: 16 bpm

HR: 108 bpm

BP: 108/65 mmHg

SpO$_2$: 99% on air

Blood sugar: 5.4 mmol/L

Lead II ECG: sinus rhythm

Temp: 38.9 °C

Exposure

Systemically warm to touch.

TASK

Look through the information provided in this case study and highlight all of the information that might concern you as a paramedic.

Using what you currently know about the case at this point, including what you may have seen and how the patient is presenting to you, which vital signs should you undertake first?

The airway is clear, so no intervention is required there; the breathing and pulse are within normal limits, but the child is warm to touch. Measure the child's temperature and complete the primary survey.

Once you have undertaken the essential vital signs and completed the primary survey, what would be your diagnosis?

Pyrexia of unknown origin. The elusiveness of the cause of a patient's PUO may lie with the myriad of conditions that can present this way and the variability with which these conditions may present.

Which of the following non-technical skills do you think are the most important to be able to safely treat this patient?
a. Effective verbal communication.
b. Effective non-verbal communication.
c. Empathy.
d. Reassurance.
e. Situational awareness.
f. All of the above.

f. All of the above.

Case Progression

The mother explains that her son has been feeling generally unwell with an intermittent temperature for the last few weeks, occasionally he has a headache and muscle aches, but he has been sleeping lots once he arrives home from school. She thought it was because he was doing a lot of sports. The child has not received any analgesia in the last 4 hours. You administer 1 g paracetamol via the oral route to manage his pain.

Patient assessment triangle
General appearance
The patient is alert and talks freely to you. He looks uncomfortable on movement of his left leg.

Circulation to the skin
Normal.

Work of breathing
Normal, quiet breathing.

SYSTEMATIC APPROACH
Danger
Nil.

Response
Alert on the AVPU scale.

Airway
Clear.

Breathing
Rate: 17 bpm. Effort: normal. Accessory muscle use: no. Auscultation: clear, no added sounds.

Circulation
Heart rate: 104 bpm. Effort: strong. Heart regularity: regular. Capillary refill time: 1 second.

Vital signs
RR: 17 bpm
HR: 104 bpm

BP: 125/85 mmHg
SpO$_2$: 99%
Blood sugar: 5 mmol/L
Lead II ECG: sinus rhythm
Temperature: 38.4 °C

Exposure
Left knee is reddened, slightly swollen and warm to touch in comparison to right knee. He is unable to straighten the leg fully and has difficulty weight bearing.

What kinds of questions would you ask this patient and his mother specifically related to pyrexia of unknown origin as part of the history-taking process?

See Table 9.1.

Table 9.1 History-taking questions

Knee pain
Any history of trauma?
Does the pain get worse at a particular point of the day?
What provokes or lessens the pain?
Does the pain radiate elsewhere?
What type of pain is it?
Pain score
Has there been an effect on the range of motion (ROM)?

Pyrexia
Do you think the patient has an infection?
When did this episode start? (How long have you been like this today?) When did the previous episodes start?
What were you doing when this started?
Do you know what your triggers are?
When did you last visit your GP about these symptoms?
Have you ever been admitted to hospital before due to this temperature (taken to the Emergency Department and admitted into the hospital system)?
Any other symptoms associated with the temperature?

Medication history
Do you take any medications?
If so, which ones and how frequently?
Have there been any changes to the way they work?
Has your prescription changed at all?
Do you take any medications for any other condition?

F/SH (family and social history)
Does anyone else in your family have any medical conditions?
Who do you live with?
Any other siblings with illnesses?
Recent travel or open water exposure?
Any pets at home?

Past medical history (PMH)
Do you have any other medical conditions?

Differential diagnosis (DDx) – What else could this be?
Infective causes – ?septic arthritis
Viral causes
Neoplastic causes – acute myeloid leukaemia
Miscellaneous causes

Given the patient's history, and now that you have ruled out any immediately life-threatening concerns, what are you going to do next?

a. Take him to hospital.
b. Refer him back to his GP for further review.
c. Discharge on scene with advice for pain management.

a. Take him to hospital.

That with a differential of septic arthritis then he should be taken to hospital as SA is an orthopaedic emergency. It may not be life-threatening at present, but can lead to sepsis and cartilage destruction and growth damage.

LEVEL 1 CASE STUDY
Toothache

Information type	Data
Time of origin	09:10
Time of dispatch	14:40
On-scene time	14:59
Day of the week	Saturday
Nearest hospital	20 minutes
Nearest backup	EMT crew, 35 minutes
Patient details	Name: Sachi Glenine
	DOB: 09/05/2004

CASE
You have been called to a private address for reports of a 16-year-old female with toothache.

Pre-arrival information
The patient is conscious and breathing.

Windscreen report
The area outside the house appears to be safe. The house is well kept from the exterior with a small garden. No obvious activity outside.

Entering the location
You are greeted by a female who appears distressed. She tells you that three days ago she was eating a mint polo when she realised she had broken her tooth. She states her jaw aches and she can't get on top of the pain.

Patient assessment triangle
General appearance
The patient is alert and she guides you through into the kitchen. She states her parents are at work and she is unable to get hold of them.

Circulation to the skin
Pink and well perfused. Blotchy from crying.

Work of breathing
No difficulty.

SYSTEMATIC APPROACH
Danger
Nil.

Response
Alert on the AVPU scale.

Airway
Clear, pale.

Breathing
Rate: 14 bpm. Effort: mildly increased. Accessory muscle use: no.

Circulation
Heart rate: 90 bpm. Effort: normal. Heart regularity: regular. Capillary refill time: <2 seconds.

Vital signs
RR: 14 bpm
HR: 90 bpm
BP: 130/85 mmHg
SpO_2: 99%
Blood sugar: 4.2 mmol/L
Lead II ECG: sinus rhythm

Exposure
No swelling or bleeding noted inside mouth.

TASK

Look through the information provided in this case study and highlight all of the information that might concern you as a paramedic.

Case Progression

The patient states that she has taken paracetamol and ibuprofen every 4–6 hours since yesterday morning when the pain started to get bad, but now the pain is unmanageable and she is unable to chew and swallow.

Most commonly, are teeth damaged in the maxillary jaw or the mandibular jaw?

Maxillary jaw.

Case Progression

On detailed examination of the patient's mouth, you note that one of the patient's teeth in her upper jaw is broken. You note a fracture of the enamel and secondary dentine, with a slight reddening to the middle of the tooth.

What are the risk factors for this injury?

Local infection such as an abscess; systemic infection such as infective endocarditis.

What is your management plan for this patient?

The patient's pain is unable to be managed with over-the-counter medication. Due to the reddening and initial bleeding, it is likely that the pulp of the tooth and therefore the nerve root are exposed. The patient requires urgent referral to a dentist for cleaning, exposure and fixation of the tooth to manage the infection risk and the pain.

LEVEL 2 CASE STUDY
Febrile convulsions

Information type	Data
Time of origin	11:19
Time of dispatch	11:20
On-scene time	11:28
Day of the week	Monday
Nearest hospital	16 minutes
Nearest backup	Paramedic crew, 9 minutes
Patient detail	Name: Simon Says
	DOB: 01/06/2018

CASE
You have been called to a domestic address for reports of a 2-year-old child having a seizure. The caller states the child has been unwell for a 3 days with an intermittent temperature. Two other children are present at the property.

Pre-arrival information
The patient is unconscious and having a seizure. It is a second-floor apartment.

Windscreen report
The building is well kept from the outside and is gate controlled with remote access. No obvious activity outside.

Entering the location
You are greeted by a male who shows you into the living area. He tells you that his son has had a temperature for a few days with coryzal symptoms.

On arrival with the patient
The child is laid on his side on the sofa.

Patient assessment triangle
General appearance
The patient is not alert and is visibly shaking.

Circulation to the skin
Pink cheeks. Clothes in situ, so unable to assess peripheral colour.

Work of breathing
Fast, grunting.

SYSTEMATIC APPROACH
Danger
Nil.

Response
Unresponsive on the AVPU scale.

Airway
Saliva ++, jaw clenched.

Breathing
Rate: 28 bpm. Effort: increased. Auscultation: good air entry to all lung fields.

Circulation
Heart rate: 130 bpm. Effort: strong. Heart regularity: regular. Capillary refill time: <2 seconds.

Vital signs
RR: 28 bpm
HR: 130 bpm
BP: unable to obtain during the seizure
SpO$_2$: 94% on air
Blood sugar: 6.2 mmol/L
Lead II ECG: unable to obtain during the seizure
Temp: 39.2 °C

Exposure
Systemically warm to touch.

TASK
Look through the information provided in this case study and highlight all of the information that might concern you as a paramedic.

Using what you know about the case at this point, including what you may have seen and how the patient is presenting to you, what are your immediate actions?

The patient is having a convulsion. He requires supportive airway management and, given the timeframe, control of the seizure.

How will you control the seizure?

First-line management in the paediatric cohort with a febrile seizure following airway protection is removal of clothing in order to cool the child. In the absence of IV access, rectal administration of diazepam with age-appropriate dosing.

Case Progression

You gain further history from the father, who advises that the patient has not had a seizure before. The oldest child has been home from school all week with chickenpox and since then this child has become unwell with flu-like symptoms. You remove the child's clothes and administer benzodiazepines.

Patient assessment triangle
General appearance
The patient is not alert, but the shaking has stopped.

Circulation to the skin
Pink cheeks and normal peripheral colour, no mottling.

Work of breathing
Fast, no grunting.

SYSTEMATIC APPROACH
Danger
Nil.

Response

Unresponsive on the AVPU scale.

Airway

Clear after suctioning, supported with manual manoeuvres only.

Breathing

Rate: 24 bpm. Effort: increased. Auscultation: good air entry to all lung fields.

Circulation

Heart rate: 118 bpm. Effort: strong. Heart regularity: regular. Capillary refill time: <2 seconds.

Vital signs

RR: 24 bpm

HR: 118 bpm

BP: unable to obtain during the seizure

SpO$_2$: 100% on 15 Lpm O$_2$

Blood sugar: not recorded again

Lead II ECG: unable to obtain

Temp: 39.3 °C

Exposure

Systemically warm to touch.

What are the side effects and possible complications of this medication?

The main concern with benzodiazepine administration is respiratory depression, although cardiovascular depression may also occur with larger doses. The pre-hospital practitioner should be prepared to manage the airway and provide supportive ventilations if the child becomes apnoeic.

Case Progression

You continue to monitor the child post-seizure.

Patient assessment triangle

General appearance

The patient is not alert, but the shaking has stopped.

Circulation to the skin

Pink cheeks and normal peripheral colour, no mottling.

Work of breathing

Fast, no grunting.

SYSTEMATIC APPROACH

Danger

Nil.

Response

Unresponsive on the AVPU scale.

Airway

Clear after suctioning, supported with manual manoeuvres only.

Breathing

Rate: 24 bpm. Effort: increased. Auscultation: good air entry to all lung fields.

Circulation

Heart rate: 118 bpm. Effort: strong. Heart regularity: regular. Capillary refill time: <2 seconds.

Vital signs

RR: 24 bpm

HR: 118 bpm

BP: 95/56 mmHg

SpO_2: 100% on 15 Lpm O_2

Blood sugar: 6.2 mmol/L

Lead II ECG: sinus tachycardic rhythm

Exposure

Systemically warm to touch.

LEVEL 2 CASE STUDY

Trauma

Information type	Data
Time of origin	15:21
Time of dispatch	15:22
On-scene time	15:30
Day of the week	Friday
Nearest hospital	16 minutes
Nearest backup	EMT crew, 20 minutes
Patient details	Name: Simone Checka
	DOB: 06/05/2015

CASE

You have been called to reports of a road traffic collision outside a school. A 5-year-old child has been hit by a car.

Pre-arrival information

The patient is unconscious.

Windscreen report

Cars line both sides of the street and reduce access to a single vehicle at any one time. A police car blocks the scene. There are numerous bystanders lining the streets, who appear panicked.

Entering the location

You park in the fend-off position and don your reflective jacket and protective helmet. You are greeted by a female, who shows you where the patient is. You see two police officers performing CPR. The woman tells you that the girl was hit by the black BMW 4×4 that you can see distant to the scene, and thrown into the air; she landed in the road. The woman begins to cry.

On arrival with the patient

The scene is loud. Two adults are crouched next to the patient, crying and screaming at you to help her.

Patient assessment triangle
General appearance:
The patient looks lifeless. There are grazes all over her body.

Circulation to the skin
Her body is pale, she is bleeding from her head.

Work of breathing
Her chest inflates as the police officer breathes into her mouth.

SYSTEMATIC APPROACH

Danger
Street is blocked in both directions, by a police car on one side and the BMW 4×4 on the other. The scene is loud and chaotic. There is shouting in the background.

Response
Unresponsive.

Airway
There is blood in the airway, some teeth are missing. The police officer has blood around their mouth.

Breathing
The child is not breathing.

Circulation
The child does not have a pulse. Capillary refill time >2 seconds.

Vital signs
The child is unresponsive. You attach your monitor and find the child is in asystole.

Exposure
She has multiple noticeable injuries after her clothes are cut off.

TASK

Look through the information provided in this case study and highlight all of the information that might concern you as a paramedic.

What are your immediate clinical actions?

Complete a trauma primary survey and concurrently address the immediate clinical needs. The child is in traumatic cardiac arrest. Your immediate actions should be to address the HOT principles of Hypovolaemia, Oxygenation and Tension/obstructive pathology.

Case Progression

You introduce yourself to the immediate bystanders and establish that the adults crouched next to the patient are the girl's parents. They explain she got out of the car into the road and was hit by the BMW. She has been unconscious since.

You find there is no catastrophic haemorrhage. You manage the airway by suctioning the bloody secretions, insert a size 2 iGel and connect a BVM connected to 15 L of flowing oxygen. You instruct the police officer to stop CPR. The patient's chest inflates slightly with each breath. On auscultation, breath sounds are limited on both sides.

What are the likely causes of limited chest rise and fall in this context?

The most likely causes in this situation are bilateral pneumothoraces ± haemothoraces, which are tensioning; the lower airways are obstructed with secretions; or the child has pulmonary contusions.

How would you manage these findings in this context?

The child's chest should be decompressed bilaterally as both a diagnosis and a treatment intervention. The oral cavity should be suctioned concurrently.

What are the landmarks for needle chest decompression in this age group?

Second intercostal space in the mid-clavicular line above the third rib.

Case Progression

You undertake a needle chest decompression. There is air release from the cannula on the right side. You note bruising across the abdomen and the right anterior superior iliac spine, and she has a closed femoral fracture and open distal tibula/fibula fracture to her right leg.

SYSTEMATIC APPROACH

Danger
Street is blocked in both directions, by a police car on one side and the BMW 4×4 on the other. The shouting has decreased.

Response
Unresponsive.

Airway
Managed with an iGel, minimal secretions.

Breathing
Bag-valve mask ventilation is easier following needle decompression. No crepitus noted.

Circulation
The child does not have a pulse. Capillary refill time >2 seconds. The child is still in asystole. There is no active bleeding from her lower right leg you bind the pelvis, pull the long bones straight and out to length, providing manual traction to the femur fracture, and dress the open lower limb fracture.

Vital signs
Blood sugar: 4.6 mmol/L

Exposure
Systemically she is cool to touch. Following exposure to assess for injury, you cover the child with a blanket to keep her warm.

How much fluid do you wish to administer as part of the resuscitation?

5 mL/kg boluses.

Where would you take this patient?

A major trauma centre.

Which additional support do you require to scene to manage this patient?

Scene commander, critical care clinician/team.

LEVEL 3 CASE STUDY
Unintentional overdose

Information type	Data
Time of origin	07:13
Time of dispatch	07:22
On-scene time	07:40
Day of the week	Monday
Nearest hospital	6 minutes
Nearest backup	Paramedic crew, 45 minutes
Patient details	Name: Zac Orion
	DOB: 05/08/2017

CASE
You have been called to reports of a 3-year-old child who has been found with an empty bottle of his grandma's medication.

Pre-arrival information
The patient is conscious.

Windscreen report
Call is to a neighbourhood in an affluent area of town.

Entering the location
You park on the drive and are welcomed at the door by the caller, who introduces herself as the patient's mother. She appears anxious and distressed. You can hear shouting in the background. The mother advises you that she is the primary carer for her mother, who suffers with Alzheimer's disease. She states that her mother has become worse over the last few months and is requiring more frequent supervision. The house is untidy, with toys on the floor, washing laid out in a heap, dirty food plates visible from breakfast, but it appears grossly clean.

On arrival with the patient
The child is in the downstairs living room watching an animated TV series and drinking from his cup. The grandmother is sat in the next room and watches you come in. She questions who you are.

Patient assessment triangle
General appearance
The patient looks well.

Circulation to the skin
He is pink and well perfused.

Work of breathing
His work of breathing appears adequate and he looks comfortable.

SYSTEMATIC APPROACH
Danger
Nil.

Response
The child is alert.

Airway

Patent, able to swallow his juice, no dribbling.

Breathing

Appears to be without effort. Respiration rate 26 bpm, no added sounds.

Circulation

No external haemorrhage visible. Pink and well perfused. Abdomen looks normal, no tenderness. Radial Pulse.

Vital signs

The child is interacting normally with mum. Pupils are a normal size for the environmental conditions and are accommodating.

Exposure

Systemically the patient is warm to touch, but not hot.

TASK

Look through the information provided in this case study and highlight all of the information that might concern you as a paramedic.

From the history of events you know so far, have you identified any risk factors regarding the safeguarding of this child?

Demands on the mother are increasing. The house is a little unkempt, but given the demands on the mother's time, it is not abnormal to struggle to stay on top of running the home. There are no signs of evident neglect and the child appears to be interacting normally with his mother.

What history would you like to gain from the mother?

See Table 9.2.

Table 9.2 History-taking questions

History of the event

The mother explains that every morning her son watches television while she helps her mother wash and dress in the downstairs bathroom. Her mother slipped this morning in the bathroom, which meant that the child was alone for longer than normal. She could hear him singing along to the television and so didn't think anything of it. When she had finished helping her mother, she returned to the living room to find the pill tray for his grandmother's medication on the floor; the lids to the pill tray were open. She recalls administering the Monday medication that morning and then placing the tray back on the dining table in the living room prior to assisting her mother.

Medication history

Which medications does your mother take?
How frequently? What are the doses?
Are there any other medications he could have taken?
Where are the medications normally kept?

F/SH (family and social history)

Does anyone else in your family have any health conditions?
Who do you live with?
Any other siblings with illnesses?
Names, GP and school details of child and other siblings

Past medical history (PMH)

Does the child have any medical conditions?

Differential diagnosis (DDx) – What else could this be?

No ingestion has taken place

What is your management plan?

The area should be searched for evidence of the missing tablets and as a precaution the child should be transferred to hospital for observation. You could also contact your local poisons unit if you have access to this service to determine how urgent the situation may be.

LEVEL 3 CASE STUDY
Meningococcal disease

Information type	Data
Time of origin	07:13
Time of dispatch	07:22
On-scene time	07:40
Day of the week	Monday
Nearest hospital	6 minutes
Nearest backup	Paramedic crew, 45 minutes
Patient details	Name: Steven Brightside DOB: Not established

CASE
You are dispatched to a school where there are reports of a 6-year-old male looking unwell. No further information available.

Pre-arrival information
The patient is not conscious.

Windscreen report
A staff member greets the ambulance at the gates.

Entering the location
A clean, tidy, safe environment.

On arrival with the patient
The child is in the first-aid room with the first-aider who is also a maths teacher.

Patient assessment triangle
General appearance
Tired, looks asleep

Circulation to the skin
Pale, but warm to touch

Work of breathing
Strained.

SYSTEMATIC APPROACH
Danger
Nil.

Response
The child moves slightly to pressure on the AVPU scale.

Airway
Patent, dry.

Breathing
Appears laboured. Respiration rate 32 bpm, no added sounds.

Circulation
Pink and well perfused, cold peripheries, radial pulses are weak but fast.

Vital signs
The child is limp. Pupils are a normal size for the environmental conditions.

Exposure
No exposure yet.

Previous medical history
Nil, usually fit and healthy.

TASK
Look through the information provided in this case study and highlight all of the information that might concern you as a paramedic.

List as many differential diagnoses for this condition as possible with the information you have right now.

Meningococcal septicaemia, hypoglycaemia, post-seizure, accidental overdose, trauma.

Case Progression

OPA inserted, high flow O2 administered, complete primary survey, move to ambulance rapidly.

Vital signs
RR: 32 bpm, laboured, accessory muscle use
HR: 140 bpm, regular, weak
BP: not taken
SpO$_2$: 90% on high-flow O$_2$
Blood sugar: 5 mmol/L
Temperature 39.9 °C

List as many signs of meningococcal disease as possible.

Fever, food refusal, irritability, grunting, vomiting, diarrhoea, convulsions, neck stiffness, aching, sore muscles, photophobia.

What does a non-blanching rash indicate?

Meningococcal septicaemia.

What makes this case time critical?

The patient is acutely unwell with signs of compensation, probably as a result of meningococcal septicaemia causing shock.

What drugs can you administer for this patient?

Antibiotics such as ceftriaxone, Benzylpenicillin and IV fluids.

Would you transport this child to hospital under emergency conditions or routine conditions? Explain your answer.

Emergency conditions, as he has a GCS of 3 and is showing signs of shock.

References and further reading

Chiappini, E., Bortone, B., Galli, L. et al. (2017) Guidelines for the symptomatic management of fever in children: Systematic review of the literature and quality appraisal with AGREE II. *BMJ Open*, 7: e015404. doi: 10.1136/bmjopen-2016-015404

Ishimine, P. (2019) Assessment of fever in children. *BMJ Best Practice.* https://bestpractice.bmj.com/topics/en-gb/692 (Accessed 9 July 2020).

Mewasingh, L. & Morrison, F. (2019) Febrile seizure. *BMJ Best Practice.* https://bestpractice.bmj.com/topics/en-us/566 (Accessed 9 July 2020).

Mitchell, C., Hall, G. & Clarke, R.T. (2009) Acute leukaemia in children. *British Medical Journal*, 338: b2285. doi: 10.1136/bmj.b2285

NICE (2020) Leukaemia. National Institute for Health and Care Excellence. https://pathways.nice.org.uk/pathways/blood-and-bone-marrow-cancers/leukaemia (Accessed 8 September 2019).

NICE (2020) Clinical knowledge summaries. National Institute for Health and Clinical Excellence. https://cks.nice.org.uk (Accessed 9 July 2020).

Niehues, T. (2013) The febrile child: Diagnosis and treatment. *Deutsches Arzteblatt International*, 110(45): 764–774. doi: 10.3238/arztebl.2013.0764

Wadjdowicz, M. (2019) Overview of dental emergencies. *Merck Manual: Professional Version.* https://www.merckmanuals.com/professional/dental-disorders/dental-emergencies/overview-of-dental-emergencies (Accessed 12 September 2019).

Chapter 10 Patient-centred care in complex cases

Yasaru Gunaratne and David Krygger
Queensland Ambulance Service, Gold Coast, QLD, Australia

CHAPTER CONTENTS

LEVEL 1 CASE STUDY
Transgender persons

Information type	Data
Time of origin	17:00
Time of dispatch	17:36
On-scene time	17:57
Day of the week	Saturday
Nearest hospital	15 Minutes
Nearest backup	None available
Patient details	Name: Tina DOB: Not available

CASE

Third-party caller states a girl of unknown age is sitting on the road in front of her house crying, with blood coming from her wrist. Caller states patient is always on the street doing this.

Pre-arrival information

The patient is conscious and breathing. The patient is flagged for mental health (anxiety and depression), but nil history of weapons or violence at the address.
Special instructions: Crew to proceed with caution.
Message from the police: Police will not be in attendance, no units available.

Windscreen report

Patient is seated on the driveway of an unkempt house with overgrown grass. The patient is compliant and non-threatening to ambulance staff.

Clinical Cases in Paramedicine, First Edition. Edited by Sam Willis, Ian Peate, and Rod Hill.
© 2021 John Wiley & Sons Ltd. Published 2021 by John Wiley & Sons Ltd.

Entering the location

As you disembark from the vehicle, an elderly woman dashes over to you from across the road. As you greet her, she begins to speak to you loudly. 'This girl is a nuisance, playing her loud music and that barking dog. They ought to straighten her out. In my day, girls like this would get a good beating. She should be cleaning this filthy house like a good girl.' The elderly woman then remembers she left the kettle on, and rushes back to her house.

On arrival with the patient

As you approach the patient, they are crying profusely. They raise their head and state, 'Please leave, you can't help me.' The patient is of feminine appearance, but has significant facial hair with a shaved head and is wearing a singlet and trackpants.

Patient assessment triangle
General appearance

As described.

Circulation to the skin

Skin is normal in colour with no clamminess.

Work of breathing

Normal.

SYSTEMATIC APPROACH
Danger

Nil.

Response

Alert on the AVPU scale.

Airway

Clear and patent, able to speak normally.

Breathing

Rate 18 bpm. Nil increase in effort and is a regular rhythm. Auscultation is normal.

Circulation

Pulse 90 bpm. Regular and strength normal. Capillary refill time 2 seconds.

Vital signs

RR: 18 bpm
HR: 90 bpm
BP: 119/63 mmHg
SpO_2: 99% on room air
Blood sugar: 5.2 mmol/L
GCS: 15/15
ECG: normal sinus rhythm

Exposure

Three superficial lacerations to right wrist, nil active bleeding. Evidence of extensive scarring from previous self-harm attempts. Nil other abnormalities detected.

TASK

Look through the information provided in the case and highlight all of the information that might concern you as a paramedic.

PRACTICAL TIP

The paramedic should relocate the patient to somewhere with more privacy, such as the ambulance or inside the house.

What are some strategies for de-escalating the situation with the neighbour? What are the risks of not de-escalating?

Effective communication relies on clear verbal and non-verbal cues, which when contradictory can negatively influence interaction. A formula developed by Mehrabian and Ferris outlines the total impact of a message, which consists of 0.07% verbal, 0.38% vocal (e.g. tone, pitch, speed, etc.) and 0.55% facial (e.g. eye contact, facial expressions, etc.; Vogel et al., 2018). In the context of this case, it is imperative for the clinician to maintain composure by projecting an image of calmness, assertiveness and confidence while being respectful. Use empathy where possible and reflect the patient's emotions without repeatedly asking: for example, 'I can see you are upset, help me understand why' rather than 'How are you feeling?' (Ambulance Tasmania, n.d.). The use of a clear, low pitch and monotonous tone with neutral facial expressions and an open stance/position can make a patient more receptive. The choice of words can have a significant impact on certain groups of people due to the societal connotations or inherent disrespect attached to them, therefore be mindful of the patient's reactions. Additionally, strive to offer choices where possible, avoid responding to insults (remember they are not angry at you, but the situation) and avoid rushing the exchange. If possible, remove the patient from the situation when safe to do so (i.e. relocate to ambulance or house; Eilers, 2017). Throughout the interaction maintain a physical buffer between you and the patient (e.g. increased distance), be vigilant and plan for a rapid egress. Your safety is paramount.

PRACTICAL TIP

A failure to effectively de-escalate the situation may exacerbate the issues, which may potentially endanger you, the patient or bystanders.

What are some strategies for initially approaching a transgender patient?

The principles discussed above are essential for building rapport with all patients. The use of respectful language and supporting their autonomy will assist in developing an open relationship. All interactions between the patient and the health professional must involve the use of the patient's chosen name and their preferred pronouns (Speck, 2016). If unsure of these details, make a conscious effort to establish how they would like to be referred to from the initial interaction. It may be reasonable to plead ignorance rather than mislabel them.

What impact would the neighbour's outburst be likely to have on the patient?

Language that purposefully and/or ignorantly misgenders is known to have a significantly detrimental outcome for a transgender person's mental health. The neighbour's outburst is certainly cruel and generally abusive, but more significantly it will be interpreted by the patient as particularly offensive due to the obvious gender mislabelling and reaffirming of gender stereotypes (Speck, 2016). Several studies have found that individuals with low levels of family support experience a greater proportion of adverse outcomes, which could be expanded to include other community members (Simons et al., 2013). Studies involving transgender individuals have found that use of their chosen name and preferred pronouns was associated with relief and elation, with one individual stating: 'It made my whole day' (Gridley et al., 2016).

What impressions can you get from the state of the house?

It is evident that the house is not well looked after, potentially due to ongoing social issues. Paramedics have a unique opportunity to have a glimpse into someone's life and gather a plethora of information that can assist other clinicians later down the track. For example, having a look in their fridge, the boxes of medication and examining other artefacts can suggest a patient's diet, medication compliance or drug/alcohol use. Paramedics can also gauge the level of family support available to patients within the home setting, which as mentioned is a significant confounding factor of illness (Simons et al., 2013).

Case Progression

After the initial interaction, the patient advises you that they prefer to be called 'he' and that they identify as a man. He states to you that his parents wanted nothing to do with him, and he was forced to move out to this halfway house till he could get a job. He has been unable to find work, and is constantly harassed by his roommates and the neighbours. He is continually called a 'freak' and continues to be misgendered. He hasn't been eating or sleeping well.

Secondary survey

Pain assessment: no abnormalities detected (NAD).

Signs and symptoms: anxious and thoughts of self-harm.

Allergies: nil.

Medications: Aveed (testosterone undecanoate) commenced 1/12; Pristiq and Valium.

Past medical history: anxiety, depression, gender dysphoria.

Last in/out: toasted cheese sandwich this morning; normal bowel motions and urine output.

Events prior: He was involved in an altercation with a roommate this morning where he was told 'go die'. Patient states he made the lacerations to 'feel something'.

No change in vital signs survey.

What do you consider to be the most important issues revealed by this case?

This case explores the challenges of communicating with a transgender individual with concurrent mental illness. It highlights the importance of using chosen names and preferred pronouns, which can often be overlooked in some healthcare settings. It further examines the negative impact of lack of family support and societal stigma on the health outcomes of these individuals. The clinical care provided to the patient is secondary to the larger mental health issues, and some vital signs or other assessments could be omitted. It is important to build rapport, be respectful and gather information/history that can be used to refer the patient to the appropriate services.

What immediate management would you consider for your patient?

Bandaging of right wrist, and consider transport to an appropriate facility where a mental health assessment can be conducted.

LEVEL 1 CASE STUDY
Homelessness

Information type	Data
Time of origin	18:28
Time of dispatch	18:30
On-scene time	18:40
Day of the week	Saturday
Nearest hospital	15 minutes
Nearest backup	10 minutes
Patient details	Name: Suzie
	DOB: Not available

CASE

You have been called to a unit complex for reports of a female lying underneath a flight of stairs. Caller states he does not want to approach the patient and does not know if she is conscious or breathing.

Windscreen report

The area is a large metropolitan suburb. On arrival you see a conscious female patient holding a sleeping bag and pillow, sitting underneath a staircase.

Entering the location
The female appears to be alone. The ambulance is able to be parked close to the scene, with only a small distance to walk.

On arrival with the patient
The female appears emotional, shivering and has limited personal supplies.

Patient assessment triangle
General appearance
The patient is alert, looking at the crew, shaking mildly.

Circulation to skin
She appears pale.

Work of breathing
Breathing appears mildly rapid, with obvious condensation being expelled from her mouth on expiration.

SYSTEMATIC APPROACH
Danger
Cold weather, small environment (under stairs).

Response
Alert on the AVPU scale.

Airway
Patent.

Breathing
Rate: 22 bpm, slightly shallow.

Circulation
Heart rate: 100 bpm, regular, normal strength on radial palpation. Capillary refill time 2.5 seconds.

Vital signs
RR: 22 bpm
HR: 100 bpm
BP: 105/65 mmHg
SpO2: 93% (hands very cold)
Blood sugar: 4.8 mmol/L
Temperature: 34.2 °C
ECG: sinus tachycardia

CHAPTER 10: PATIENT-CENTRED CARE IN COMPLEX CASES

PRACTICAL TIP

For vulnerable patients such as the homeless or in acute emotional situations, be careful of their personal space. Spend some time gaining rapport first before approaching them for vital signs or other treatments – unless a time-critical medical or safety issue is obviously identified.

TASK

Look through the details of the case that you already know. Highlight the pieces of information that are concerning you as a paramedic. What are your differential diagnoses?

What questions would you ask this patient to find out more information?

See Table 10.1.

Table 10.1 History-taking questions with typical responses

Social history questions	Typical responses
Introduce yourself and explain why you have been called	
How are you feeling?	I am feeling cold and tired
How long have you been here for?	This is my second night here
Where were you before then?	With my partner in his house
May I ask how you ended up here?	My husband has been abusing me and I ran away last night, but I don't know where to go. I have nothing and I'm scared he'll hurt me if I return
Medication history	
Do you take any current medications?	No
Medical history	
Have you got any medical issues, or are you allergic to anything?	No
Family and social history	
Do you currently work, or have you been working recently?	No
Are there any medical conditions in your family?	No
May I please ask your age?	28 years old
Have you been taking any alcohol or drugs recently?	No
I would like to help you, may I conduct some vital signs on you?	Yes, that's fine

Once the vital signs have been conducted, what will your next actions be?

- Active warming of the patient (warm blankets, ambulance heater, etc.).
- Maintain an empathetic and reassuring approach.
- Use clear verbal and non-verbal communication to ensure the patient feels safe.

Case Progression

The paramedics warm the patient in the ambulance and use blankets to raise her body temperature.

Patient Assessment Triangle

General appearance

The patient is sitting in a warmed ambulance feeling slightly better, but still shivering mildly. She is conversing well with the crew.

Circulation to the skin

She is still pale, but her colour has improved.

Work of breathing

Eased, she is breathing normally.

SYSTEMATIC APPROACH

Danger
Nil.

Response
Alert on the AVPU scale.

Airway
Patent.

Breathing
Respiration rate 18 bpm.

Circulation
Heart rate 90 bpm, regular, normal strength on radial palpation. Capillary refill time 2.5 seconds.

Vital signs
RR: 18 bpm
HR: 90 bpm
BP: 110/70 mmHg
SpO_2: 98%
Blood sugar: 4.8 mmol
Temperature: 35.0 °C
ECG: sinus rhythm

Consider the general improvement of the patient and her current condition. Reassess what concerns you most about the patient currently.

The patient has presented with acute homelessness and hypothermia, secondary to domestic violence. Being empathetic, calm and approachable as well as providing active warming has improved the patient's condition, and she is now calmer, but still mildly hypothermic.

Now the patient has improved slightly, what care should you consider for this patient? What are the pros and cons of each option?

- Option 1: Non-transport (with or without advice to access social support services).
  - Pros: Nil.
  - Cons: Patient at risk of further medical deterioration this evening due to poor current support.
- Option 2: Emergency Department admission.
  - Pros: Will keep patient warm this evening; social work referral possibly available. Likely will get some food/water.
  - Cons: Busy, patient will likely have to wait some time before being seen; being around other acutely unwell patients exposes patient to disease.
- Option 3: Other shelter options for this evening (homeless shelter/women's refuge/ friends or family).
  - Pros: Will keep patient warm this evening, homeless shelter could link patient with specific support services. Likely will get some food/water.
  - Cons: Urgent homeless services may not be available this evening.

PRACTICAL TIP

Consider patients who are victims of domestic violence or homelessness as being extremely vulnerable. These patients may have poor health literacy and are at high risk of a range of medical and mental health issues. Extreme care and empathy should be used when caring for these patients.

LEVEL 2 CASE STUDY
Religion and sensitive examinations

Information type	Data
Time of origin	11:15
Time of dispatch	11:30
On-scene time	11:50
Day of the week	Thursday
Nearest hospital	20 minutes
Nearest backup	10 minutes
Patient details	Name: Barbara Bundita DOB: Not available

CASE

You have been called to a home in an urban neighbourhood for a 15-year-old female complaining of hypogastric pain and discomfort. The neighbourhood is well known to local ambulance crews and has a largely African immigrant population.

Windscreen report

The mother and father meet you at the front door. They appear welcoming and usher you into the patient's bedroom. The patient is sitting on her bed appearing to be guarding her abdomen.

Entering the location

No access issues, you are able to comfortably bring any equipment into the home and to the patient's bedroom door.

On arrival with the patient

The patient appears to be in moderate discomfort and she is guarding her abdomen. Her parents have entered the room with you and are standing by the wall. The patient and her family appear to be of Sudanese descent.

Patient assessment triangle
General appearance

The patient is alert, looking at the crew, mildly tearing.

Circulation to the skin

She appears well perfused.

Work of breathing

No abnormalities, she appears to be breathing normally.

SYSTEMATIC APPROACH
Dangers

Nil.

Response

Alert on the AVPU scale.

Airway

Patent.

Breathing

Normal work (effort), rate approx. 15 bpm

Circulation
Heart rate 82 bpm, regular, normal strength on radial palpation. Capillary refill time 1.5 seconds.

Vital signs
RR: 15 bpm
HR: 82 bpm
BP: 105/60 mmHg
SpO_2: 100%
Blood sugar: 5.4 mmol/L
Temperature: 37.7 °C
ECG: sinus rhythm
Pain: 6/10

PRACTICAL TIP

Assessing and questioning minors should be conducted with an appropriate guardian where possible. However, be aware that patients may guard their answers if they don't want their guardian to hear a truthful response. Work to gain good rapport with both the patient and the guardian present, and consider asking for privacy with the patient at an appropriate time.

What questions would you ask the patient to find out more information?

See Table 10.2.

Table 10.2 History-taking questions with typical responses

Medical history questions	Typical responses
What seems to be the problem today?	I have a bad pain in my belly
Do you mind showing me where this pain is and does it refer anywhere?	Patient gestures to her hypogastrium – 'It doesn't move anywhere else'
How long has the pain been there?	Worsening for 4 days
What does it feel like?	Feels like a cramping pain
How severe is it on a scale of 1 to 10?	6/10
Does anything make it better?	No
Have you got any medical issues, or are you allergic to anything?	No
Have you seen a doctor?	We have newly immigrated and I don't have a current doctor.
Have you had any urinary or bowel symptoms?	No, I have been regular and normal
Have you had any abdominal trauma?	No
Have you had this pain before?	No
Have you been eating normally?	Yes, I had breakfast this morning

(Continued)

Table 10.2 (Continued)

When was your last menstrual period?	I am 5 days late, this is unusual
May I ask if you're sexually active and if so, when was the last time you had sexual intercourse?	Please don't tell my parents, but I had intercourse 2 weeks ago without protection.
Have there been any other symptoms?	Yes, I had had some clear vaginal discharge, but no bleeding.

Social history
Patient attends a well-known local religious Christian school

Family and social history

Are there any medical conditions in your family?	No
May I please ask your age?	15 years old
Have you been taking any alcohol or drugs recently?	No

During your history taking, the patient appears to be reserved with her answers and is obviously avoiding eye contact with her parents. You suspect that there is more information that she doesn't want her parents to know. How would you ask her parents for some privacy with the patient to explore her condition more?

Case Progression

On further abdominal examination, the patient's abdomen does not feel distended or rigid. She complains of mild increased pain on deep palpation over the hypogastrium, has normal percussive notes and active bowel sounds on auscultation.

Now that you have undertaken a history and vital signs survey, what will your next actions be?

- Invite the parents back into the room, but be careful to respect the wishes of the patient not to inform them of her sexual history.
- Consider analgesia for the patient, *but* you should seek parental permission to do so.
- Consider multi-modal analgesia options.

Case Progression

Analgesia is administered.

Patient assessment triangle
General appearance
Patient appears more comfortable, no longer guarding abdomen.

Circulation to the skin
Skin normal.

Work of breathing
Patient is breathing normally.

SYSTEMATIC APPROACH

Dangers
Nil.

Response
Alert on the AVPU scale.

Airway
Patent.

Breathing
Normal.

Circulation
Heart rate 72 bpm. Capillary refill time 1.5 seconds.

Vital signs
RR: 18 bpm
HR: 72 bpm
BP: 105/60 mmHg
SpO$_2$: 100%
Blood sugar: 5.6 mmol/L
Temperature: 37.5 °C
ECG: sinus rhythm
Pain: 1/10 (post-analgesia)

With the improvement of the patient, what are your choices now? What would you like to do next?

The patient should be transported to an Emergency Department for review. It would be appropriate for a parent to escort the patient if possible. Continue standard clinical care and observations and ensure that identified cultural challenges are handed over to medical staff.

LEVEL 2 CASE STUDY
Rural communities and social determinants of health

Information type	Data
Time of origin	23:05
Time of dispatch	23:06
On-scene time	23:58
Day of the week	Tuesday
Nearest hospital	65 minutes
Nearest backup	Intensive care unit, 90 minutes
Patient details	Name: Isaiah
	DOB: Not available

CASE

You are called to a 7-year-old male, inconsolable, ongoing ear infection.

Pre-arrival information
The child is conscious, but not breathing normally.

Windscreen report

You arrive at a well-kept house with multiple cars parked outside that obstruct the driveway. The crew is unable to get a stretcher up to the house, but can navigate through the cars with other equipment. One dim light is flickering, and you are met by a distressed woman.

Entering the location

On arrival you are greeted by the patient's sister. She states the patient has been experiencing an ear infection for several days and nothing is helping. She tells you that he has been inconsolable all day, not eating and is very hot to touch. She also says: 'I don't think he's doing so good, he won't stop crying.' She continues: 'Please help Isaiah! He's not doing good,' and she begins to cry uncontrollably.

You provide her with reassurance and enter the house to find a large group of people surrounding a small boy who is irritable and crying. The house is filled with overwhelming sensory stimuli. Some people appear to be cooking in the kitchen, there are children playing in front of the television, you can hear loud snoring coming from the bedrooms and several people are asking you to help Isaiah.

The family appears to be of Indigenous Australian descent. There are several small bottles of various colours on the table next to the child, which seem to be oils.

On arrival with the patient

You manage to control the scene and gain access to the patient. He appears to be relatively small in stature for his age and cachexic. He is alternating between coughing and crying while clutching his left ear. The patient does not respond normally to your questions, but ceases crying when his grandmother holds him. He communicates with his grandmother, but refuses to engage with you.

The grandmother tells you 'Yeah, his hearing is not good. Normally when he gets sick, we put some tea tree oil in his ear and he becomes good again. We've never had to call you lot, we don't want no hospital, it's too far away and we can't get home. Can you just make him good?'

Patient assessment triangle
General appearance

Distressed, crying, but the grandmother says the delay in his responses is normal for the patient.

Circulation to the skin

Skin is normal in colour, and no clamminess.

Work of breathing

Elevated respiratory rate, but normal depth and rhythm.

SYSTEMATIC APPROACH
Danger

Nil.

Response

Alert on the AVPU scale.

Airway

Clear and patent. Verbal responses not appropriate for a 7-year-old.

Breathing

Respiration rate 22 bpm. Nil increase in effort. Auscultation is normal.

Circulation

Pulse 88 bpm, regular and strength normal. Capillary refill time 1.5 seconds.

Vital signs
RR: 22 bpm
HR: 88 bpm
BP: 109/72 mmHg
SpO$_2$: 100% on room air
Blood sugar: 4.8 mmol/L
Temperature: 37.9 °C
GCS: 15/15 (grandmother states patient is orientated to person and place, able to follow her instructions, eyes are spontaneous)
Basic ECG: normal sinus rhythm

Exposure
Purulent discharge from left ear, obvious signs of inflammation. Tender to touch. No other abnormalities detected.

TASK
Look through the information provided in the case and highlight all of the information that might concern you as a paramedic.

What strategies could be used for achieving and maintaining scene control during a chaotic scene?

Achieving scene control is essential to ensure that appropriate assessment and management of the patient can be undertaken. In ordinary circumstances when presented with a chaotic scene, it may be appropriate to relocate the patient to a more controlled environment (e.g. the ambulance) along with the carer. Additionally, if the patient is stable, consider delaying any non-visual observations until scene control is achieved.

In this context, it may be inappropriate to remove the child from the communal care environment without exacerbating the distress to the family and the patient. High-context cultures, including Indigenous Australians, may recognise rigid directions or questioning as disrespectful and in turn withhold information from you and/or ask you to leave. Instead, it may be advisable to involve the family in the assessment and management of the patient. For example, distract individuals with simple tasks like gathering medications, finding immunisation records and other medical documents, asking for the television to be switched off and so on. In this case, Isaiah is presenting with an acute exacerbation of a chronic condition, therefore assessment and management can be undertaken slowly. However, if it is a time-critical emergency, it would be useful to clearly, concisely and respectfully convey the severity of the situation to the family, including the potential consequences of their not listening to you.

What might Isaiah be suffering from? What are the potential complications?

Indigenous Australians, particularly those in rural communities, are disproportionately burdened with certain infectious diseases. It is likely that Isaiah is suffering from chronic suppurative otitis media (CSOM), which is a recurrent bacterial infection of the middle ear structures with persistent discharge and perforation of the tympanic membrane (Thornton et al., 2017). CSOM can progress to sepsis, which is associated with significant mortality. It may also lead to inflammatory necrosis of middle ear structures, resulting in hearing loss. Several studies have suggested that hearing loss associated with CSOM can lead to developmental delays, particularly social and cognitive deficiencies (Leach & Morris, 2017).

The grandmother states that the patient is acting normally, but he appears developmentally delayed. What might be some developmental milestones you would expect to see at 7 years that Isaiah might not have met?

As already mentioned, hearing loss as a result of CSOM has been associated with major physical, cognitive, emotional and social developmental delays. From the case, it is evident that Isaiah is small in stature, and displays significant attachment issues and language deficiencies.

Normal developmental milestones at 7 years old (Brennan, 2019; Great Schools, 2019):

- Physical: continued growth at ~6 cm/year and up to 3 kg/year; slow replacement of baby teeth with permanent teeth.
- Language: able to begin forming sentences with increasing complexity, distinguish between differences and similarities as well as tell the time.
- Social/emotional: increasing independence from caregivers; values peer acceptance, makes friends and recognises the importance of sharing and teamwork; association with same-gender play groups; improved ability to articulate events and feelings; curious exploration of boundaries and establishment of right/wrong.

What are likely to be the challenges to overcome when advocating for transport to hospital in this case?

Rural and remote communities are often under-served by healthcare services due to logistical restrictions such as remoteness/geography, small populations and lack of infrastructure. Aside from the limited access to primary healthcare, these communities may not have any access to medical specialists, diagnostic testing and treatments without travelling significant distances away from their homes and families.

When travelling these distances, patients will also need to consider the availability and affordability of transportation to larger health services, as well as accommodation away from home. This could easily turn into an expensive, isolating and arduous logistical challenge. If you find yourself in one of these instances, it may be worth speaking to the local hospital regarding financial or logistical support that could be provided to the patient. Social workers could be of immense assistance to these patients, and the role of a paramedic may be to put the patient/family in contact with them (Victoria State Government, 2015).

Case Progression

You are still unable to communicate with the patient, but he is compliant with the grandmother. She says he is crying because he is in pain. She tells you that this is Isaiah's fifth ear infection, but normally the oils help the pain. She states: 'This is the worst one, I think he had some fevers last night too.'

Secondary survey
Pain assessment: Pain in left ear for the past week, gradual increase in intensity. Pain is severe but patient can easily be calmed by grandmother. Nil radiation.
Signs and symptoms: Crying, irritable, pain, purulent discharge/inflammation of left ear and fever.
Allergies: Nil.
Medications: Tea tree oil and other natural remedies.
Past medical history: Chronic suppurative otitis media.
Last in/out: Hasn't been eating normally or drinking over the past week, had some porridge this afternoon; runny bowel motions and decreased urine output.
Events prior: Generally unwell for the past week.

Vital signs
No changes in the vital signs survey.

What would be your treatment options at this point?

- Administer paracetamol for temperature reduction and possible pain relief.
- Consider referring to the paediatric sepsis tool and transport to hospital for immediate assessment.
- Consider referring to a social worker regarding ongoing social care.

What do you need to bear in mind when communicating with high-context cultures?

A cultural exchange is influenced by a multitude of obvious (e.g. communication style and appearance) and discreet (e.g. beliefs, assumptions, values, expectations and attitudes) factors (Springer, 2019). The impact of these factors can vary depending on the cultural context.

High-context cultures such as Middle Eastern, French, Asian, African and South American can differ significantly from low-context cultures such as mainstream Australian, North American and Western European. Low-context cultures value logic, facts and action in decision making; they often rely on a linear and individualistic approach rather than intuition. Communication with low-context cultures is most effective when straightforward, factual, concise and action orientated. Contrastingly, high-context cultures are less dependent on reason/facts and more influenced by intuition or feelings. They are often collectivist, and communication can be indirect but more formal. Effective communication relies on building trust, and an exaggerated emphasis on non-verbal communication (e.g. tone of voice, facial expressions, gestures, posture), as well as the authority of the person speaking (e.g. an older clinician or a senior member of the community may be afforded greater respect). Descriptive language, formal address and humility can contribute to building rapport.

LEVEL 3 CASE STUDY
Disability care and compassion fatigue

Information type	Data
Time of origin	20:06
Time of dispatch	21:02
On-scene time	21:34
Day of the week	Sunday
Nearest hospital	15 minutes
Nearest backup	Intensive care unit, 8 minutes
Patient details	Name: Simon Dady
	DOB: Not available

CASE
You are called to a private residential address for a 10-year-old male in distress. The caller states that her son has been increasingly agitated and aggressive today. She is unable to calm him down. He has a history of autism spectrum disorder, but no history of violence or weapon use. He has been compliant with ambulance crew in the past, with no history of police assistance.

Pre-arrival information
Patient is conscious and breathing.

Windscreen report
You arrive at a well-kept suburban house with a pristinely manicured lawn and an adjacent garden.

Entering the location
An elderly woman is sitting on the porch in front of the house, she appears exhausted with her hands covering her face. She remains seated as you approach, and she responds in a soft voice: 'Thank you for coming, I know you've been busy tonight.'

You can hear screaming from inside the house, the door is open. The woman states: 'He has been like this all day; I just can't deal with it today. I haven't been able to get anything done.' From her description, it appears that the patient is in his normal mental state, with a slight increase in agitation.

On arrival with the patient
As you walk into the house with her, there is shattered glass and a broken table. The woman begins to cry. The patient is sitting in a chair, and as you attempt to introduce yourself, the patient interrupts with inaudible screeching. The mother states: 'I just can't do it any longer. I can't keep up with him, my health isn't so good any more. I'm all alone.'

She tells you that she has recently registered for a care service, but is awaiting a nursing assessment. She states that her husband also recently passed away. The patient is extremely difficult to assess, but you manage to gather some information.

Patient assessment triangle
General appearance
Normal mental state and appears well.

Circulation to the skin
Normal.

Work of breathing
Normal.

SYSTEMATIC APPROACH
Danger
Nil to crew.

Response
Alert on the AVPU scale.

Airway
Clear and patent; able to speak at normal level for patient.

Breathing
Rate 18 bpm with normal effort. Auscultation is normal.

Circulation
Pulse 98 bpm, regular and strength normal. Capillary refill time: 2 seconds.

Vital signs
RR: 18 bpm
HR: 98 bpm
BP: 100/79 mmHg
SpO$_2$: 99% on room air
Blood sugar: 6.3 mmol/L
Temperature: 36.8 °C
Basic ECG: normal sinus rhythm

Exposure
No abnormalities detected.

TASK
Look through the information provided in the case and highlight all of the information that might concern you as a paramedic.

What are some strategies for communicating with intellectually or developmentally impaired individuals?

Patience is the most crucial element in effective communication and rapport building with intellectually impaired individuals, but other suggestions include (Smeltzer et al., 2017):

- Treat adults with intellectual impairment with the same respect that you extend to other adult patients.
- Attempt to speak directly to the patient, and avoid completely ignoring them to speak with the carer.
- Adjust your manner of communication depending on the patient's responsiveness.
- Try speaking to them in a normal tone of voice, avoid shouting, but slow your speech to an appropriate level and introduce information gradually.
- Simple, direct sentences, careful repetition, visual aids and gestures may be useful.

- Avoid directional terms, abstract language and complicated instructions.
- Maintain standard non-verbal communication such as talking at eye level, making eye contact, but avoid excessive hand gesturing.
- Take all necessary precautions to eliminate distractions, and minimise background noise or excessive sensory stimulus.

What is your primary concern with this patient? Why has the ambulance been called?

The mother appears to be experiencing some difficulty in being her son's primary carer, following some recent changes to her circumstances (e.g. the passing of her husband and the decline in her health). She has finally reached out to some 'respite care' services, but is still awaiting an assessment.

The patient is potentially in his normal behavioural state, but the mother is unable to cope, with recent events having forced her to reluctantly accept that fact. Sedation may not be appropriate for the patient as a result. The role of paramedics in this scenario may be to expedite and facilitate access to urgent respite care.

Case Progression

You are still unable to communicate effectively with the patient, but he appears to have calmed down. The mother informs you that the patient hasn't been unwell recently, and has been eating, drinking and sleeping normally. When speaking to the mother you notice that she is short of breath on exertion and appears to have significant arthritic deformities in her hands. You offer to examine her, which she consents to. She is in her mid-60s. She has been experiencing these symptoms over the past few months, but hasn't been able to visit the doctor due to carer commitments, including not being able to leave her son alone at home.

SYSTEMATIC APPROACH

Airway
Clear and patent; able to speak normally.

Breathing
Respiration rate 20 bpm with increase in effort. Auscultation is normal.

Circulation
Pulse 88 bpm, irregular and strength normal. Capillary refill time: 3 seconds.

Vital signs
RR: 20 bpm
HR: 88 bpm
BP: 165/90 mmHg
SpO_2: 97% on room air
Blood sugar: 10.2 mmol/L
Temperature: 36.4 °C
Basic ECG: normal sinus

Exposure
No abnormalities detected.

Secondary survey
Pain assessment: Chronic osteoarthritic pain of knees and back, gradually increasing in intensity.
Signs and symptoms: shortness of breath, generalised joint pain.
Allergies: Phenergan (anaphylaxis).
Medications: Nil.
Past medical history: Hysterectomy, meningitis.
Last in/out: Normal food intake; normal bowel motions but increased urine output.
Events prior: Unable to determine cause.

What does your assessment of the mother indicate?

The mother has spent a good portion of her life caring for her son, which has evidently been at the expense of her own health. It is a common phenomenon among carers to strive to be independent and self-sufficient; this often leads to overburdening themselves, resulting in poor health outcomes. Carers may also only have limited opportunities to improve their education and income, which can lead to poor health literacy (Hussain et al., 2016).

From the assessment, the mother may be exhibiting several signs and symptoms of heart failure. It will be important to treat the symptoms, as well as refer to other services for investigation, with a focus on expediting at-home assistance.

What could you do in the short term to make the mother feel better about her situation?

Being a caregiver often involves a significant emotional, mental and physical commitment to another individual. Prolonged care can become overwhelming for caregivers, and may result in a state of exhaustion, often referred to as carer fatigue. Caregivers may experience feelings of anger, depression, anxiety, isolation and apathy (Day & Anderson, 2011).

It is unreasonable to expect a paramedic to alleviate carer fatigue during a single callout. However, some small gestures may result in a big impact downstream. Suggestions include:

- Encouraging the caregiver to celebrate small victories.
- Get them to appreciate their incredible efforts and bravery in balancing it all.
- Comment on how beautiful the house/garden is.
- Comment on how caring and generous they are to go over and beyond to support their loved one.
- Remind them that if their loved one could tell them, they would say 'thank you'.
- Help the caregiver to find a silver lining.
  Other practical suggestions include:
- Exploring respite care options and caregiver support groups (local and online forums).
- Encouraging mental and physical self-care.
- Pending operational demand, some small gestures such as changing a lightbulb, loading the dishwasher or taking out the trash might just be enough to put a smile on an exhausted caregiver's face (Smith, 2019).

What would be some alternatives to transport to the Emergency Department in this case?

It is clear that there are two patients, therefore appropriate management of both is essential. As both patients are suffering from a chronic issue, it may be worthwhile exploring some other referral services aside from the Emergency Department.

- Contacting nursing care/support services directly may expedite the process of organising care. You may be better able to advocate for these patients and effectively convey their situation. Remember that when patients contact these services, they are often reluctant and may not divulge the entirety of the situation due to embarrassment, pride or other misconceptions.
- Contacting the patient's GP and bringing them into the loop may assist in streamlining any long-term management. If possible, organise transport to the clinic for assessment of both mother and son.
- Organising a mental health referral for both patients is essential, and it may be worthwhile discussing this with the GP. Avoid the Emergency Department mental health referrals where possible, due to the inability to sustainably manage conditions following cessation of emergency care.

LEVEL 3 CASE STUDY
End-of-life care

Information type	Data
Time of origin	14:59
Time of dispatch	15:00
On-scene time	15:10

Information type	Data
Day of the week	Wednesday
Nearest hospital	15 minutes
Nearest backup	10 minutes
Patient details	Name: Bailey Briersley DOB: Not available

CASE

You are called to a 90-year-old male who is unconscious and not breathing. The family are on scene and no CPR is being conducted.

Windscreen report

A family member meets you outside saying she thinks her father has died.

Entering the location

Easy access for stretcher and all required bags. Single-floor home.

On arrival with the patient

Patient appears catatonic, cachectic. He is lying in a hospital-type bed with multiple medications around him.

Patient assessment triangle
General appearance
Pale, catatonic, unresponsive.

Circulation to the skin
Pale.

Work of breathing
Reduced, shallow respirations.

SYSTEMATIC APPROACH
Dangers
Nil.

Response
Nil.

Airway
Patent, pale, dry.

Breathing
Shallow respirations noticed with gurgling sounds heard without auscultation. Respiration rate 12 bpm.

Circulation
Carotid pulse present, bradycardic and weak, radial pulses absent.

Vital signs
RR: 12 bpm
HR: 50 bpm with regular unifocal PVCs
BP: 70/45 mmHg
SpO_2: 88%
Blood sugar: 4.3 mmol/L
Temperature: 36.9 °C
ECG: sinus bradycardia
Pain: no obvious pain

> **TASK**
>
> The patient appears to be in a critical state. Based on what you know about the patient's history, what options exist to care for this patient? Is resuscitation and/or transport required? What services or assistance could you engage with to care for this patient appropriately?

> **PRACTICAL TIP**
>
> When assessing critically ill or dying patients, it is important to include the family who may be on scene. Don't forget to communicate effectively and walk through what is happening and why you are performing assessments or clinical skills.

What might you ask the family members who are present in order to establish the situation?

See Table 10.3.

Table 10.3 History-taking questions with possible responses

Current history	Possible responses
What has been happening today?	We have seen the patient deteriorate over the past 2 days. He has not eaten or drunk for 2 days, has been doubly incontinent and became unresponsive a few hours ago.
How long has the patient been unwell for?	The patient has been unwell for a few years, but has significantly declined in the past 2 days.
Does the patient have any advanced care wishes?	Yes, the patient has a documented 'Not for Resuscitation Order' and has expressed wishes to remain at home to die. Documentation can be provided.
Medical history	
What medical history does the patient have?	Terminal bowel cancer, Alzheimer's dementia, hypertension
What medications is he taking?	Amlodipine, oxycodone, Exelon
Social history	
Who has been providing care recently?	Cared for by family at home.
Has the patient been receiving health services at home?	Yes. The patient has been seeing the local palliative care team, who saw him a few days ago. They let us know that they expect him to die within the next week.

> **PRACTICAL TIP**
>
> Try to consult with the patient's medical team when making treatment or transport decisions for patients with complex medical histories. In this case, consulting with the palliative care team will give you a deeper understanding of the patient's condition and care options.

Case Progression

The patient becomes grey and appears to stop breathing. The family identify that something has occurred, become worried and start to ask what is happening.

Vital signs
RR: 0 bpm
HR: 0 bpm
BP: unrecordable
SpO$_2$: unrecordable
Temperature: 36.9 °C
ECG: ventricular fibrillation deteriorating to asystole shortly after

What are your actions? Do you attempt resuscitation? If so, why? If not, why not, and how would you proceed with the case?

Resuscitation would not be indicated in this scenario. Documented Not for Resuscitation (NFR) or Do Not Attempt Resuscitation (DNAR) wishes and a strong history suggest the patient is expected to die and that this process should be respected.

Talk to the family, explain what has happened/is happening. Talk openly, respectfully and allow them to start to grieve. Field any questions they have (expect repetitive questioning as family members adjust emotionally to the situation).

It would be appropriate to make a call to the palliative care team to inform them of the patient's death. They will be able to guide you through the process that needs to happen next.

Follow local ambulance guidelines or protocols with regard to reporting the death. Are police required or not? What documentation needs to be completed by the paramedics?

Case Progression

The family indicate that they are Jewish and custom dictates that the patient is buried within a day. They ask you if you could call their local rabbi and inform him of the death so the appropriate processes can start.

A family member also asks if you could call the patient's other daughter who lives interstate to inform her of the death.

If the crew decides to call the palliative care team, they are told that all death certificates will be signed before the end of the day by the doctor and that a team of palliative care nurses will attend the home in the next two hours.

TASK
At what point is it appropriate to leave the scene? What are your local work practices around this question? Is it OK to leave the body in the home before palliative care or the funeral home arrives?

References and further reading

Ambulance Tasmania (n.d.). De-escalation techniques. http://www.ambulance.tas.gov.au/community_information/handsoff/de-escalation_techniques (accessed 14 October 2019).

Bai, H. (2016) A cross-cultural analysis of advertisements from high-context cultures and low-context cultures. *English Language Teaching*, 9(8): 21–27.

Bratianu, P. (2015) Facing the fear: Working with dying patients. *Ausmed*, 16 June.

Brennan, D. (2019) Your child at 7: Milestones. *WebMD*. https://www.webmd.com/parenting/guide/child-at-7-milestones#1 (accessed 16 October 2019).

Day, J. & Anderson, R. (2011) Compassion fatigue: An application of the concept to informal caregivers of family members with dementia. *Nursing Research and Practice*, Article ID 408024.

Eilers, E. (2017) De-escalation tip of the day: Use nonthreatening nonverbals. Crisis Prevention Institute. https://www.crisisprevention.com/Blog/September-2017/De-Escalation-Tip-of-the-Day-Use-Nonthreatening-N (accessed 14 October 2019).

Great Schools (2019) Developmental milestones: Your 7-year-old child. Greatschools.org. https://www.greatschools.org/gk/articles/developmental-milestones-your-7-year-old-child/ (accessed 18 November 2019).

Gridley, S., Crouch, J., Evans, Y. et al. (2016) Youth and caregiver perspectives on barriers to gender-affirming health care for transgender youth. *Journal of Adolescent Health*, 59(3): 254–261.

Homelessness Australia (n.d.) Homelessness statistics. https://www.homelessnessaustralia.org.au/about/homelessness-statistics (accessed 9 July 2020).

Hussain, R., Wark, S., Dillon, G. & Ryan, P. (2016) Self-reported physical and mental health of Australian carers: A cross-sectional study. *BMJ Open*, 6(9): e011417.

Institute of Medicine (US) Committee on Health Care for Homeless People (1988) Health problems of homeless people. In *Homelessness, Health, and Human Needs*, Washington, DC: National Academies Press, Ch. 3. https://www.ncbi.nlm.nih.gov/books/NBK218236/ (accessed 9 July 2020).

Leach, A. & Morris, P. (2017) Otitis media and hearing loss among Aboriginal and Torres Strait Islander children: A research summary. Centre of Research Excellence in Ear and Hearing Health of Aboriginal and Torres Strait Islander Children. https://www.aph.gov.au/DocumentStore.ashx?id=10703288-84e1-4581-84c2-2fc851a3d5a8&subId=511822 (Accessed 9 July 2020).

Simons, L., Schrager, S., Clark, L. et al. (2013) Parental support and mental health among transgender adolescents. *Journal of Adolescent Health*, 53(6): 791–793.

Smeltzer, S., Mariani, B. & Meakim, C. (2017) Communicating with people with disabilities. National League for Nursing. http://www.nln.org/professional-development-programs/teaching-resources/ace-d/additional-resources/communicating-with-people-with-disabilities (accessed 29 September 2019).

Smith, M. (2019) Caregiver stress and burnout. *HelpGuide.org*. https://www.helpguide.org/articles/stress/caregiver-stress-and-burnout.htm (accessed 29 September 2019).

Speck, K. (2016) Initial assessment: Trans primary care guide. *Rainbowhealthontario.ca*. https://www.rainbowhealthontario.ca/TransHealthGuide/gp-initialassess.html (accessed 14 October 2019).

Springer, S. (2019) Effective cross-cultural communication. Lecture notes. https://ilearn.bond.edu.au

Thornton, R., Kirkham, L., Corscadden, K. et al. (2017) Australian Aboriginal children with otitis media have reduced antibody titers to specific nontypeable haemophilus influenzae vaccine antigens. *Clinical and Vaccine Immunology*, 24(4) :e00556-16.

Victoria State Government (2015) Rural and regional healthcare. *Better Health Channel*. https://www.betterhealth.vic.gov.au/health/servicesandsupport/rural-and-regional-healthcare (accessed 16 October 2019).

Vogel, D., Meyer, M. & Harendza, S. (2018) Verbal and non-verbal communication skills including empathy during history taking of undergraduate medical students. *BMC Medical Education*, 18(1): 157.

Zanchetta, P. (2006) Health literacy within the reality of immigrants' culture and language. *Canadian Journal of Public Health*, 97(Supp 2): S26–S30.

Chapter 11

Legal and ethical cases

Ruth Townsend

Charles Sturt University, Bathurst, NSW, Australia

LEVEL 1 CASE STUDY
Consent

Information type	Data
Time of origin	18:25
Time of dispatch	18:30
On-scene time	18:42
Day of the week	Thursday
Nearest hospital	15 minutes
Nearest backup	Intensive care crew, 15 minutes
Patient Details	Name: John Evans
	DOB: 12/12/1970

CASE
You have been called to a private address for reports of a male in distress.

Pre-arrival information
The patient is conscious and breathing.

Windscreen report
The area outside the house appears to be safe. The house is well kept from the exterior with a small garden. No obvious activity outside.

Entering the location
You are greeted by a middle-aged female who appears distressed. She tells you that her partner, John, has come home from work intoxicated and has put a nail through his hand with a nail gun.

Clinical Cases in Paramedicine, First Edition. Edited by Sam Willis, Ian Peate, and Rod Hill.
© 2021 John Wiley & Sons Ltd. Published 2021 by John Wiley & Sons Ltd.

On arrival with the patient

John is sitting in his shed in the back yard with a beer in one hand. His left hand is covered in blood and you can see that a piece of metal is impaled through it.

Patient assessment triangle
General appearance
Alert and orientated to time and place.

Circulation to the skin
Mild pallor to the face.

Work of breathing
No obvious deficits.

SYSTEMATIC APPROACH

Danger
No immediate dangers.

Response
The patient is alert on the AVPU scale.

Airway
Clear.

Breathing
By observation, approximately 17 bpm, regular.

Circulation
John refuses to allow palpation of the radial pulse.

Disability
Hand injury.

Exposure
Not necessary.

After conducting a full assessment, you determine that John has had at least six cans of full-strength beer in the last 2 hours. This is not an unusual number for John. He says that he is not in pain. You assess that he will need to go to hospital for treatment. This is primarily because John uses his hands for his work and you are concerned there may be some permanent damage if the nail is not removed surgically.

John refuses consent for treatment. He does not want to go to hospital. He says, 'Nah, she'll be right, mate.'

TASK

Look through the information provided in this case study. Use the PRECARE model (Townsend & Luck, 2019) to identify the legal, ethical and professionalism issues with this case.

- **P**roblem – identify the issue.
- **R**econnaissance – get the facts.
- **E**thics – consider the four principles of bioethics (autonomy, beneficence, non-maleficence, justice).
- **C**ode – consider the Code of Conduct for Paramedics.
- **A**lternative – is there another option?
- **R**egulations – consider the law.
- **E**valuate – evaluate all the information and make a decision.

What is the problem for the paramedics in this case?

The patient is refusing to go to hospital even though that would be best for him. There is some doubt that he has the capacity to make such a decision because he is intoxicated.

List the four bioethical principles and consider how they apply in this case.

- Autonomy – it is ethical to uphold the patient's right to choose what happens to him for himself, even if it results in a harm.
- Beneficence – there are two actions that could benefit the patient: upholding his autonomy and leaving him at home, or transporting him to hospital for further medical care.
- Non-maleficence – do no harm. There are two actions that could harm John: not upholding his autonomy and taking him to hospital, or upholding his autonomy and risk something worse happening to his health.
- Justice – access to health resources. There is no issue of justice in this case. John has access to healthcare.

What does the Paramedicine Board of Australia Code of Conduct say about consent?

Section 3.5 of the Code says, 'Informed consent is a person's voluntary decision about healthcare that is made with knowledge and understanding of the benefits and risks involved.

Good practice involves: a) providing information to patients or clients in a way they can understand before asking for their consent; b) obtaining informed consent or other valid authority before undertaking any examination or investigation, providing treatment; d) when working with a patient or client whose capacity to give consent is or may be impaired or limited, obtaining the consent of people with legal authority to act on behalf of the patient or client and attempting to obtain the consent of the patient or client as far as practically possible; and f) documenting consent appropriately' (Paramedicine Board of Australia, 2018).

What does the law say about consent?

A patient over 18 years of age is legally entitled to make decisions about themselves for themselves. This requires the paramedic to give the patient *all* the information needed to make such a decision. Consent should be informed. It should be voluntary (that is, not coerced by another person) and the person giving it should have capacity to make an informed decision for themselves. Sometimes patients are not capable of making a decision. If the paramedic doubts the patient's capacity to make a decision, then the onus is on the paramedic to undertake an assessment to establish the patient's capacity. This would involve an assessment of the patient's capacity to understand the information given, believe the information, weigh up the information and communicate a decision. If the patient is able to demonstrate capacity, then no matter how irrational the decision may appear to the paramedics, the paramedics should work to support the patient's choice.

If the patient is assessed as not competent because they cannot understand the information you have given, they do not believe the information you have given them or they cannot communicate to you that they have weighed up the pros and cons of their decision and told you what they want to do anyway, then the patient is likely to be incompetent to make decisions. The decision making can then sit with a surrogate decision maker, who may be the patient's guardian, spouse, carer or other family member. In this case, the patient's partner is likely to be his surrogate decision maker. The paramedics are required to give her all the information they would give the patient and ask her to make a decision in lieu of the patient, because the patient is not capable of making a decision. The surrogate is required to make decisions in the patient's best interest (i.e. not their own).

What do you do and why? Justify your decision with reference to law and ethics.

You need to assess John's capacity to see if he is able to make decisions for himself. If you determine that he understands all the information you have given him, he believes it and has weighed up the benefits and risks and is therefore competent to refuse treatment, then you should leave him at home. If you believe he is incompetent, then you should provide John's partner with all the information so that she can make a decision as his surrogate decision maker. This approach upholds both legal and ethical principles of autonomy and self-determination.

LEVEL 1 CASE STUDY
Confidentiality

Information type	Data
Time of origin	21:05
Time of dispatch	21:10
On-scene time	21:21
Day of the week	Sunday
Nearest hospital	10 minutes
Nearest backup	Intensive care crew, 15 minutes
Patient details	Name: Raj Rodriguez
	DOB: 27/09/2000

CASE
You have been called to a young male threatening suicide.

Pre-arrival information
The patient is conscious, breathing, talking, but standing with his head close to a noose around a tree in the backyard.

Windscreen report
The area outside the house appears to be safe and it is a quiet suburban house. The police arrive on scene as you do.

Entering the location
You are greeted by a female who appears distressed. She tells you that her friend has been 'threatening to kill himself'. He is a young doctor who has had a complaint made against him at work. You walk out the back of the house where the police are with the patient.

On arrival with the patient
The man is walking back and forth around the noose, which is hanging from a tree about 10 metres from you.

Patient assessment triangle
General appearance
The patient is well dressed, agitated, crying and saying 'I just can't do it.'

Circulation to the skin
Unable to assess in detail, but looks well perfused from where you are standing.

Work of breathing
Unable to assess.

SYSTEMATIC APPROACH
Danger
Nil.

Response
Alert on the AVPU scale.

Airway
Clear.

Breathing
Unable to assess in detail.

Circulation

Unable to assess in detail.

Disability

Unable to determine.

Exposure

Not yet appropriate.

You commence talking with the patient, whose name is Raj. He eventually removes the noose from the tree. He approaches you with the rope and you are able to hand it to the police, who then leave. You sit with the patient a little longer and manage to learn a little bit about him and what has happened in the last few months to trigger the episode today. His behaviour is entirely rationale given the circumstances and you have assessed the patient as being competent. The man agrees to voluntarily come with you to hospital to be seen by another doctor to be assessed for depression and anxiety. You assure him that you will maintain his confidence and that all the information you have seen and heard tonight is confidential. The patient is terrified that his threatened suicide will get back to his family, who frown on that sort of behaviour.

As you are leaving, the patient's brother arrives at the house. You recognise him as a friend from school, Aditya. He is shocked to see you here and says with genuine concern, 'Oh my God, Raj, is everything alright, are you OK?' Raj doesn't answer. You tell Aditya that everything is OK. You accompany Raj to the ambulance, but you have left something in the house. Adi approaches you and says, 'Hey, what is happening with my brother? Please tell me. You know me, we're old friends. I love my brother and I am just concerned.'

TASK

Look through the information provided in this case study. Use the PRECARE model (Townsend & Luck, 2019) to identify the legal, ethical and professionalism issues with this case.

- **P**roblem – identify the issue.
- **R**econnaissance – get the facts.
- **E**thics – consider the four principles of bioethics (autonomy, beneficence, non-maleficence, justice).
- **C**ode – consider the Code of Conduct for Paramedics.
- **A**lternative – is there another option?
- **R**egulations – consider the law.
- **E**valuate – evaluate all the information and make a decision.

What is the problem in this case?

The brother is asking what is happening and what has happened. Your patient has asked you not to disclose any details to his family. You think that you have a responsibility to protect the confidentiality of the patient, but you also wonder if you should tell the brother so that he can help the patient.

What are the ethical considerations in this case?

Upholding the autonomy of the patient requires that the patient's confidence is protected as he has asked. Beneficence means acting to benefit the patient, and in this case acting to benefit the patient is to do as the patient has asked and not share any information with his brother. Non-maleficence means to do no harm, and in this case that means not sharing information with the brother of the patient, because to do so would be to cause harm to the patient. Justice means doing what is fair and ensuring the patient has access to resources. In this case it means having access to a paramedic who will act with professionalism and in a legal and ethical way for the patient's benefit.

What does the Paramedicine Board of Australia Code of Conduct say about confidentiality?

Section 1.5 of the Code on Professional Values and Qualities says that 'Patients rely on practitioners to protect their confidentiality.' Section 3.2 on Partnership says that a 'good partnership between a practitioner and the person they are caring for requires high standards of personal conduct including protecting the privacy and right to confidentiality of patients or clients, unless release of information is required by law or by public interest considerations'. Section 3.4 on Confidentiality and privacy says that 'Practitioners have ethical and legal obligations to protect the privacy of people requiring and receiving care. Patients or clients have a right to expect that practitioners and their staff will hold information about them in confidence, unless release of information is required by law or public interest considerations'. Good practice involves 'treating information about patients or clients as confidential; seeking consent from patients or clients before disclosing information, where practicable; and sharing information appropriately about patients for their healthcare while remaining consistent with privacy legislation and professional guidelines about confidentiality'. The requirement to share information 'appropriately about patients for their healthcare' means that those treating the patient should have patient information shared with them. It does not mean that patient information can be shared with family members, unless the patient has given consent to do so, or the patient is incapable of giving consent and the family member is the surrogate decision maker and is therefore required to have all the information about the patient in order to make a decision about the care of the patient that will be in the patient's best interest.

What does the law say about confidentiality?

Under privacy law, a person's health information is considered to be sensitive information that is afforded a higher level of protection than other types of information. The reason for this is that this type of information has the potential to embarrass and exploit a patient, be used in a discriminatory way against them or in some other way create a harm for the patient. For example, in this case the sharing of the patient's information with his brother risks the patient being ostracised from his family. There is a risk that if this information were revealed to the patient's employer, the patient might be at risk of losing his job. Under the Health Practitioner Regulation National Law Act that regulates paramedics in Australia (State of Queensland, 2020), there is a mandatory obligation for registered health practitioners to notify the regulator if they treat a patient who is also a registered practitioner, but only if the treating practitioner forms a reasonable belief that the patient practitioner poses a risk of harm to the public. Remember, the primary purpose of the regulator is to protect the public from harm. In this case there is no obligation on the paramedic practitioner to report the patient to the regulator, because the patient does not appear to pose a risk to anyone other than himself and has voluntarily agreed to seek help.

What do you do and why? Justify your decision with reference to law and ethics.

Although you believe that the brother of the patient has the patient's best interest at heart, you are not legally or ethically able to share the patient's health information with the brother unless the patient gives you consent to do so.

LEVEL 2 CASE STUDY
Clinical negligence

Information type	Data
Time of origin	13:40
Time of dispatch	14:00
On-scene time	14:03
Day of the week	Tuesday
Nearest hospital	10 minutes
Nearest backup	Intensive care crew, 15 minutes
Patient details	Name: Philippina Caruthers DOB: 10/10/2000

CASE

You have been called to a private address for reports of a female in her 20s with difficulty in breathing. The caller states the patient is a known asthmatic.

Pre-arrival information

The patient is conscious and breathing.

Windscreen report

The area outside the house appears to be safe. The house is well kept from the exterior with a small garden. No obvious activity outside.

Entering the location

You are greeted by a female who appears to be distressed. She tells you that her friend has 'bad asthma' and that she has tried to take her inhaler, but it is not working.

On arrival with the patient

The female patient is lying down with an obvious decreased level of consciousness (LOC) at GCS 11/15. She appears confused.

Patient assessment triangle

General appearance

The patient is distressed and cannot complete a sentence without taking a breath.

Circulation to the skin

Pale with central cyanosis.

Work of breathing

Pursed lips, tachypnoea, silent bilateral breath sounds due to minimal air movement.

SYSTEMATIC APPROACH

Danger

Nil.

Response

Verbal on the AVPU scale.

Airway

Clear, cyanosed.

Breathing

Respiration rate: 44 bpm, poor tidal volume, appears to be panting. Effort: patient appears exhausted. No breath sounds due to minimal air movement.

Circulation

Heart rate: 133 bpm, weak, regular. Capillary refill time: >2 seconds.

Vital signs

RR: 44 bpm
HR: 133 bpm
BP: 160/100 mmHg
SpO_2: 91%
Blood sugar: 3.2 mmol/L
GCS: 11/15
Lead II ECG: sinus tachycardia

Exposure

Difficulty exhaling, no accessory muscle use.

After checking your Clinical Practice Guidelines you notice they state:

WHEN THERE IS A RISK OF IMMINENT ARREST

If GCS <12, bradycardia/absent pulse then 100% O_2, assist ventilation with prolonged expiratory phase, consider adrenaline IV/ETT/IM, transport without delay.

OR

SEVERE ASTHMA ATTACK

If minimal air movement, 1 or 2 words per breath, cyanosed, SpO_2 <93% on 50% O_2, then high concentration O_2 and consider salbutamol IV and nebulised. Move from IV to nebulised when SpO_2 >93%.

You think the patient is at risk of imminent arrest. Your more senior partner thinks the patient does not meet the criteria for imminent arrest because she is not bradycardic as per the guidelines, and is concerned about acting outside the guidelines. You commence treatment with salbutamol, which appears to have no effect. The patient continues to deteriorate. Now you administer intramuscular adrenaline, support her breathing and rapidly transport the patient to hospital. Upon arrival the patient is not breathing and as a result of a period of time without oxygen suffers brain damage.

TASK

Look through the information provided in this case study. Identify the legal, ethical and professionalism issues with this case.

What is the problem in this case?

There is confusion about the application of the guideline between the treating paramedics. One is concerned about what will happen to them and the patient if they do not apply the guideline strictly verbatim. The other paramedic has made an assessment of the patient's condition that anticipates the clinical path the patient is on (i.e. that she is tachycardic because she is compensating before she becomes bradycardic) and wants to act in the patient's interest by administering the 'Imminent Arrest' protocol. As paramedics you have a duty of care to the patient. Because you are registered, each of you individually is held to a legal and ethical standard of care. That standard includes being able to use guidelines with a degree of discretion that allows paramedics to work in the best interests of the patient.

What is the legal standard of care expected of a registered paramedic?

The legal standard of care owed by a paramedic to a patient is the standard expected of a 'reasonable' paramedic. A 'reasonable' paramedic is one who would act in accordance with the standard of care and treatment that their paramedic peers would say was required for a paramedic in a similar situation.

What is negligence and where did the negligence occur in this case?

Negligence is when a practitioner breaches their duty of care by failing to meet the standard of care required and in so doing harms the patient. There is a causal link between what the practitioner did or did not do but should have done (or not) that results in harm to the patient. In this case the negligence occurred when the paramedic failed to identify the seriousness of the case and in so doing failed to administer adrenaline, support the patient's breathing and rapidly transport the patient to hospital early enough. A 'reasonable' paramedic would have identified the seriousness of the patient's condition sooner and *not* have been concerned about their own wellbeing, but placed the patient's interests first.

What is vicarious liability?

Vicarious liability is when an employee is found to have been liable for an offence, for example negligence, but rather than the employee being required to pay compensation to the victim for the breach of duty of care, the employer pays the compensation to the victim. In this way the liability is shifted from the paramedic to their employer, who takes on that liability vicariously. Vicarious liability does not protect a negligent paramedic from sanction by the Paramedicine Board of Australia.

Can the Paramedicine Board of Australia hold me responsible and impose a punishment for negligence?

Yes. The law that regulates paramedics in Australia says that '"Unprofessional conduct" is professional conduct that is of a lesser standard than that which might reasonably be expected of the health practitioner by the public or the practitioner's professional peers' (State of Queensland, 2020, Section 5). However, the matter would have to be referred to a professional standards committee to be reviewed. The paramedic would be afforded procedural fairness, which means they would have the opportunity to defend themselves and let the committee know if there were any mitigating circumstances that should be taken into account.

LEVEL 2 CASE STUDY
Healthcare records

Information type	Data
Time of origin	12:00
Time of dispatch	15:45
On-scene time	15:51
Day of the week	Thursday
Nearest hospital	15 minutes
Nearest backup	Intensive care paramedic crew, 5 minutes
Patient details	Name: Bron Lacey DOB: 07/09/1983

CASE
You have been called to a local bank where a 37-year-old female has had a syncopal episode and is now complaining of severe lower abdominal pain.

Pre-arrival information
The patient is conscious and breathing, but in a great deal of pain.

Windscreen report
The bank is busy with a large number of customers. You are able to park in the street outside.

Entering the location
You are taken by a member of staff to the staff bathroom, where you find the patient lying on the floor. Another bank employee tells you that the patient had been complaining of sudden left-sided abdominal pain before she fainted (syncope). The syncopal episode lasted about 10 seconds. When she awoke, she said she needed the bathroom and so staff assisted her to the toilet, where she vomited and then lay down on the floor in the foetal position, with her knees to her abdomen. Her abdominal pain has been increasing and she is now in obvious discomfort, moaning loudly.

On arrival with the patient
The patient's name is Bron. She is 37 years old. She is lying on the floor. She is awake but in pain and she is clutching at her lower abdomen. She weighs approximately 55 kg. She says she has been having IVF therapy and that she may be around 8 weeks pregnant.

Patient assessment triangle
General appearance
The patient is alert and in severe discomfort with abdominal pain. Her abdomen appears slightly distended. You note a small blood stain on the back of her skirt.

Circulation to the skin
Pale.

Work of breathing
No evidence of shortness of breath.

SYSTEMATIC APPROACH

Danger
Nil.

Response
Alert on the AVPU scale.

Airway
Clear, patent, slightly dry with furring of the tongue.

Breathing
Respiration rate: 24 bpm. Effort: no increased effort. Accessory muscle use: no. Auscultation: clear air entry throughout on auscultation.

Circulation
Heart rate: 120 bpm, regular, radial pulses strong bilaterally. Capillary refill time: 2 seconds.

Vital signs
RR: 24 bpm
HR: 120 bpm
BP: 100/60 mmHg
SpO_2: 99%
Blood sugar: 5.2 mmol/L
Temperature: 36.8 °C
Lead II ECG: sinus tachycardia
Allergies: Nil

Exposure
10/10 sharp left lower abdominal pain, non-radiating.

Your provisional diagnosis is an ectopic pregnancy, ovarian torsion or ruptured ovarian cyst. You rapidly transport the patient to hospital and on the way administer analgesia, along with an anti-emetic that shows some effect. Fluids are administered and a second set of vital signs are recorded; however, you are so busy treating the patient that you are unable to keep contemporaneous records of the treatment or the vital signs. You don't worry too much about it because you know you will have time to complete the case report once you have handed her over to Emergency Department staff.

After handover you sit down to complete the case sheet. You are called to another case – baby not breathing. You respond without having completed the paperwork on the previous case. It isn't until a few hours later that you get another chance to complete your paperwork on that case.

TASK
Look through the information provided in this case study and identify the legal and ethical issues.

What is the problem in this case?

The problem is that the paramedic has moved on to another case before completing the case sheet. This is potentially problematic, because it means that until the case sheet is completed there is no written record of what treatment the paramedics gave to Bron, when, how effective it was and why they gave it. This may pose a problem for continuity of care for the patient and place her at risk. Additionally, it means that when the paramedic does complete their case sheet at a later time, there is a risk that the information that is recorded will not be accurate.

What does the Code of Conduct say about record keeping?

The Paramedicine Board of Australia Code of Conduct (Interim) at Section 8.4 says: 'Maintaining clear and accurate health records is essential for the continuing good care of patients or clients. Good practice involves keeping accurate, up-to-date, factual, objective and legible records that report relevant details of clinical history, clinical findings, investigations, information given to patients or clients, medication and other management in a form that can be understood by other health practitioners; ensuring that records are sufficient to facilitate continuity of care; making records at the time of events or as soon as possible afterwards.'

What are the benefits of keeping accurate, contemporaneous, objective healthcare records?

The benefits of keeping accurate, contemporaneous, objective records is that not only does it mean information is made available from the paramedics to the next treating team to ensure that there is continuity of care for the patient, but that any risks associated with a lack of transference of accurate assessment or treatment information are minimised. For example, if the paramedic had administered an opiate as analgesia, it is important for the Emergency Department treating team to be aware of the dose, time administered and effect. So good healthcare records are an important part of keeping patients safe.

What are the legal issues associated with keeping accurate, contemporaneous, objective healthcare records?

The maintenance of good healthcare records is an important part of paramedic professionalism, and not just because they help protect the patient. Healthcare records can also be used as evidence in an investigation, disciplinary hearing or court case and may be used to establish names, dates, times, places, actions and justifications for decisions, or to establish what was seen and heard by paramedics at a particular moment in time. From time to time complaints are made about paramedics and an accurate, contemporaneous, objective healthcare record helps provide evidence that the paramedic engaged in satisfactory professional performance 'by exercising the knowledge, skill or judgment, or care required to be exercised to the standard reasonably expected of a paramedic of an equivalent level of training or experience' (State of Queensland, 2020, Section 5) and thus helps provide a defence against such complaints.

LEVEL 3 CASE STUDY
Mental health and cultural sensitivities

Information type	Data
Time of origin	20:50
Time of dispatch	21:00
On-scene time	21:11
Day of the week	Sunday
Nearest hospital	35 minutes
Nearest backup	Unknown
Patient details	Name: Maria Stacey DOB: 21/03/1977

CASE

You have been called to an agitated female.

Pre-arrival information

The patient is conscious. The neighbours called the 'job' in because the patient is in the front yard of her home, half-naked and wailing.

Windscreen report

On arrival you see a woman in the front yard. She has a skirt on, but no top. She is holding her hands to the sky. You can hear her saying, 'God, why are you doing this to me, why? My babies, my babies.'

On arrival with the patient

You approach the woman by introducing yourself and asking her name. She replies, 'Maria, my name is Maria.'

Patient assessment triangle
General appearance

The patient appears healthy. There are no obvious signs of injury or illness.

Circulation to the skin

Within normal limits (WNL).

Work of breathing

WNL.

SYSTEMATIC APPROACH

Danger

Nil.

Response

Alert on the AVPU scale.

Airway

Clear, as she is talking, but unable to perform any additional assessments.

Breathing

WNL.

Circulation

WNL.

Disability

Nil physical injury.

Exposure

Not necessary.

Maria says she is 43 years old and from Tonga. She has recently separated from her husband. He has taken their two children aged 10 and 13 to live with him. She says he will not let her see them because she scares them. Maria says that she has had depression before when the children were little and she spent some time in hospital. She says that she thinks God is punishing her and that is why her kids have gone. She says that she has not had a shower in a week and that she is not eating. She says she was outside praying to God and performing a traditional dance because she is very sad. She does not want to go to hospital again because then she will never get to see her kids. She does not give any indication that she poses a risk of harm to herself or others, beyond the risk of harm to her reputation by dancing at the front of her house with no shirt on.

> **TASK**
>
> Look through the information provided in this case study. Use the PRECARE model (Townsend & Luck, 2019) to identify the legal, ethical and professionalism issues with this case.
> - **P**roblem – identify the issue.
> - **R**econnaissance – get the facts.
> - **E**thics – consider the four principles of bioethics (autonomy, beneficence, non-maleficence, justice).
> - **C**ode – consider the Code of Conduct for Paramedics.
> - **A**lternative – is there another option?
> - **R**egulations – consider the law.
> - **E**valuate – evaluate all the information and make a decision.

What is the problem in this case?

The issue is whether or not Maria is suffering from a mental illness requiring transportation to hospital for treatment because she poses a risk to herself or to others. Risk to self can include risk to reputation. However, given the circumstances, it is completely rational for Maria to feel sad and for her to express her sadness in a way that is particular to her culture. This may not be the way the paramedics would express their grief, but the expression of grief and loss in this way is not a sign, on its own, of mental illness.

What does the law say about the definition of mental illness/mental disorder?

The law varies from state to state regarding the definition of mental illness. Paramedics should be aware of the provisions of the Mental Health Act that applies in their jurisdiction. However, in order for paramedics to use any of the powers they are afforded under the Mental Health Act (e.g. sedation and restraint), they must first assess that the patient does indeed have a mental illness or disorder that places the patient at risk of harm to themselves or others. If the paramedics assess that the patient is mentally ill and in need of treatment because they pose a risk of harm to themselves or others, paramedics must then assess if there is a less restrictive alternative care pathway for this patient than transporting them to hospital. A patient's expression of political, religious, cultural or sexual views that are not consistent with the views of paramedics is not a sign of mental illness, and would not give paramedics the legal authority to use the powers ascribed to them under the Mental Health Act.

What does the Code of Conduct say about cultural good practice?

The Paramedicine Board of Australia Code of Conduct refers to good practice as culturally safe and sensitive practice. Section 3.7 says, 'Good practice involves an awareness of the cultural needs and contexts of all patients and clients, to obtain good health outcomes. This includes having knowledge of, respect for and sensitivity towards the cultural needs and background of the community practitioners serve, including those of Aboriginal and/or Torres Strait Islander Australians and those from culturally and linguistically diverse backgrounds.' Good practice also includes 'an understanding that a practitioner's own culture and beliefs influence their interactions with patients or clients', and that good practice is about 'adapting practice to improve engagement with patients or clients and healthcare outcomes'.

It is therefore very important for the paramedics in this case to assess the patient thoroughly to determine if she is suffering from a mental illness requiring treatment and transport to hospital, or if she is simply sad and requires some support from her local GP, friends and community groups.

LEVEL 3 CASE STUDY
Paediatrics and end-of-life care

Information type	Data
Time of origin	05:40
Time of dispatch	05:45

(Continued)

Information type	Data
On-scene time	05:55
Day of the week	Tuesday
Nearest hospital	55 minutes
Nearest backup	30 minutes
Patient details	Name: Stacey Sutcliffe
	DOB: 05/10/2017

CASE

You have been called to a private address in a regional town. A mother has called and reports that she requires assistance for her 3-year-old daughter who has severe congenital muscular dystrophy (CMD). The mother states that the child was found unresponsive in her bed this morning and she has noted the child's laboured breathing.

The patient is cared for at home by her parents and extended family and requires daily medication to manage her condition. Her parents have been advised that due to the severity of her illness, this is a life-limiting condition for the child.

Pre-arrival information

The patient is unconscious with laboured breathing. She has a history of CMD. More recently the patient has been managed in hospital for multiple episodes of aspiration pneumonia.

Windscreen report

On your arrival, there appear to be many people outside the house. It is assumed that these are extended family and friends of the patient.

Entering the location

You are greeted by the patient's father, who appears calm and sombre. The father clearly explains the patient's chronic and declining medical history. He is able to produce an advance care plan that outlines comfort treatment and pain management only. No lifesaving or invasive interventions are to be performed. The father states that the family has extended family and friend support and that the decline of the patient is not unexpected. He further explains that his wife is not accepting of the imminent death of their daughter and that he was initially unaware that the ambulance had been called. The father would like to follow the end-of-life care plan that both he and his wife agreed to. His wife now wants all lifesaving treatment undertaken.

On arrival with the patient

The patient is lateral on the sofa with her head cradled by her mother. The mother is sobbing and appears extremely distressed. She asks you to treat her child.

Patient assessment triangle
General appearance
The patient is pale, unconscious and has laboured, irregular breathing.

Circulation to the skin
Pale. Capillary refill time >4 seconds.

Work of breathing
Bradypnoeic. Irregular. Poor tidal volume.

SYSTEMATIC APPROACH
Danger
Nil.

Response
Unresponsive on the AVPU scale.

Airway
Obstructed due to positioning of the patient.

Breathing
Respiration rate: 10 bpm. Increased effort. On auscultation: breath sounds bilaterally diminished. Poor tidal volume.

Circulation
Heart rate: 82 bpm. Effort: weak. Heart regularity: regular. Capillary refill time: >4 seconds.

Vital signs
RR: 10 bpm
HR: 82 bpm
BP: 55/40 mmHg
SpO_2: 82%
Blood sugar: 3.1 mmol/L
Lead II ECG: regular
Temperature: 38.3 °C (febrile)

Exposure
Pale.

TASK
Look through the information provided in this case study. Use the PRECARE model (Townsend & Luck, 2019) to identify the legal, ethical and professionalism issues with this case.
- **P**roblem – identify the issue.
- **R**econnaissance – get the facts.
- **E**thics – consider the four principles of bioethics (autonomy, beneficence, non-maleficence, justice).
- **C**ode – consider the Code of Conduct for Paramedics.
- **A**lternative – is there another option?
- **R**egulations – consider the law.
- **E**valuate – evaluate all the information and make a decision.

What is the problem in this case?

The problem in this case is that the legal and ethical issues are unclear. Time is a critical factor in clinical decision making and, as such, the paramedics need to know what their legal and ethical requirements are in order to act quickly and professionally in this case. The paramedics will be considering the following questions:

- What does the advance care plan say? A copy is required so the paramedics know what has been agreed between the family and the patient's doctor.
- What should happen when a parent wants to ignore the advance care plan?
- Should/can the paramedics commence treatment while they are undertaking their 'reconnaissance', i.e. getting the facts?
- Even if the family asks for the child to be treated, do paramedics have to commence treatment if they know that treatment will be futile?

How do the four ethical principles apply in a case like this?

- Autonomy: In this case the patient is too young to be competent to make decisions about end-of-life care for herself. Her parents are her legal guardians and have the power at law to do so unless an alternative decision maker has been appointed by the court. Guardians have an obligation to act in the best interest of their ward. In this case, the parents have an obligation to act in the best interest of their daughter. The issue is when one parent's view of what is best differs from the view of the other parent.

- Beneficence: Beneficence means acting for the benefit of the patient. Traditionally medicine (and paramedicine by extension) has been paternalistic. Paternalism is where a healthcare practitioner makes a decision about the patient based on what the practitioner thinks is 'best' for the patient. Paternalism is not consistent with the ethical principle of autonomy or the legal right of an individual to choose what they wish to do for themselves. In order to avoid a 'hard' paternalism where the practitioner makes decisions for the patient based on what the practitioner believes is best, or, in this case, where the parents make a decision for the child based on what they believe is best for the child, the decision maker should make a decision that the patient would make if they had the capacity to do so.

  Sometimes there is conflict between the parents, or the parents and the practitioners, as to what action would benefit the patient. In this case, it is unlikely to be beneficial to the patient for active treatment to be commenced, because the child has a life-limiting illness and the condition she has presented with today is as a result of that illness. If she was sick due to another cause (e.g. a fall with a broken arm), then paramedics may treat that condition because it is treatable. However, in this case, the action that would benefit the patient is for paramedics to provide palliative care to the patient and support to her parents.

- Non-maleficence: In this case it is likely that there is a paradox confronting the paramedics. To treat the patient would ordinarily be the action that does 'no harm' or the least harm, but in this case it is likely that active treatment of the patient may cause more harm and distress than the provision of palliative care.

- Justice: The issue of justice in this case is about ensuring that the patient has access to appropriate care. That does not necessarily mean active care.

What does the code of conduct say about such situations?

Section 3.6 of the Paramedicine Board of Australia Code of Conduct says, 'Caring for children and young people brings additional responsibilities for practitioners. Good practice involves placing the interests and wellbeing of the child or young person first. It involves recognising the role of parents or guardians. However, good practice also includes remaining alert to situations where a parent or guardian is refusing treatment for their child or young person and this decision may not be in the best interests of the child or young person.'

In this situation, the parents have been made aware of the life-limiting nature of the patient's illness and, in partnership with their daughter's doctors, have agreed to develop an advance care plan to ensure that at the end of their daughter's life, she is not subject to unnecessary treatment that would likely cause harm and have no benefit. Advance care plans are written, as the name suggests, in advance of the patient's condition deteriorating, so that when the high emotion of the end of a patient's life approaches, the patient's best interests are able to be protected.

In addition, Section 3.12 of the Code refers to good practice for end-of-life care. It says, 'Practitioners have a vital role in assisting the community to deal with the reality of death and its consequences. In caring for patients or clients towards the end of their life, good practice involves: a) taking steps to manage a person's symptoms and concerns in a manner consistent with their values and wishes; b) when relevant, providing or arranging appropriate palliative care; c) understanding the limits of services in prolonging life and recognising when efforts to prolong life may not benefit the person; and d) for those practitioners involved in care that may prolong life, understanding that practitioners do not have a duty to try to prolong life at all cost but do have a duty to know when not to initiate and when to cease attempts at prolonging life, while ensuring that patients or clients receive appropriate relief from distress.'

What does the law say about advance care directives?

Advance care directives should be followed because they are a document that sets out the patient's wishes for their end-of-life health care. In essence, the document acts as the patient's voice when they no longer have one. The legal right for individuals to make these decisions for themselves is captured in the legal principle of bodily inviolability. The exception to this principle is when the patient is incompetent to make decisions for themselves. The law says that children under 16 are incompetent to make decisions for themselves. They are therefore appointed a guardian, usually their parent(s), to act as surrogate decision makers. The obligation of the surrogate decision maker is to act in the best interests of the patient; that is, as the patient would have acted if they had been competent.

The law allows advance care plans to be changed because the plans are supposed to act as an extension of the patient. So if the patient changes their mind about treatment at the end of their life, they can change the plan. Likewise, if the surrogate decision maker acting on behalf of the patient changes their mind, they are able to. In this case, the advance care directive may not be binding because one of the decision makers has changed their mind about treatment. This now becomes a question of where the duty of care for the paramedics rests; that is, who is their patient? Although the mother is lawfully the surrogate decision maker for the child, the child is still a legal entity in her own right and the paramedics' duty of care is to her. The paramedics are legally able to treat the patient with active measures if they deem it clinically necessary to do. The paramedics are also legally able to withhold active treatment and instead provide palliative treatment as per the advance care plan, but also in accordance with their clinical assessment of the patient's needs.

What would you do and why? Justify your decision with reference to law and ethics.

When as a paramedic you are unsure about the patient's treatment goals because there is no advance care plan or there is conflict between surrogate decision makers, you could treat actively until such time as advice from the patient's medical practitioner and/or palliative care team is made available. Paramedics should be mindful of the harm active treatment may cause to the patient and weigh up the benefit of providing that treatment for the patient. Alternatively, paramedics may choose to rely on the advance care plan and the decision of the father of the child to provide palliative care to the patient, because this is in the patient's best interest. Either way, the paramedics must base their decision on what is best for the patient, not what is best for themselves in terms of their relationship with the mother, the father or their employer.

References and further reading

Australian Commission on Safety and Quality in Health Care (2016) *National Consensus Statement: Essential Elements for Safe and High Quality Paediatric End of Life Care.* Sydney: ACSQC.

Australian Government (2014) Privacy Act 1988. https://www.legislation.gov.au/Details/C2014C00076 (accessed 10 July 2020).

Feudtner, C. (2007) Collaborative communication in pediatric palliative care: A foundation for problem-solving and decision-making. *Pediatric Clinics of North America*, 54(5): 583–607. doi: 10.1016/j.pcl.2007.07.008

Paramedicine Board of Australia (2018) Interim Code of Conduct. AHPRA. https://www.paramedicineboard.gov.au/Professional-standards/Codes-guidelines-and-policies/Code-of-conduct.aspx (accessed 10 July 2020).

Queensland Ambulance Service (2020) Clinical Practice Manual (CPM). https://www.ambulance.qld.gov.au/clinical.html (accessed 10 July 2020).

Queensland Government (2020) Advance health directive. https://www.qld.gov.au/law/legal-mediation-and-justice-of-the-peace/power-of-attorney-and-making-decisions-for-others/advance-health-directive (accessed 28 January 2020).

State of Queensland (2020) Health Practitioner Regulation National Law Act 2009. https://www.legislation.qld.gov.au/view/pdf/inforce/current/act-2009-045 (accessed 10 July 2020).

Townsend, R. & Luck, M. (2019) *Applied Paramedic Law, Ethics and Professionalism*, 2nd ed. Chatswood: Elsevier.

Victoria State Government (2020) Advance care planning forms. *health.vic.* https://www2.health.vic.gov.au/hospitals-and-health-services/patient-care/end-of-life-care/advance-care-planning/acp-forms (accessed 25 January 2020).

Chapter 12 | Mental health cases

David Davis[1], Tom Hewes[2], Lynne Walsh[2] and Brian Mfula[2]
[1] College of Paramedics, Bridgewater, UK
[2] Swansea University, Wales, UK

CHAPTER CONTENTS

LEVEL 1 CASE STUDY
Anxiety

Information type	Data
Time of origin	11:30
Time of dispatch	12:00
On-scene time	12:08
Day of the week	Tuesday
Nearest hospital	10 minutes
Nearest backup	Paramedic team leader solo responder, 15 minutes
Patient details	Name: Catherine Rhymes DOB: 04/08/2005

CASE

You are called to a 15-year-old female who is suffering with breathing difficulties, chest pain and circumoral paraesthesia.

Pre-arrival information

The patient is sitting in the school lavatory, where she has been since morning break; she is with one of her friends and the school first aid and welfare staff are on scene. It is reported that she takes a blue inhaler for asthma.

Windscreen report

You arrive at the school, which you have not seen before, it is a large boarding school with impressive grounds. You are directed by the security staff to one of the female boarding houses, where you are met by four other students, who tap on the window to tell you that the patient's boyfriend 'dumped her' this morning and that has caused her to suffer an asthma attack.

Clinical Cases in Paramedicine, First Edition. Edited by Sam Willis, Ian Peate, and Rod Hill.
© 2021 John Wiley & Sons Ltd. Published 2021 by John Wiley & Sons Ltd.

Entering the location
You are met by teaching and pastoral care staff, who take you to the patient's location, the female student's lavatories, toilet and tell you that the patient, who has a history of asthma, is in a bad way and can barely breathe.

On arrival with the patient
When you arrive at the patient's side, one of the staff says that she is having an asthma attack. The patient is sat on the toilet with tears pouring down her face, a pile of tissues on her lap. She has a picture of a teenage boy open on her smartphone. The first aider says that she is not sure whether the patient is suffering from an asthma attack because she did not seem to have a wheeze.

Patient assessment triangle
General appearance
Other than the tears already observed, you notice that the patient is red-eyed. She otherwise looks well, her clothes are well maintained, and she is generally well presented. The patient is very distressed, crying and wailing.

Circulation to the skin
Slight pallor to the face and the patient has cold hands.

Work of breathing
You can see and hear that she is breathing very fast and moving a large amount of air with each breath, despite tears and mucous secretions running from her nose. She is complaining that she has pain in her chest and that her face and arms are numb and have a pins-and-needles sensation in them. Though she is given her salbutamol inhaler by one the staff, she says she does not need it between breaths and pushes it away.

SYSTEMATIC APPROACH
Danger
Nil.

Response
Alert on the AVPU scale.

Airway
The patient's airway is clear and patent, observed through breathing and speaking, albeit in broken sentences as a result of the rapidity of her breathing.

Breathing
Respiratory rate 38 bpm, high volume of air being moved with the use of accessory muscles. No audible adventitious breath sounds to hear or on auscultation. Equal movement of chest wall, not possible to percuss the chest due to the distress of the patient.

Circulation
The patient looks well perfused with no circumoral cyanosis observed. However, capillary refill in her fingertips is delayed at around 3 seconds and her hands are cold to touch. The pulse oximeter is at first unable to secure a reading, although it eventually settles.

Vital signs
RR: 38 bpm, reducing to 32 bpm after initial assessment
HR: 112 bpm
BP: 109/69 mmHg
SpO_2: 100%
Blood sugar: 4.9 mmol/L
Temperature: 37.5 °C, tympanic
Lead II ECG: not assessed

Exposure
As described within the earlier narrative. You also notice some spasticity in the patient's hands.

TASK

Look through the information provided in this case study and highlight all of the information that might concern you as a paramedic

What is an anxiety disorder and how does it present?

An anxiety disorder describes a feeling of fear, dread and apprehension, which leads to a deterioration of one's ability to function even when there are no identified dangers. The range of anxiety disorders includes generalised anxiety disorder (GAD), panic disorder and phobias.

What is the epidemiology of anxiety disorders?

On a global scale, incidence of anxiety disorders varies from between 2.5% and 7% of the population, with females being more likely to experience anxiety disorders than males. Specifically, incidence is 9.3% for the UK and 13.1% for Australia (Ritchie & Roser, 2018).

What are the different ways in which anxiety can present in the out-of-hospital setting?

The World Health Organisation's (WHO) International Classification of Diseases (ICD-10) notes frequent symptoms of:

'(a) apprehension (worries about future misfortunes, feeling "on edge", difficulty in concentrating, etc.);

(b) motor tension (restless fidgeting, tension headaches, trembling, inability to relax);

(c) autonomic overactivity (light headedness, sweating, tachycardia or tachypnoea, epigastric discomfort, dizziness, dry mouth, etc.' (WHO, 2016).

Case Progression

It is apparent from your systematic assessment that there is no evidence of asthma, owing to the large volume of air being moved and absence of adventitious breath sounds. You talk to the patient and notice that her respiratory rate is decreasing while you are talking with her. She tells you that her life is over because her boyfriend has dumped her, and she is really worried that she will never, ever find anyone to love her again, and she is worried that this will adversely affect her results when she takes her GCSE exams next month.

SYSTEMATIC APPROACH

Danger
Nil.

Response
Alert on the AVPU scale.

Airway
Clear.

Breathing
Nothing has changed, other than rate is now slower.

Circulation
The patient remains well perfused and looks well, her hands are now warming up and she has a normal capillary refill time.

Vital signs
RR: 16 bpm
HR: 92 bpm

BP: 100/65 mmHg

SpO$_2$: 100%

Blood sugar: not taken

Temperature: not taken

Lead II ECG: not observed

Exposure

Patient is complaining of pins and needles in her face and all over her body, she says it is improving but it is painful.

Mental health assessment

You are coaching the patient to manage her breathing to a normal rate and find that the best way to achieve this is to talk with her.

She tells you that she has been worried a lot recently and not sleeping properly. Not only has she separated from her boyfriend, but she has been very worried about body image and her work at school – it is final exams year for senior school and she does not want to let her family down. She is worried about the money that her parents have paid for the school and thinks she is a failure compared with her siblings.

She says that she keeps feeling dizzy and worrying about everything, she is lacking in energy and just cannot stop thinking about things. She has not been eating properly and says her hands are trembling all the time. She says that the only time she feels better is at drama class, when she is acting in the school play.

What is a panic attack?

A panic attack is a distinct and separate episode of overwhelming fear and discomfort that develops abruptly within a short space of time and manifests through palpitations, derealisation (feeling unreal), sweating, trembling, shortness of breath, dizziness, chest pain, and hot flushes/chills (American Psychiatric Association, 2019).

What are the referral requirements for a patient suffering with anxiety and a resolve episodes of hyperventilating associated with a panic attack?

All interventions for the patient with an anxiety disorder should be delivered by a competent practitioner. A comprehensive assessment for the child or young person should enable them to be interviewed alone at some point of the assessment, and if possible include a responsible adult known to the patient who could provide further information about current or past behaviours.

What is the out-of-hospital treatment for this patient?

Calm the patient, helping her to slow her breathing to reduce her anxiety and prevent respiratory alkalosis. Thorough history taking and making an appropriate referral to services that can meet her needs. A delayed referral is probably appropriate in this case where the panic attack symptoms are abated.

LEVEL 1 CASE STUDY
Depression

Information type	Data
Time of origin	22:30
Time of dispatch	00:00
On-scene time	00:30
Day of the week	Friday night/Saturday morning
Nearest hospital	40 minutes
Nearest backup	None available
Patient details	Name: Dion Smythe DOB: 12/12/1950

CASE

A call is received via the urgent care system for an ambulance regarding a 70-year-old man who reports to the emergency call handling staff that he 'can't take care' of his disabled wife any longer. The caller is his wife, who states her husband is crying and upset and keeps repeating 'I can't do this any more'. She is worried as he is getting breathless.

Pre-arrival information

The additional information from the dispatch system states that the case has been reviewed by a senior paramedic within the call centre, who has manually upgraded the case to a medium-priority emergency call due to welfare concerns for all parties.

Windscreen report

You arrive at a street of bungalows in a small town. You find the house in question that has the lights on, where you notice an adapted entrance and wheelchair ramp.

Entering the location

You ring the doorbell and there is no reply; you try the front door, which is unlocked, and quietly say that you are a paramedic. Still there is no reply. You walk into the front room of the property and find an elderly woman in a wheelchair; she says hello and tells you that she is sorry to waste your time, but she is worried about her husband because after getting her up this morning, he went back to bed and has not spoken with her all day. She tells you she is fine, since her daughter is coming over to give her a hand to get to bed and that she is going to stay with her.

On arrival with the patient

You enter the bedroom and find the patient lying in the bed. There are various bottles of tablets on his bedside locker. You can see that he is breathing and that it looks to be a normal rate. You introduce yourself to him and he does not reply, instead shrugs his shoulders. You ask if it is OK if you take his pulse, he does not answer but instead once again shrugs his shoulders, although he does not pull away when you take his arm – you assume consent and take his pulse, which is normal. You notice that the patient is unshaven, unkempt and has dirty hands. He appears very tired and lethargic.

SYSTEMATIC APPROACH

Danger

There is a hoist lift hanging over the bed and you move this to one side to allow access to the patient. Various bottles of tablets on his bedside locker – are they his? Has he taken anything more than usual?

Response

Alert on the AVPU scale.

Airway

Assumed to be clear and patent given the colour of the patient and his breathing.

Breathing

Respiration rate 16 bpm and appears normal.

Circulation

Present, normal capillary refill, heart rate 60 bpm.

Vital signs

RR: 16 bpm
HR: 60 bpm
BP: not taken, in line with patient's wishes
SpO_2: 97%
Blood sugar: Not taken, in line with patient's wishes
Lead II ECG: Not taken, in line with patient's wishes

Exposure

After initially not speaking, the patient reluctantly says a few words, asking who called you to him and why you are wasting your time with him. It is apparent from an initial physiological assessment that his observations appear normal. You continue to patiently interact and engage with him. Through observing and speaking to him, from a psychological perspective you have some significant concerns.

TASK

Look through the information provided in this case study and highlight all of the information that might concern you as a paramedic.

How would you recognise depression in a patient?

- Poor hygiene, self-neglect, lack of food in the house, disturbed sleep and poor appetite.
- Reduced attention and concentration, loss of interest, low mood, reduced energy.
- Ideas of self-harm or suicide, ideas of guilt, feelings of unworthiness and poor self-esteem.

What is your priority when attending a call to a patient with depression?

- Showing clear communication skills and understanding, being non-judgemental, demonstrating listening skills and self-awareness of the situation.
- Assess the risk of suicide/self-harm.
- Gain a patient history regarding recent life events and stress, past life events, any previous suicide attempts.

What policies and guidance are available on depression to guide your practice?

National Institute for Health and Care Excellence (NICE) Clinical Guidance:

- Depression in adults, recognition and management (CG90).
- Depression in adults with a chronic physical health problem (CG91).
- Stepped-care model (in CG90).
- Depression in children and young people: identification and management (CG28).

See also the Welsh Government's, Together for Mental Health strategy (2018).

Case Progression

You spend an hour with the patient, during which time you build trust. He tells you that he has been a carer for his wife, who has a muscle-wasting disease, for the last 40 years. He tells you that he is tired and fed up. He says that all they do is argue and he has lost all of his friends. His dog died and now he has little contact with anyone other than his wife. He believes his children do not like him any more and that is why they stay away from him and his wife. He says he loves her and is letting her down because he has lost appetite for all of his life and has decided he is going to stay in bed forever. He tells you that he knows it is stupid, but it is how he feels. He tells you he sees no way out from this situation and has considered taking all the tablets on his bedside locker.

SYSTEMATIC APPROACH

No physiological observations have changed since the first examination, although the patient has now consented to measurement of blood pressure, a blood sugar test and to give details of his medical history, which includes high blood pressure for which he takes an ACE inhibitor.

BP: 164/94 mmHg

Blood sugar: 6.4 mmol/L

Mental health assessment

Key findings include:
- Potential risk of suicide.
- Reduced self-esteem.
- Increased fatigue.
- Lack of motivation to engage in usual activities.

How would you assess the risk in a patient experiencing signs and symptoms of depression?

- Can the patient rate their mood between 1 and 10, 1 being very good and 10 being very low?
- Ask about their sleep pattern, appetite, feelings and enjoyment.
- Do they feel life is worth living and have they considered taking their life or harming themself?

What are the complexities in managing depression in the elderly population?

- Loneliness, isolation, vulnerability and stress.
- Potential risk of suicide, alcohol abuse.
- Stigma associated with mental illness.

Note: In this case study there is further complexity arising from the patient's caring responsibilities and the need to safeguard both parties.

LEVEL 2 CASE STUDY
Bipolar disorder

Information type	Data
Time of origin	07:00
Time of dispatch	07:15
On-scene time	07:23
Day of the week	Friday
Nearest hospital	43 minutes
Nearest backup	None available
Patient details	Name: Noah Bates
	DOB: 15/01/2003

CASE

You have been called to a private address for reports of a 17-year-old male who is highly agitated. The caller states the patient is erratic and they fear he is going to 'do something stupid'.

Pre-arrival information

Just as you pull up outside the house, ambulance control contact you to state that they have requested police attendance as they can hear raised voices during the call and want to ensure the ambulance crew's safety.

Windscreen report

The area outside the house appears to be quiet. An adult male has seen you pull up to the house. He wants you to come in, but you are hesitant as the police have not yet arrived. He tells you the patient, who is his son, is not dangerous any longer and directs you into the house. The father states he cannot deal with his son's mood swings any more.

Entering the location

You are greeted by the patient's mother, who appears very distressed. She tells you that her son is now in his bedroom. He has broken crockery and pictures and although only 17 years old, he is too big for them to deal with on their own.

On arrival with the patient

The male is in his bedroom. He is smoking a cigarette and looking with a fixed stare at the wall. He then laughs out loud and appears to be talking to someone and giggling. He turns to look at you and starts talking non-stop, of which much appears to be gibberish and not making any sense. He jumps off the bed and starts pacing back and forth, still talking very fast and getting louder.

Patient assessment triangle

General appearance

The patient is alert and looks at you as you enter the room, but then looks away. He appears dissociated and distant. His behaviour is very bizarre with rapid speech and his thoughts seem to be racing.

Circulation to the skin

Appears normal.

Work of breathing

Appears a little erratic.

SYSTEMATIC APPROACH

Danger

The patient is sitting on a sofa, there is nothing obvious near him that he could use as a weapon. He appears to have a high BMI for his age. Initially he was not hostile, but you become more aware of his rapid speech and pacing up and down the bedroom. This leads you to become more cautious in your approach. His behaviour is bizarre and periodically he appears to be talking to someone and laughing loudly.

Response

Alert on the AVPU scale.

Airway

Clear.

Breathing

From a distance it appears to be of adequate rate and depth.

Circulation

From a distance the patient seems to have adequate circulation.

Vital signs

RR: not gained, the patient does not give consent to be touched
HR: not gained
BP: not gained
SoO$_2$: not gained
Blood sugar: not gained
Lead II ECG: not gained

Exposure

The patient's fingers show signs of nicotine staining. There are no obvious signs of injury or physical restriction. He looks dishevelled and unclean and seems to be irritable.

TASK

Look through the information provided in this case study and highlight all of the information that might concern you as a paramedic.

How would you recognise the signs of mania in a patient with bipolar disorder?

- Rapid speech and thoughts; elation and excitability; irritability.
- Bizarre behaviour; flights of ideas; hearing voices.
- Lack of sleep; restlessness.

What is your priority when attending a patient who is showing signs of mania?

- Talking calmly and slowly with clear communication; observing patient's non-verbal as well as verbal communication; awareness of your own verbal and non-verbal communication; keeping a safe distance.
- Awareness of potential trigger factors that may cause further irritation.
- Assessment of risk: to others, patient and self.

What policies/guidance are available on bipolar disorder to guide your practice?

NICE clinical guidance – Bipolar disorder: Assessment and management (CG185).

What factors must you consider in a patient experiencing signs of mania?

- Safety to the patient and others and early intervention.
- Patient's lack of insight, paranoia, lowered inhibitions, lack of contact with reality.
- Patient making risky/harmful decisions (Walsh, 2009).

Case Progression

You speak to the mother, asking her what has happened in the lead-up to this event. You ask if her son is known to have any medical conditions, taken illicit drugs, or sustained a head injury. The mother says no to all of these questions. She asks to speak to you out of earshot of the patient and tells you that he has been having similar mood swings for the last couple of years. He is their only child and they have thought his behaviour was simply the 'normal mood swings of a teenager'. Tonight, however, they have decided they cannot cope with his outbursts any more.

The police arrive and when he sees them outside his bedroom, your patient allows you to take a set of observations.

SYSTEMATIC APPROACH

Danger
Nil acute, but you remain on your guard.

Response
Alert and irritable.

Airway
Clear.

Breathing
Respiration rate 22 bpm.

Circulation
Heart rate 90 bpm.

Vital signs
RR: 22 bpm
HR: 90 bpm
BP: 140/80
SpO_2: 98% on air
Blood sugar: 5.7 mmol/L

Temperature: 37.1 °C
Lead II ECG: sinus tachycardia

Exposure
Patient appears to have normal colour.

Mental health assessment
The patient lacks capacity. He shows distrust towards his parents for calling the emergency services. He lacks insight and appears disorientated to time, date and space. On arrival the police do not think he is a risk to others. However, you take him to the hospital and arrange for him to have a further mental health assessment with a psychiatrist.

What are the complexities of managing mania in the out-of-hospital setting?

- Patient's non-compliance with medication caused through lack of insight into their deteriorating mental health.
- Reckless behaviour and lowered inhibitions making patient vulnerable to abuse from others.
- Increasing irritation and excitability leading to potential physical problems and potential cardiac arrest (Walsh, 2009).

LEVEL 2 CASE STUDY
Schizophrenia

Information type	Data
Time of origin	23:00
Time of dispatch	00:50
On-scene time	00:55
Day of the week	Friday
Nearest hospital	N/A
Nearest backup	N/A
Patient details	Name: Danny Boyd DOB: 12/03/1975

CASE
You are a paramedic, working with a non-paramedic, ambulance assistant crew member, called to undertake a transfer of a 45-year-old male from the custody centre of a police station to a forensic mental health hospital.

Pre-arrival information
You are told that the patient is believed to be suffering acute psychosis and is involuntarily detained for treatment under the Mental Health Act, having been found committing petty crimes at the international airport in a state of undress. Due to his condition he requires an ambulance transport from the police custody centre with police and social worker escorts.

Windscreen report
You arrive at a busy city police station and enter the secure custody centre, wait for 10 minutes to be let through the security gates and back up to the ambulance bay. The roller shutter closes behind the ambulance and you are met by the civilian detention staff.

Entering the location
You walk into a busy detention centre, with a number of individuals being checked into custody; one young, obviously drunk man is in the process of being physically restrained, having spat at the custody officer, before being carried into a cell. In the background you can hear dull thuds coming from one of the cells; the custody centre clinician waves you over.

On arrival with the patient

As you are taken to the cell the dull thuds are coming from, the custody centre clinician explains that the patient has been assessed by a psychiatrist and independent advocate and found to be suffering from acute psychosis, and is currently under the belief that he is being spied on by aliens. You are told that the patient is a workaholic, high achiever who is chief executive of an international company operating out of New Zealand and Australia and across Asia. He travels extensively across time zones and had been reported as missing by his colleagues and family. You are told that he was arrested at the airport in his underclothes while stealing food from a shop on the concourse. You are advised that the patient is ethnically a Pacific Islander, and that he has a family history of schizophrenia. You are also told that he is tall and strong and very anxious and suspicious of others, and has been getting agitated and threatening violence. You are advised to approach with caution, and where possible to avoid the need for police restraint, since this exacerbates his agitation.

The clinician tells you that the patient's physiological measurements are within normal ranges, given his acute agitation, and that he has refused to take benzodiazepines orally since he does not want to be poisoned.

The cell door is opened and the patient, who is lying in the corner of the cell, is under a blanket and is gently banging his head against the metal toilet bowl. As you approach him you introduce yourself as a paramedic. The patient does not reply, so you approach closer and the clinician introduces you and tells the patient that he can trust you.

The patient says he is scared, and you explain that you are there to help him feel better and that you have come to take him to the hospital to get some treatment. The patient says that he is not unwell, just being spied on. He tells you to close the cell door, so that he can have a private conversation with you. The custody staff shake their heads to say that would be a bad idea. You ask him who he is worried will overhear your conversation. He replies, 'the aliens.'

TASK

Look through the information provided in this case study and highlight all of the information that might concern you as a paramedic.

What is schizophrenia and how does it present?

Schizophrenia affects a person's ability to feel, think and act. Diagnostic criteria include two or more of the following symptoms being present for at least six months: delusions, hallucinations, disorganised speech, disorganised or catatonic behaviour, or negative symptoms such as diminished emotional expression or avolition (Marel et al., 2016). Around 1% of the population will develop psychosis and schizophrenia. The first symptoms usually start in early adulthood, but can occur at any age (NICE, 2014).

Do any symptoms increase the chances of the condition being schizophrenia rather than other psychotic disorders?

The following negative symptoms are associated with schizophrenia, but are less prominent in other psychotic disorders:

- Less emotional expression.
- Decreased interest in initiating or continuing activities.
- Difficulty communicating, through difficulty keeping track of conversations, switching between unrelated topics, or incoherent words or sentences.
- Restricted ability to experience pleasure from positive stimuli.
- Decreased interest in social interactions (Marel et al., 2016).

What are the treatments and can people recover?

There are several treatment options available for the treatment of psychotic disorders, including psychotherapy, pharmacotherapy and physical activity (Marel et al., 2016). Most people will recover, although some will have lasting difficulties or remain vulnerable to future episodes (NICE, 2014).

Case Progression

After some time, you build trust with the patient and he agrees to go to the ambulance with you. The custody centre is cleared and you and the police officer accompanying you walk slowly to the back of the ambulance.

The patient's trust in you is built up because of your empathy and understanding around his concerns about the aliens spying on him. Before he gets into the ambulance, he asks to check it over and is reassured that the vehicle is in a locked metal compound.

Eventually you start the journey and after just a few minutes, as you are driving down a major road at speed, the patient starts shouting and reaching for the ambulance doors. He manages to open the back doors and lunges to jump out. Fortunately your colleague, who is driving, has undertaken an emergency stop and the police officer and you have managed to restrain the patient. You know only a week before in a similar case a patient had died jumping from the back of an ambulance.

After some considerable time, the patient agrees to get into the back of the ambulance again. He explains that the ambulance was not secure. You agree a plan to blanket and tape the windows and create a secure tent around the trolley cot with a blanket, sheet and foil thermal sheet, which the patient insists will prevent the spies from seeing him.

The patient lays on the floor of the ambulance under the 'tent' for the remainder of the journey, which is uneventful. He is much calmer and is transferred into the care of the hospital staff with no further events. Whilst this approach is uncustomary, the police officer and your colleague agree that this is the best way to keep the patient safe.

What are the potential risk factors for schizophrenia from a family history and ethnicity perspective?

The Framework for Mental Health in Multicultural Australia (2014) states that compared to the general community, those from culturally and linguistically diverse communities (which include refugees) receive poorer-quality mental healthcare and are more likely to be exposed to adverse safety risks (Galletly et al., 2016).

How should you manage a situation like the one described in this case?

Focus on the things the patient is good at, or what they enjoy. Remind them that they are important within their family and community. Ask them who they trust, and try to get in touch with this person, so that they can help calm the situation (RANZCoP, 2017).

LEVEL 3 CASE STUDY
Post-traumatic stress disorder (PTSD)

Information type	Data
Time of origin	16:37
Time of dispatch	17:03
On-scene time	17:22
Day of the week	Monday
Nearest hospital	15 minutes
Nearest backup	None currently available
Patient details	Name: Jade Fox
	DOB: 17/04/1981

CASE

You are asked to attend a 39-year-old female who has attempted to take her own life.

Pre-arrival information

The initial call came through 45 minutes ago. The patient is unconscious and the caller has stated 'there's blood everywhere'. Family members on scene say that the patient is an off-duty paramedic.

Windscreen report

You arrive at a semi-detached house in a rural part of your area. The house looks well maintained and safe. Ambulance control report that the police have been mobilised, but the patient's family have advised that the area is now safe.

Entering the location

You are met by the patient's family. They are very distressed at the condition of the patient, and they are upset due to the circumstances leading up to the call and the slow ambulance response time. They quickly guide you up to the master bedroom.

On arrival with the patient

The patient is in the recovery position on the floor. There is evidence of alcohol consumption on the bedside table and blood visible on the bed. Her husband states that he found her. He has dressed her self-inflicted wounds and gives you the tool that he believes was used to make them. He says she has been struggling with her mental health for some time now.

Patient assessment triangle

General appearance

You vaguely recognise the patient, but she is not well known to you. She normally works in a different area, but you know she has a good number of years' experience as a paramedic. The patient is unresponsive.

Circulation to the skin

Pale, showing peripheral cyanosis.

Work of breathing

From a distance you can see that she is breathing. Her respirations look shallow.

SYSTEMATIC APPROACH

Danger

Nil.

Response

Unresponsive on the AVPU scale.

Airway

Airway clear, you can smell alcohol on her breath.

Breathing

Equal bilateral air entry with no added sounds. Respiration rate of 23 bpm.

Circulation

Weak radial pulse. Tachycardia of 130 bpm. Capillary refill time >2 seconds. Cyanosis evident at her lips.

Vital signs

RR: 23 bpm
HR: 130 bpm
BP: 80/60 mmHg
SpO_2: 89% on air
Blood sugar: 4.3 mmol/L
Lead II ECG: sinus tachycardia

Exposure

The patient has what appear to be self-inflicted wounds on her wrists and neck.

TASK

Look through the information provided in this case study and highlight all of the information that might concern you as a paramedic.

What is post-traumatic stress disorder (PTSD)?

Harvey et al. (2015) state that PTSD is a persistent, severe mental health impairment that can happen after being exposed to a single or multiple traumatic events. PTSD regularly presents with other conditions such as major depressive disorder and alcohol use disorder (Harvey et al., 2015). Risk factors include being in the emergency services, the armed forces, nursing or medicine, and also having multiple major life stressors or previous experience of trauma (NICE, 2019b). It can affect people of any age (NICE, 2019b). Causes include directly experiencing or witnessing a traumatic event, learning that one happened to someone very close, or repeated exposure to traumatic events (NICE, 2019b).

What are the signs and symptoms of PTSD?

There are a range of symptoms:

- Re-experiencing symptoms (including intrusive thoughts, nightmares, flashbacks).
- Arousal symptoms (such as hypervigilance, insomnia, irritability, anger, sleeping or concentration difficulties).
- Avoidance symptoms (such as actively avoiding thoughts, reminders, memories or situational reminders of the trauma).
- Negative symptoms (such as emotional numbing, inability to recall details of the event, dissociation or interpersonal difficulties) (NICE, 2019b; Harvey et al., 2015).

What is the incidence of PTSD?

Shalev et al. (2017) state that the prevalence of PTSD varies according to social background and country of residence, ranging from 1.3 to 12.2%. Bennett et al. (2004) studied the prevalence of PTSD in a sample of emergency ambulance personnel working in the UK. They found the overall rate of PTSD was 22%. A more thorough review conducted among Australian emergency workers identified the prevalence of PTSD to be 10%. Fear et al. (2010) found that in a study of UK armed forces personnel, the probable prevalence of PTSD was 4%. Although these studies involve different methodologies and are therefore non-comparable, they may suggest that the prevalence of PTSD among emergency services workers is greater than that found within the military.

Those with PTSD are six times more likely to attempt suicide and five times more likely to self-harm compared to the general population (Harvey et al., 2015). Paramedics within England have a higher incidence of suicide than in the broader population (Office for National Statistics, 2017). However, a link between suicide and PTSD has not been established.

Case Progression

One wound is still bleeding heavily through the dressing that is not stopping through direct pressure, so you apply a tourniquet and note the time. You insert a supra-glottic airway and administer oxygen therapy 100% at 15 Lpm. While you're doing this your colleague gains IV access and administers tranexamic acid and sodium chloride as per local guidelines. During treatment the husband states, 'She's not been right mentally since going to a really nasty job in work – but that was about 8 months ago now. Everything used to be so good, she loves being a paramedic.'

The patient's vital signs improve while you transport her to the Emergency Department under emergency driving conditions. During the journey, you ask the husband more questions. You identify that she has been experiencing many of the symptoms of PTSD for months. She has been reluctant to seek help, as she was sceptical of the effectiveness of treatment and afraid she would lose her job and be referred to her professional regulator if identified.

What is the treatment for PTSD and does it work?

When someone is diagnosed with PTSD, they should be assessed for the presence of comorbid problems such as anxiety, substance misuse and depression. If any of these are present they should be addressed. The patient should also be assessed for risks of suicide, self-harm, violence or aggression. The presence of these factors may indicate inpatient care. Trauma-focused psychological therapy sessions, such as cognitive behavioural therapy or eye movement desensitisation and reprocessing, may then be initiated. Pharmacological treatments may also be considered. These include antidepressant medications such as selective serotonin reuptake inhibitors (SSRIs) or venlafaxine a selective serotonin and norepinephrine reuptake inhibitor (SSNRI), which have evidence to support their effectiveness in treating PTSD (NICE, 2018b). Other medications that may be considered are alpha-blockers, anti-psychotics or benzodiazepines (Harvey et al., 2015).

How do you access help for the patient?

Clinical assessment for PTSD is necessary if there is at least one symptom from each of the following categories: re-experiencing symptoms, arousal symptoms, avoidance symptoms and negative symptoms; *and* the person experiencing these has been exposed to a single or multiple traumatic events. Assessment can be sought from primary care, such as a GP, or through an organisation's Occupational Health Department (OHD).

Work-related PTSD has a return-to-work rate of 85% (Stergiopoulos et al., 2011). Patients can return to work if their symptoms improve, even if they are still undergoing active treatment. However, it should be noted that some activities (such as emergency driving) may need special consideration by the workplace's OHD and Human Resources Department. The use of modified duties may be necessary. Work-related triggers should be identified through the patient's psychological therapy and these should be monitored on return to work (Harvey et al., 2015).

PTSD is a treatable condition. Preventing mental health disorders can include wellbeing checks, post-trauma interventions, peer support schemes and resilience training.

LEVEL 3 CASE STUDY
Drug-induced psychosis

Information type	Data
Time of origin	09:44 hrs
Time of dispatch	09:45 hrs
On-scene time	10:12 hrs
Day of the week	Thursday
Nearest hospital	22 minutes
Nearest backup	Non-paramedic crew, 35 minutes
Patient details	Name: Nigel Grindle DOB: 27/12/1988

CASE

A young woman has called for an ambulance as she thinks her partner has 'gone mad'. She says he is speaking to the wall and having hallucinations. She is scared.

Pre-arrival information

The patient is reportedly aggressive. Police have been requested. Stand-off advised until their arrival.

Windscreen report

On arrival you park a distance from the property to await police presence before continuing. When they arrive, you tell them the limited information you know and agree to follow them the short distance to the caller's flat.

Entering the location

The police and you walk towards an open front door. A woman wearing a dressing gown and slippers meets you at the door. She looks scared, but relieved that you have arrived. She says her partner is in the lounge. He is seeing things and talking to voices in his head. He has not hurt her, but he is a body builder and his demeanour at the moment is frightening.

On arrival with the patient

The patient looks at the police and you with distrust. He is extremely big, a muscular athlete. You are glad the police are with you, but their presence makes the patient turn angry. He launches into a deluge of verbal abuse towards the police. The police and you try to calm the patient down. You notice one officer putting her hand on her Taser pistol.

SYSTEMATIC APPROACH

Danger

The patient is a highly agitated bodybuilder. He is in a state of emotional turmoil, pacing his lounge and shouting.

Response

Alert on the AVPU scale.

Airway

Clear.

Breathing

From a distance his respiration appears to be of adequate rate and depth.

Circulation

From a distance the patient seems to have adequate circulation.

Vital Signs

RR: not gained, the patient is currently too dangerous to approach
HR: not gained
BP: not gained
SpO$_2$: not gained
Blood sugar: not gained
Lead II ECG: not gained

Exposure

The patient is showing no signs of trauma, he is moving freely, he keeps banging his temples with his hands.

Task

Look through the information provided in this case study and highlight all of the information that might concern you as a paramedic.

What is drug-induced psychosis and how does it present?

Psychosis significantly alters a person's perception, thoughts, mood and behaviour. Sufferers can experience unique combinations of symptoms, which can include delusions, hallucinations, apathy, lack of drive, social withdrawal and self-neglect (NICE, 2014). Drug-induced psychosis can occur as a direct physiological consequence of intoxication, or from withdrawal (Marel et al., 2016).

Stimulants including amphetamine or methamphetamine can directly induce this condition (McKetin, 2018). Cocaine (NEPTUNE, 2015), novel psychoactive substances (Bonaccorso et al., 2018) and severe GHB withdrawal (NEPTUNE, 2015) are also known to induce psychosis.

What additional information would it be helpful to provide at handover?

- If the patient is intoxicated or withdrawing.
- The type of drug potentially responsible.
- Any known comorbid mental health conditions.
- Details of any care package already in place.

What can you do on scene?

Remain alert to your personal safety. Create a safe environment with few distracting factors (Gael, 2017) and set boundaries concerning behaviour. For example, 'You are welcome to express your anger with words and emotions, just not with violence.' Provide a grounded and compassionate approach that allows the patient to believe they are safe and everything that they experience is going to be OK. Ask them to share their experiences (Gael, 2017). Employ active listening skills.

Patients with new-onset psychosis, or suspected psychosis, including those who are suspected of coexisting substance misuse, should go to either secondary care mental health services or child and adolescent mental health services for assessment and further management (NICE, 2011).

Case Progression

You speak to the woman who called you, asking her what has happened in the lead-up to tonight's event. You specifically ask if her partner has taken illicit drugs or sustained a head injury. The woman states he has not taken anything for the last few days. He usually takes GHB when training, but has tried to cut this out of his daily routine. He has no history of any trauma.

You speak to the patient in a calm voice saying that you are there to help, the police are only there to make sure everyone remains calm and safe. You ask the police to back away slightly so that the focus of the patient's attention is on you. The patient gradually becomes less agitated. He begins to trust you and tentatively allows you to take some observations. He answers some of your questions and agrees to being taken in your ambulance for further assessment.

SYSTEMATIC APPROACH

Danger
Possibility of physical assault from the patient.

Response
Alert.

Airway
Clear.

Breathing
Respiration rate 20 bpm.

Circulation
Heart rate 110 bpm.

Vital signs
RR: 20 bpm
HR: 110 bpm
BP: 180/80 mmHg
SpO_2: 98% on air
Blood sugar: 5.7 mmol/L
Temperature: 37.3 °C
Lead II ECG: sinus tachycardia

Exposure
Pale, withdrawn.

Mental health assessment
The patient says he is hearing voices. He also says he is seeing things written on the wall (which are not there). He has moments of clarity where he may be deemed to have capacity, but then moments of heightened agitation.

How do you manage someone who is having delusions/hallucinations?

Importantly, practitioners should not go along with a psychotic person's delusions or hallucinations. However, they should not dismiss them either. For example, if someone is saying they can fly, do not go along with it, in case they jump from a height truly believing they can. Also, do not dismiss it and tell them they cannot, in case they jump to prove you wrong. Instead, distract the patient from these delusions and take the patient to receive specialist care.

Can the condition be cured?

Symptoms of substance-induced disorders tend to reduce over time with a period of abstinence (Marel et al., 2016). If symptoms persist for a substantial period, patients should be suspected of having a psychotic mental health impairment (McKetin, 2018).

References and further reading

American Psychiatric Association (2019) *Diagnostic and Statistical Manual of Mental Disorders: DSM-5*. Washington, DC: APA. https://www.psychiatry.org/psychiatrists/practice/dsm (accessed 19 December 2019).

Barley, E. & Lawson, V. (2016) Using health psychology to help patients: Common mental health disorders and psychological distress. *British Journal of Nursing*. 25(17): 966–973.

Bennett, P., Williams, Y., Page, N. et al. (2004) Levels of mental health problems among UK emergency ambulance workers. *Emergency Medicine Journal*, 21: 235–236. doi: 10.1136/emj.2003.005645

Bonaccorso, S., Metastasio, A., Ricciardi, A. et al. (2018) Synthetic cannabinoid use in a case series of patients with psychosis presenting to acute psychiatric settings: Clinical presentation and management issues. *Brain Sciences*, 8(7): 133. doi: 10.3390/brainsci8070133

Cerimele, J.M., Chwastiak, L.A., Chan, Y.F. et al. (2013) The presentation, recognition and management of bipolar depression in primary care. *Journal of General Internal Medicine*, 28(12): 1648–1656. doi: 10.1007/s11606-013-2545-7

Fear, N., Jones, M., Murphy, D., et al. (2010) What are the consequences of deployment to Iraq and Afghanistan on the mental health of the UK armed forces? A cohort study. *The Lancet*, 375: 1783–1797 doi: 10.1016/S0140- 6736(10)60672-1

Gael, S. (2017) Understanding and working with difficult psychedelic experiences. *Global Drug Survey*. https://www.globaldrugsurvey.com/past-findings/gds2017-launch/understanding-and-working-with-difficult-psychedelic-experiences/ (accessed 29 August 2019).

Galletly, C., Castle, D., Dark, F., et al. (2016) Royal Australian and New Zealand College of Psychiatrists clinical practice guidelines for the management of schizophrenia and related disorders. *Australian and New Zealand Journal of Psychiatry*, 50(5), 410–472. doi: 10.1177/0004867

Global Drug Survey (2014) *The High-Way Code: The Guide to Safer, More Enjoyable Drug Use*. https://www.globaldrugsurvey.com/wp-content/uploads/2014/04/COMPLETE-High-Way-Code.pdf (accessed 10 July 2020).

Harvey, S.B., Devilly, G., Forbes, D. et al. (2015) *Expert Guidelines: Diagnosis and Treatment of Post-traumatic Stress Disorder in Emergency Service Workers*. Sydney: Black Dog Institute.

Karam, M., Friedman, M., Hill, E. et al. (2014) Cumulative traumas and risk thresholds: 12-month PTSD in the World Mental Health (WMH) surveys. *Depression and Anxiety*, 31(2): 130–142. doi: 10.1002/da.22169

Marel, C., Mills, K.L., Kingston, R. et al. (2016) *Guidelines on the Management of Co-occurring Alcohol and Other Drug and Mental Health Conditions in Alcohol and Other Drug Treatment Settings, 2nd edition*. Sydney: Centre of Research Excellence in Mental Health and Substance Use, National Drug and Alcohol Research Centre, University of New South Wales.

Mazza, D., Brijnath, B., Chakraborty, S.P.; Guideline Development Group (2019) *Clinical Guideline for the Diagnosis and Management of Work-Related Mental Health Conditions in General Practice*. Melbourne: Monash University. https://research.monash.edu/en/publications/clinical-guideline-for-the-diagnosis-and-management-of-work-relat-4 (accessed 10 July 2020).

McKetin, R. (2018) Methamphetamine psychosis: Insights from the past. *Addiction*, 113: 1522–1527. doi: 10.1111/add.14170.

Mental Health in Multicultural Australia (2014) *Framework for Mental Health in Multicultural Australia: Towards Culturally Inclusive Service Delivery*. MHiMA, Queensland, Australia.

NEPTUNE (2015) *Guidance on the Clinical Management of Acute and Chronic Harms of Club Drugs and Novel Psychoactive Substances*. London: Novel Psychoactive Treatment UK Network. http://neptune-clinical-guidance.co.uk/wp-content/uploads/2015/03/NEPTUNE-Guidance-March-2015.pdf (accessed 11 August 2019).

NICE (2006) *Bipolar Disorder: The Management of Bipolar Disorder in Adults, Children and Adolescents, in Primary and Secondary Care (CG38)*. London: National Institute for Health and Care Excellence. https://www.nice.org.uk/guidance/cg38 (accessed 2 September 2019).

NICE (2010) *Depression in Adults with a Chronic Physical Health Problem (CG91)*. London: National Institute for Health and Care Excellence. https://www.nice.org.uk/guidance/cg91/evidence/full-guideline-243876061 (accessed 26 November 2019).

NICE (2011) *Coexisting Severe Mental Illness (Psychosis) and Substance Misuse: Assessment and Management in Healthcare Settings (CG120)*. London: National Institute for Health and Care Excellence. https://www.nice.org.uk/guidance/cg120 (accessed 2 September 2019).

NICE (2013) *Social Anxiety Disorder: Recognition, Assessment and Treatment (CG159)*. London: National Institute for Health and Care Excellence. https://www.nice.org.uk/guidance/cg159 (accessed 9 December 2019).

NICE (2014) *Psychosis and Schizophrenia in Adults: Prevention and Management (CG178)*. London: National Institute for Health and Care Excellence. https://www.nice.org.uk/guidance/cg178 (accessed 2 September 2019).

NICE (2018a) *Depression in Adults: Recognition and Management (CG90)*. London: National Institute for Health and Care Excellence. https://www.nice.org.uk/guidance/cg90 (accessed 10 July 2020).

NICE (2018b) *Post-traumatic Stress Disorder (NG116)*. London: National Institute for Health and Care Excellence. www.nice.org.uk/guidance/ng116 (accessed on 19 August 2019).

NICE (2018c). *Bipolar Disorder: Assessment and Management (CG185)*. London: National Institute for Health and Care Excellence. https://www.nice.org.uk/guidance/cg185 (accessed 2 September 2019).

NICE (2019a) *Depression in Children and Young People: Identification and Management (NG134)*. London: National Institute for Health and Care Excellence. https://www.nice.org.uk/guidance/ng134 (accessed 26 November 2019).

NICE (2019b) *Post-traumatic Stress Disorder*. London: National Institute for Health and Care Excellence. https://cks.nice.org.uk/post-traumatic-stress-disorder (accessed 19 August 2019).

NICE (2019c) *Generalised Anxiety Disorder and Panic Disorder in Adults: Management (CG113)*. London: National Institute for Health and Care Excellence. https://www.nice.org.uk/guidance/cg113 (accessed 2 September 2019).

NICE (2019d) *Anxiety Disorders (QS53)*. London: National Institute for Health and Care Excellence. https://www.nice.org.uk/guidance/QS53 (accessed 2 September 2019).

Office for National Statistics (2017) Suicide by occupation, England: 2011 to 2015. https://www.ons.gov.uk/releases/suicidesbyoccupationengland2011to2015 (accessed 10 July 2020).

RANZCoP (2017) Helping someone with schizophrenia. *Your Health in Mind*. https://www.yourhealthinmind.org/mental-illnesses-disorders/schizophrenia/helping-someone (accessed 11 December 2019).

Ritchie, H. & Roser, M. (2018) Mental health. *Our World in Data*, April. https://ourworldindata.org/mental-health (accessed 10 July 2020).

Shalev, A., Liberzon, I. & Marmar, C. (2017) Post-traumatic stress disorder. *New England Journal of Medicine*, 376: 2459–2469. doi: 10.1056/NEJMra1612499

Stergiopoulos, E., Cimo, A., Cheng, C. et al. (2011) Interventions to improve work outcomes in work related PTSD: A systematic review. *BMC Public Health*, 11: 838.

Walsh, L. (2009) *Depression Care across the Lifespan*. Oxford: Wiley-Blackwell.

Welsh Government (2012) *Together for Mental Health Strategy: A Strategy for Mental Health and Wellbeing in Wales*. Cardiff: Llywodraeth Cymru. https://gov.wales/sites/default/files/publications/2019-04/together-for-mental-health-summary.pdf (accessed 10 July 2020).

World Health Organisation (2016) *International Statistical Classification of Diseases and Related Health Problems, 10th Revision (ICD-10)*. Geneva: WHO. https://icd.who.int/browse10/2016/en (accessed 19 December 2019).

Chapter 13 Older adults

Sam Taylor
Air Ambulance Kent Surrey Sussex, Chatham, UK

CHAPTER CONTENTS

Level 1: Fractured neck of femur (NOF)
Level 1: Pelvic fracture
Level 2: Drug overdose
Level 2: Fall, minor injury
Level 3: Loss of balance
Level 3: Safeguarding concerns

LEVEL 1 CASE STUDY
Fractured neck of femur (NOF)

Information type	Data
Time of origin	10:55
Time of dispatch	11:00
On-scene time	11:15
Day of the week	Tuesday
Nearest hospital	15 minutes
Nearest backup	Intensive care crew, 25 minutes
Patient Details	Name: Elsie Convenor
	DOB: 12/03/1946

CASE

You have been called to outside a coffee shop for a 74-year-old female who has fallen.

Pre-arrival information

The patient is conscious and breathing, but unable to get up.

Windscreen report

It is a cold day on a busy road in the centre of town; there is an area to park outside the coffee shop. A small crowd has gathered around the woman who is lying on the floor outside the main entrance to the coffee shop (which has two steps leading up to it), with a couple of blankets placed on top of her. The area appears safe and the road has some light traffic movement on it.

Entering the location

You are met by the coffee shop owner and the woman's friend, who explain that she was walking out of the shop, missed her footing on the last step and fell onto her left side. She has been unable to get herself up and has pain in her left hip.

On arrival with the patient

The patient is lying on the floor, with a couple of blankets over her and a cushion under her head. She is awake and talking to a member of staff from the coffee shop, who is holding her hand.

Patient assessment triangle

General appearance

The patient is alert and she looks up as you approach, she smiles and says 'Hello, I think it's my leg that is the problem' (she touches her left leg).

Circulation to the skin

Hands appear well perfused, slightly cold to touch, as she has been on the floor for a while.

Work of breathing

Appears normal, no obvious difficulty.

SYSTEMATIC APPROACH

Danger

None.

Response

Alert on the AVPU scale.

Airway

Clear.

Breathing

Normal, equal bilateral chest rise and air entry on auscultation.

Circulation

Radial pulse palpable, regular.

Disability

GCS 15/15, able to move all limbs but reports pain to her left hip, which radiates down her leg and is worse on movement.

Vital signs

RR: 20 bpm
HR: 100 bpm
SpO2: 99% on air

Exposure

On cutting the patient's trousers off and comparing her left leg to her right, you notice the left is shorter and externally rotated. A pedal pulse is present bilaterally with a capillary refill time of <2 seconds in both feet. Sensation is normal in both legs and feet.

TASK

Look through the information provided in this case study. What are your immediate thoughts or concerns? What injury do you suspect this patient has?

What specific questions would you like to ask this patient relating to her fall and the leg injury?

- How did she fall?
- Did she feel unwell before the fall?
- Does she recall falling?
- Did she hit her head when she fell?
- Does she have any pain? If so, where is the pain?
- Consider using a pain mnemonic such as PQRSTA (Pain/Quality/Radiates/Severity/Timings/Associated symptoms) or SOCRATES (Severity/Onset/Character/Radiation/Alleviating factors/Timings/Exacerbating factors/Severity).
- Can she move all her limbs?
- Does she have pain anywhere else?

Case Progression

The patient explains that she was walking out of the coffee shop and chatting to her friend; not concentrating properly, she missed her footing on the last step, lost her balance and fell. She felt fine before the fall, having just had a coffee and slice of cake with her friend. She remembers falling and landing on the floor on her left side; she did not hit her head. Her left hip area is painful, she describes the pain as a dull ache that radiates down her left leg and is worse when she tries to move that leg. The pain started after she fell and she scores it 7/10 on a numerical scale (0 = no pain, 10 = worst pain she has ever experienced). She can move all her limbs, but on moving her left leg slightly she experiences more severe pain in her hip; she has no pain anywhere else.

Vital signs
RR: 20 bpm
HR: 98 bpm
BP: 130/85 mmHg
SpO2: 99% on air
Blood sugar 6.3 mmol/L

Having performed a primary survey and gained information from the patient, what differential diagnoses should you consider?

Suspected fractured neck of femur (left); soft tissue injury; severe bruising.

What is your plan of action? How do you propose to move the patient and what equipment would be best considering her injury?

Address her analgesic requirements in a structured manner and then formulate a plan to lift her off the floor and transport her for further assessment at hospital. Once appropriate control of pain has been achieved, consider using a scoop to lift her and place her onto your trolley bed, then remove the scoop and make her comfortable for transport.

Consider your analgesic options:
- What would you like to administer?
- In which order?
- By which route?
- At what dose?
- What is your reasoning behind this?
- What other factors need to be considered before administering your chosen medication?

- Entonox; inhaled as required.
- IV morphine, 2.5 mg, re-assess pain every 5–10 minutes and consider repeat doses.
- IV paracetamol, 1 g, administered over 10–15 minutes by slow infusion.
- Reasoning: Entonox to manage immediate pain, while preparing morphine. Suspected fracture, with a pain score of 7/10, therefore not unreasonable to consider strong analgesia, started at a low dose considering the patient's age. IV paracetamol to maintain analgesia throughout journey to hospital. IV paracetamol and morphine have a synergistic relationship; using these together may reduce the quantities of morphine required to achieve pain relief, which may be beneficial in reducing the side effects often associated with morphine.
- Other factors: Does the patient have any allergies? Does she have any contraindications or cautions to the medicines you would like to give?

En route to hospital, what re-assessment is required? Are there any other relevant questions you would consider asking the patient?

Assess how well the analgesia has worked, using a pain scale, and administer further amounts if needed. Also obtain a more detailed history (see Table 13.1).

Table 13.1 History-taking questions

Past medical history (PMH)
Are you normally fit and well?
Do you have any medical conditions?

Medication history
Do you take any regular medications?
If so, what are they and what are they for?

Family and social history (FSH)
Who do you live with?
What do you do/did you used to do for work?
Do you use a walking aid(s)?
Do you have any assistance at home, such as carers, meals delivered etc.?
Do you smoke? If so, how much and how often?
Do you drink alcohol? If so, how much and how often?

LEVEL 1 CASE STUDY
Pelvic fracture

Information type	Data
Time of origin	12:50
Time of dispatch	13:00
On-scene time	13:15
Day of the week	Saturday
Nearest major trauma centre	20 minutes
Nearest trauma unit	10 minutes
Patient details	Name: Megan Smith DOB: 12/09/1948

CASE

You have been called to a farm for a 72-year-old female who has been rolled on by a horse.

Pre-arrival information

The patient is conscious and breathing, but cold and scared to move.

Windscreen report

A muddy field on a farm. The patient is lying on the ground with a friend by her side and covered in a blanket. Her helmet has been removed and a stable hand is holding her head, controlling her C-spine.

Entering the location

You are met by the farmer, who explains the patient was walking her horse back into the stables after a ride, when the horse was scared by something and reared up. The patient fell backwards, hitting her head before the horse fell, rolling on top of her. The horse suffered no injury and has been removed from the scene safely by a stable hand.

On arrival with the patient

The patient is lying on the floor, with a blanket over her, and her C-spine is being controlled correctly. She is awake and talking to the person holding her head.

Patient assessment triangle

General appearance

The patient is alert and talking, but appears pale and in some discomfort.

Circulation to the skin

Hands are pale and cold.

Work of breathing

Appears normal, no obvious difficulty.

SYSTEMATIC APPROACH

Danger

None.

Response

Alert on the AVPU scale.

Airway

Clear.

Breathing

Normal, equal bilateral chest rise and air entry on auscultation, no pain on palpation.

Circulation

Radial pulse palpable, irregular.

Disability

GCS 15/15, pupils equal and reactive to light; haematoma noted to occiput of head when palpated, no boggy mass, no bleeding. Pain on palpation to pelvic region, legs appear 'splayed open', able to move arms well, pain on attempting to move legs; reports no altered sensation in arms or legs. Reports no C-spine tenderness, has not been drinking alcohol or drugs.

Vital signs

RR: 20 bpm

HR: 60 bpm
BP: 105/60 mmHg
SpO2: 99% on air, 100% on oxygen
Temperature: 36.5 °C

Exposure
No other obvious sign of injury,

What injuries do you suspect this patient may have sustained or that cannot be ruled out?

Head injury; intra-cranial haemorrhage; C-spine fracture; spinal fracture; pelvic fracture; potential internal haemorrhage.

What age-specific concerns do you have for this patient?

As an older patient, physiology needs to be considered. Older patients have a higher risk of fractures due to degenerative conditions such as arthritis/osteoarthritis. Head injury: older patients with significant head injury can present with a higher GCS compared to younger patients; do not always be reassured by a high GCS. Medication: older patients are more likely to be taking medications that may mask signs/symptoms of bleeding; also some patients may be at higher risk of haemorrhage due to the medications they are taking, e.g. anti-coagulants.

Case Progression

On further questioning, the patient is able to tell you that she suffers with atrial fibrillation (AF) and is taking 10 mg biso-prolol for rate control. She is also taking warfarin for her AF and atorvastatin for high cholesterol. She is mildly allergic to nuts, but no medication that she is aware of. She lives with her husband and is fully independent. She used to work as a riding instructor and tries to ride her horse at least 3 times a week. She has never smoked and has a glass of wine on special occasions, but does not drink alcohol regularly.

Vital signs
RR: 20 bpm
HR: 98 bpm
BP: 100/60 mmHg
SpO$_2$: 99% on air
Blood sugar: 4.8 mmol/L
Pupils: PEARL – 5 mm

Based on the history you have obtained from the patient, is there anything from this that now concerns you? Why? How does this relate to her current physiology?

She is taking a beta blocker, which will slow her heart rate, and as a result she will be unable to mount a compensa-tory tachycardia in response to potential haemorrhage. She is also taking warfarin, an anticoagulant, which means her blood clotting ability will be affected. In relation to her injuries, she is therefore at higher risk of intra-cranial haemorrhage and internal haemorrhage from fractures or vascular injury. Masking of symptoms such as tachy-cardia may lead the clinician into a false sense of security for these patients, who can deteriorate rapidly.

TASK
In a younger healthy patient with the same suspected injuries, how would you expect their observations to differ from those seen in this case?

How would you immobilise the patient? What specific kit is required to achieve this safely and needs to be considered for her potential injuries?

Address analgesic requirements. Once appropriate control of pain has been achieved, immobilisation using a scoop and placement of a pelvic binder to manage her suspected pelvic fracture, placed at the level of the greater trochanter. A controlled roll should be used to achieve this, with the person controlling the C-spine being in control of the roll. Once binder and scoop are placed, bring the legs into the natural anatomic alignment to reduce pelvic volume. Straps can then be applied to secure the patient and head blocks placed to maintain control of C-spine and taped into position.

What is your triage decision for this patient? Why?

A major trauma centre is appropriate. With a suspected pelvic fracture, potential head injury and physiology to suggest she may be bleeding internally, this patient requires specialist trauma interventions. Also, as an older patient the threshold for transport to an MTC should be lower, as this population are more likely to sustain significant injuries.

LEVEL 2 CASE STUDY
Drug overdose

Information type	Data
Time of origin	07:57
Time of dispatch	08:00
On-scene time	08:10
Day of the week	Tuesday
Nearest hospital	15 minutes
Nearest backup	Paramedic crew, 30 minutes
Patient details	Name: Fred Burton DOB: 11/05/1934

CASE

You have been called to a residential address for an 86-year-old male who is unresponsive. No further information.

Pre-arrival information

The patient is not responding normally but is breathing.

Windscreen report

A terraced house on a residential street, with a well-kept front garden and a small path leading to the front door. A young man opens the door as you arrive and frantically waves at you.

Entering the location

The young man at the door introduces himself as the patient's carer. He said he came around as usual at 07:30 to attend to the patient and became concerned when he found him in bed, not responding. He telephoned the patient's son, who has also just arrived and is now upstairs with his father in his bedroom.

On arrival with the patient

The patient is lying in bed; his son is trying to wake him, but there is no response. A number of empty packets of tablets are lying on the bedside table and the son tells you that his father has been very down recently due to an increase in his care needs, and has felt more of a burden on his family the last couple of weeks. As a result, his GP has started him on an antidepressant. His son shows you the packets on his bedside table and says he thinks his father has taken these alongside a bottle of liquid painkiller. The patient has not done anything like this before, but his son says he has commented a few times recently that 'it would be better for his family if he wasn't here, they wouldn't have to worry so much'.

Patient assessment triangle
General appearance
The patient is pale and unresponsive.

Circulation to the skin
Hands and face are pale and cold.

Work of breathing
Appears normal, no obvious difficulty.

SYSTEMATIC APPROACH
Danger
None.

Response
Pain on the AVPU scale.

Airway
Snoring, resolved once two nasopharyngeal airways inserted; patient does not tolerate an oropharyngeal airway.

Breathing
Normal, equal bilateral chest rise and air entry on auscultation.

Circulation
Radial pulse palpable, weak and regular.

Disability
GCS 7/15 (E1; V2; M4), pupils bilaterally size 2 and pinpoint.

Vital signs
RR: 12 bpm
HR: 56 bpm
BP: 100/65 mmHg
SpO_2: 94% on air, 100% on oxygen
Blood sugar: 4.8 mmol/L
Temperature: 36.3 °C

Exposure
No obvious sign of injury,

Previous medical history (details provided by son)
- Depression.
- Insomnia.
- Chronic back pain.

Social history
- Lives alone, a carer visits twice daily to assist with washing, dressing and meals.
- Patient has become more dependent in the last 4 months, which has impacted his mental health.
- Does not leave house alone, visits son once/twice a week who also takes him food shopping.
- Uses a walking stick to mobilise.
- Ex-smoker, gave up 20 years ago, but smoked approximately 1 pack a day for 20 years prior to this.
- Rarely drinks alcohol, usually only on special occasions.

Regular medication
- Citalopram 30 mg once daily.
- Oramorph as required.
- Zopiclone 7.5 mg as required, one at night.
- Paracetamol 1 g 4 times daily.

> **TASK**
> Look through the information provided in this case study. What are your immediate thoughts and concerns?

What medication can you administer to the patient in an attempt to improve his condition? What pharmacological actions does this have and what physiological improvements would you expect to see?

Naloxone. This is an antagonist for opioid receptor sites, with a higher affinity for Mu receptors where it acts as an inverse agonist, removing opioid already bound and reversing the effects. In an opioid overdose, improvement in respiratory rate, heart rate and level of response would be expected and a change in pupil size from pinpoint to normal.

On looking at the medication the patient has overdosed on, what other investigations do you wish to perform? Why?

12 Lead ECG, as arrhythmias are associated with selective serotonin reuptake inhibitor (SSRI) overdose.

> **Case Progression**
>
> The patient's ECG shows sinus bradycardia with prolonged QTc. This is commonly seen in (SSRI) overdose, which can lead to an increased risk of arrhythmia.
>
> After you administer naloxone, the patient becomes slightly more responsive. He opens his eyes to verbal commands, localises pain and groans (GCS 10).
>
> **Vital signs**
> RR: 16 bpm
> HR: 60 bpm
> BP: 105/80 mmHg
> SpO$_2$: 100% on oxygen
> 12 Lead ECG: sinus bradycardia with long QTc

The patient is transported to hospital accompanied by his son. On handover and when completing your paperwork, what do you also need to consider in this case?

On handover, ensure staff are aware that this is a possible suicide attempt and that the patient may require mental health support and advice as part of his recovery. Also, complete a safeguarding referral according to your local protocol to ensure that appropriate support is offered once he is discharged from hospital.

What other condition is this patient at risk from and how does this present?

Serotonin syndrome (serotonin toxicity) – causes neuromuscular and autonomic nervous system excitation with altered mental state, and presents with symptoms associated with these such as rigidity, clonus, tachycardia, hyperthermia, confusion and/or agitation.

LEVEL 2 CASE STUDY
Fall, minor injury

Information type	Data
Time of origin	08:49
Time of dispatch	09:15

(Continued)

Information type	Data
On-scene time	09:45
Day of the week	Wednesday
Nearest hospital	35 minutes
Nearest backup	Paramedic crew, 40 minutes
Patient details	Name: Renuka Childs
	DOB: 05/01/1947

CASE

You have been called to a residential address for a 73-year-old female who has fallen and is unable to get up.

Pre-arrival information

The patient is conscious and breathing, but has been on the floor for about 1 hour.

Windscreen report

A bungalow on a residential estate, on a quiet road with ample parking.

Entering the location

A woman opens the door and introduces herself as the patient's daughter. Her mother is currently stuck on the floor in her bedroom and unable to get herself up.

On arrival with the patient

The patient is sitting on the floor in her dressing gown and pyjamas, she is alert and says hello as you walk in. She explains she got up about 07:30 to go to the toilet before getting dressed. As she walked back into the bedroom, her legs felt as if they would not support her any more and she slid down onto the floor, landing on her bottom. She says she feels well, has no pain, there is a small wound on her left arm from the wall, and she just does not have the strength to get herself up. She has tried a few times but unsuccessfully, and so decided to press her assist button. They called an ambulance and then her daughter, who lives nearby. Her daughter explains she has been increasingly concerned over the last few days as her mother seems less stable on her feet and has been using her walking frame more than normal, especially around the house. She also thinks she appears slightly more muddled over the last 2–3 days, which is not normal.

Patient assessment triangle
General appearance

The patient is well perfused and responding.

Circulation to the skin

Hands are warm and slightly clammy to touch.

Work of breathing

Appears normal, no obvious difficulty.

SYSTEMATIC APPROACH
Danger

None.

Response

Alert on the AVPU scale.

Airway

Clear and talking.

Breathing

Normal, equal bilateral chest rise and air entry on auscultation.

Circulation

Radial pulse palpable, regular.

Disability

GCS 15/15, pupils equal and reactive.

Vital signs

RR: 18 bpm

HR: 68 bpm

BP: 138/80 mmHg

SpO$_2$: 99% on air

Blood sugar: 4.7 mmol/L

Temperature: 37.9 °C

Exposure

Skin tear to left forearm, has been bleeding but now not actively bleeding.

Previous medical history

- Arthritis.
- High cholesterol.
- Type 2 diabetes mellitus, diet controlled.

Social history

- Lives alone, but remains independent, with support from her daughter, who assists with weekly shopping.
- Still determined to remain active, despite arthritis in her knees sometimes restricting mobility. She explains she has good and bad days, but usually tries to get out of the house a least once a day for a short walk.
- Normally she mobilises with the aid of a walking stick. The mobility frame was introduced a few months ago for when she goes out with her daughter as she finds the longer walks a bit more tiring; however, she had not used it in the house until a few days ago.
- Non-smoker.
- Alcohol: sometimes enjoys an occasional small glass of wine with dinner; has this only a couple of times a month, when she fancies it.

Regular medication (details found on prescription)

- Paracetamol 1g 4 times daily as required.
- Simvastatin 20 mg once daily at night.

TASK

Look through the information provided in this case study and highlight all of the information that might concern you as a paramedic.

Based on what you know already, what system assessments or specific questions would you like to perform or ask? What is your reasoning?

- Respiratory assessment: Any recent cough? If so, is this productive?
- Abdominal assessment: Passing urine normally? Any pain on passing? Polyuria? Any blood in urine? Does the urine have a distinct/stronger/more unpleasant odour? Bowels as normal?
- Reasoning: reduction in mobility and some confusion – could the cause be a possible infection? If so, where is this infection? Assessing the respiratory system may reveal possible signs of a chest infection. Alternatively, urinary tract infections (UTIs) can present with confusion and reduced mobility, so specific questioning here is essential.

> ### Case Progression
>
> You perform a respiratory and abdominal assessment with appropriate questioning. The patient's chest sounds normal, with equal bilateral air entry, and she reports no cough. She tells you she has found she is going to the toilet more and only passing a small amount when she does. She is not experiencing any pain when passing urine, but has noticed her urine has a strong, unpleasant odour. She also recalls she had similar symptoms about a year ago and the doctor had to prescribe some medication for her.
>
> **Vital signs**
> RR: 16 bpm
> HR: 62 bpm
> BP: 135/80 mmHg
> SpO$_2$: 100% on air
> 12 Lead ECG: normal sinus rhythm

Having performed an assessment, what do you think is the cause of the patient's fall today? What is your reasoning?

Potential urine infection, considering her history and presentation. Also, she has a slightly raised temperature, which coincides with the presence of an infection.

The wound to the patient's forearm appears to be a skin tear; it is a small wound, approximately 5–6 cm in diameter and is crescent shaped, with the skin flap covering the wound. What is your proposed management for this wound?

If the wound is to be reviewed later by a healthcare professional, clean gently with gauze and water. Pat the surrounding area dry and then cover the wound with a non-adhesive dressing that has been moistened with saline, to prevent the wound drying out. Skin in older people can be thinner and more prone to damage, therefore securing the non-adhesive dressing using a bandage rather than tape is optimum. Consider a small amount of padding under the bandage to protect from any further injury. Assess the hand for peripheral circulation to ensure the bandage is not too tight once applied.

You are able to stand the patient up with some help and sit her onto a chair. What do you need to assess before making a management plan?

Her mobility. Is she able to get herself up as normal and walk around her bungalow safely and without concern from herself/you/her daughter that she may fall again?

The patient is able to mobilise well and feels comfortable walking around the bungalow with the aid of her frame. What is your referral plan for her? What is your reasoning?

Referral to GP for a home visit, with intention to consider prescribing antibiotics for a UTI and also to review the skin tear, with a possible visit from the GP Practice Nurse or the District Nursing Team. She has mild symptoms and has only fallen once; if falls were recurrent and she was more confused or unable to manage at home without a way of summoning help or you are concerned she may fall again, then a hospital admission may be considered.

Is there anything else you need to consider before leaving this patient at home?

Worsening care advice; and if possible to leave her in the care of someone. In this case her daughter may be able to look after her. Remind the patient that she can use her assist button if she needs any further help or feels worse.

LEVEL 3 CASE STUDY
Loss of balance

Information type	Data
Time of origin	08:48
Time of dispatch	09:15
On-scene time	09:45
Day of the week	Wednesday
Nearest hospital	35 minutes
Nearest backup	Paramedic crew, 40 minutes
Patient details	Name: Walter Riley DOB: 03/03/1952

CASE
You have been called to a residential address for 68-year-old male complaining of dizziness and nausea.

Pre-arrival information
The patient is conscious and breathing, and has vomited twice.

Windscreen report
A residential estate, a semi-detached house on a quiet road; appears well kept.

Entering the location
You are met at the door by a man who introduces himself as the patient's neighbour; he had popped round for a coffee, but found the patient unwell and out of concern called the emergency services.

On arrival with the patient
The patient is lying on his sofa, and opens his eyes as you enter the room. He says he hasn't felt well for the last hour and his symptoms came on suddenly. He describes these as nausea and the room spinning, even though he is not moving. He has vomited twice, but produced only bile as he has had no food today. He is also having trouble with his balance and has to hold on to furniture if he moves. He is normally well; takes medication for high blood pressure and some other tablets for his blood; he says has not experienced anything like this before.

Patient assessment triangle
General appearance
The patient is well perfused and responding.

Circulation to the skin
Hands are warm and dry to touch.

Work of breathing
Appears normal, no obvious difficulty.

SYSTEMATIC APPROACH
Danger
None.

Response
Alert on the AVPU scale.

Airway
Clear and talking.

Breathing
Normal, equal bilateral chest rise and air entry on auscultation.

Circulation
Radial pulse palpable, regular.

Disability
GCS 15/15, pupils equal and reactive.

Vital signs
RR: 18 bpm
HR: 82 bpm
BP: 170/90 mmHg
SpO_2: 99% on air
Blood sugar: 6.2 mmol/L
Temperature: 36.5 °C

Exposure
No injuries.

Previous medical history
- High blood pressure.
- High cholesterol.
- Gastro-oesophageal reflux disease (GORD).
- Atrial fibrillation.

Social history
- Lives independently alone, used to work at the local post office up until retirement and likes to keep active, walking regularly. Independent of activities of daily living.
- Ex-smoker, gave up 5 years ago, had smoked about 5 a day since the age of 25 years prior to that.
- Consumes no alcohol.

Regular medication (details found on prescription)
- Simvastatin 20 mg once daily.
- Ramipril 5 mg once daily.
- Omeprazole 20 mg once daily.
- Rivaroxaban 20 mg once daily.

TASK
Look through the information provided in this case study and highlight all of the information that might concern you as a paramedic.

What are your initial thoughts as to the cause of this patient's symptoms? How can you exclude some of these?

- Vertigo due to viral/bacterial ear infection.
- Cerebellar stroke.
- Postural hypotension.
- Cardiac arrhythmia.
- Exclusion: Detailed history including a neurological assessment/ECG/assessment of blood pressure, seated and after standing for at least 1 minute (if patient is able to safely).

> **TASK**
> List the cranial nerves, what they control and the test for each.

Case Progression

You perform a neurological assessment. The patient is unable to walk without losing his balance and feels persistently dizzy. You note nystagmus when testing for ocular movement. He is also unable to perform dysdiadochokinesis.

Vital signs
RR: 18 bpm
HR: 84 bpm
BP: 160/85 mmHg
SpO_2: 100% on air
12 Lead ECG: atrial fibrillation

From your assessment and history, what are your differential diagnoses?

Vertigo due to viral/bacterial ear infection. Cerebellar stroke.

The patient is presenting with symptoms that could be suggestive of vertigo, but also more seriously a cerebellar stroke. From his history and assessment, what would concern you and indicate that this is more likely to be a cerebellar stroke?

Sudden onset, no history of viral or bacterial illness over the last few days. History of atrial fibrillation, which increases the risk of thrombotic stroke. Patient is also taking a novel anticoagulant and is therefore also at increased risk of intra-cranial bleed. Symptoms associated with a cerebellar stroke are varied and non-specific, including dizziness, nausea and vomiting, lethargy, nystagmus and dysarthria. Obtaining a thorough history to identify any associated risk factors and performing an appropriate examination are essential.

Would a Face Arms Speech Test (FAST) identify this type of stroke?

No. FAST tests specifically for a stroke involving occlusion of the middle cerebral artery. While speech may be affected in a cerebellar stroke, FAST is best targeted at the middle cerebral circulation, and consequently can give a false negative in strokes involving the cerebellar and posterior circulation.

What is your triage decision for this patient?

Transport to nearest hyperacute stroke unit (HASU) if highly suspicious of cerebellar stroke. These cases are complex and often diagnosis or identifying subtle symptoms can be difficult for even the experienced clinician. If unsure, call the clinical support desk or equivalent within your service for advice and/or to sense-check your decision making.

LEVEL 3 CASE STUDY
Safeguarding concerns

Information type	Data
Time of origin	14:30
Time of dispatch	15:04
On-scene time	15:56

(Continued)

Information type	Data
Day of the week	Wednesday
Nearest hospital	30 minutes
Nearest backup	Paramedic crew, 40 minutes
Patient details	Name: Jacob Jacobson
	DOB: 05/06/1933

CASE
You have been called to a residential care unit for an 87-year-old male with shortness of breath.

Pre-arrival information
The patient is conscious and breathing, and has been coughing.

Windscreen report
A large care home, with an ambulance parking bay outside, in a residential area.

Entering the location
A member of staff comes to greet you and escort you upstairs via a lift to the patient's room.

On arrival with the patient
You are introduced to the patient, who is sitting upright in a bed with padded sides to prevent him from falling out. He appears to be sleeping, but when you walk in he opens his eyes to look at you. On closer observation you notice the sheets in the bed appear to be soiled with urine. Another member of staff is with Jacob and says she came in to give him his afternoon drink, but became concerned when she noticed his breathing appeared fast.

Patient assessment triangle
General appearance
The patient is well perfused.

Circulation to the skin
Hands are warm and dry.

Work of breathing
Does not appear to be struggling, but breathing is rapid and he has a cough that sounds 'chesty'.

SYSTEMATIC APPROACH
Danger
None.

Response
Voice on the AVPU scale.

Airway
Clear.

Breathing
Rate increased, equal bilateral chest rise and air entry noted with left-sided basal crepitations on auscultation. Coughing as you listen to chest.

Circulation
Radial pulse palpable, regular.

Disability
GCS 15/15, pupils equal and reactive.

Vital signs
RR: 24 bpm
HR: 92 bpm
BP: 125/79 mmHg
SpO_2: 92% on air, 96% on nasal oxygen
Blood sugar: 8.2 mmol/L
Temperature 38.1 °C

Exposure
Bruising to left wrist and pain when you examine it. The patient is not able to move his wrist much and the pain is worse on palpation; you also notice localised swelling and a 'dinner-fork' shaped deformity.

Previous medical history
• High blood pressure.
• Left-sided weakness to left leg following a stroke 1 year ago.
• Alzheimer's dementia.

Social history
The patient has been a resident at the care home for approximately 11 months, having moved there following a stroke. Prior to this he lived at home with his wife and had a carer visiting twice daily to assist him with getting up, washing and dressing, as his wife found this a challenge alone. He suffers with mild dementia and reduced mobility, which has significantly worsened since the stroke. He now requires a frame to walk with and the care staff explain he has to be accompanied at all times due to his poor balance.

Regular medication (details found on prescription)
• Paracetamol 1 g 4 times daily as required.
• Amlodipine 5 mg once daily.
• Donepezil 10 mg once daily.
• Clopidogrel 75 mg once daily.

TASK
Look through the information provided in this case study and highlight all of the information that might concern you as a paramedic.

What type of fracture is this patient presenting with? What is the official definition of this and which mechanism of injury and abnormal shape are classically associated with it?

Colles' fracture, defined as a fracture of the distal radius with dorsal and radial displacement and impaction, sometimes with involvement of the ulnar styloid. These fractures are commonly associated with a fall onto an outstretched hand.

Case Progression

You perform a respiratory assessment and suspect the patient has a chest infection. On further examination of his wrist, you think it may be fractured and ask the staff member more about this injury. She appears surprised and says she did not know he had hurt his wrist, but explains he fell yesterday morning while walking down alone to breakfast; the staff member who was walking with him had been called away to help dress another resident. She mentions that a colleague helped the patient up and then took him down to breakfast. You also comment on the fact that his sheets are dirty; the staff member says they did not have time to change them this morning.

You decide to transport the patient to hospital for further assessment. As you move him onto the trolley bed, two red sores are visible on his buttocks; these appear to be grade 2 pressure ulcers. You approach the staff about these and they say they had not noticed them.

Vital signs
RR: 24 bpm
HR: 90 bpm
BP: 128/79 mmHg
SpO_2: 92% on air, 96% on nasal oxygen
12 Lead ECG: normal sinus rhythm

What aspects of this case are concerning?

The patient was not assessed or referred for further medical assessment following his fall and no staff member has noticed a significantly obvious injury. Also, the fact that the patient had been allowed to walk to breakfast on his own, when his care plan specifically states he should be accompanied. The patient's bed has not been changed and he has been lying in soiled bedclothes all day. Pressure ulcers were noted on moving the patient, which appear to be grade 2 and indicate that the patient has potentially been left in a sitting or lying position for a period of time and has not been encouraged to mobilise, or has been left in bed and not assisted to get up, allowing the ulcers to develop. This all suggests that the care home is not meeting the patient's care needs and he is potentially a victim of neglect.

How do you intend to raise your concerns? Who do you need to contact?

Complete a safeguarding referral according to your local protocol. Inform your line manager and discuss with them your concerns and whether police or social services need to be contacted. Is there also concern here for the welfare of other residents? Raise this within the safeguarding referral and with your line manager. Also ensure that your documentation is accurate, recording facts only and not making any inference or judgement.

The patient has what appears to be pressure ulcers. What causes these to develop?

Pressure ulcers are a result of persistent pressure on skin, usually over a bony prominence, leading to reduced capillary flow and subsequent tissue necrosis.

References and further reading

Aroor, S., Singh, R. & Goldstein, L.B. (2017) BE-FAST (Balance, Eyes, Face, Arm, Speech, Time): Reducing the proportion of strokes missed using the FAST mnemonic. *Stroke*, 48(2): 479–481. doi: 10.1161/STROKEAHA.116.015169

Aschkenasy, M.T. & Rothenhaus, T.C. (2006) Trauma and falls in the elderly. *Emergency Medicine Clinics of North America*, 24(2): 413–432. doi: 10.1016/j.emc.2006.01.005

Buckley, N.A., Dawson, A.H. & Isbister, G.K. (2014) Serotonin syndrome. *BMJ (Online)*, 348: 1–4. doi: 10.1136/bmj.g1626

Dixon, J., Ashton, F., Baker, P. et al. (2018) Assessment and early management of pain in hip fractures: The impact of paracetamol. *Geriatric Orthopaedic Surgery & Rehabilitation*, 9: 215145931880644. doi: 10.1177/2151459318806443

Isbister, G., Bowe, S.J., Dawson, A. & Whyte, I.M. (2004) Relative toxicity of selective serotonin reuptake inhibitors (SSRIs) in overdose. *Journal of Clinical Toxicology*, 42(3): 277–285.

Kehoe, A., Rennie, S. & Smith, J.E. (2015) Glasgow Coma Scale is unreliable for the prediction of severe head injury in elderly trauma patients. *Emergency Medicine Journal*, 32(8): 613–615.

Kehoe, A., Smith, J.E., Bouamra, O. et al. (2016) Older patients with traumatic brain injury present with a higher GCS score than younger patients for a given severity of injury. *Emergency Medicine Journal*, 33(6): 381–385. doi: 10.1136/emermed-2015-205180

LeBlanc, K. & Baranoski, S. (2009) Prevention and management of skin tears. *Advances in Skin and Wound Care*, 22(7): 325–332. doi: 10.1097/01.ASW.0000305484.60616.e8

Lyder, C.H. (2003) Pressure ulcer prevention and management. *Journal of the American Medical Association*, 289(2): 223–226. doi: 10.1001/jama.289.2.223

Purcell, D. (2010) *Minor Injuries: A Clinical Guide*, 2nd edn. London: Churchill Livingstone/Elsevier.

Remy, C., Marret, E. & Bonnet, F. (2005) Effects of acetaminophen on morphine side-effects and consumption after major surgery: Meta-analysis of randomized controlled trials. *British Journal of Anaesthesia*, 94(4): 505–513. doi: 10.1093/bja/aei085

Richards, A. (2009) *A Nurse's Survival Guide to Drugs in Practice*. London: Churchill Livingstone/Elsevier.

Simon, C., Everitt, H., van Dorp, F. & Burkes, M. (2014) *Oxford Handbook of General Practice*, 4th edn. Oxford: Oxford University Press.

Van Staa, T.P., Geusens, P., Bijlsma, J.W.J. et al. (2006) Clinical assessment of the long-term risk of fracture in patients with rheumatoid arthritis. *Arthritis and Rheumatism*, 54(10): 3104–3112. doi: 10.1002/art.22117

Wolf, P.A., Dawber, T.R., Thomas, H.E., Jr & Kannel, W.B. (1978) Epidemiologic assessment of chronic atrial fibrillation and risk of stroke: The Framingham study. *Neurology*, 28(10): 973–977. doi: 10.1212/wnl.28.10.973

Wright, J., Huang, C., Strbian, D. & Sundararajan, S. (2014) Diagnosis and management of acute cerebellar infarction. *Stroke*. 45(4): e56–e58. doi: 10.1161/STROKEAHA.114.004474

Zeidan, A., Mazoit, J.X., Ali Abdullah, M. et al. (2014) Median effective dose (ED$_{50}$) of paracetamol and morphine for postoperative pain: A study of interaction. *British Journal of Anaesthesia*, 112(1): 118–123. doi: 10.1093/bja/aet306

Obstetric cases

Aimee Yarrington
Shropshire, UK

CHAPTER CONTENTS

LEVEL 1 CASE STUDY
Normal birth

Information type	Data
Time of origin	22:40
Time of dispatch	23:40
On-scene time	23:45
Day of the week	Wednesday
Nearest hospital	20 minutes
Nearest backup	15 minutes
Patient details	Name: Maja Singh DOB: 27/12/1978

CASE

You are dispatched to an address for reports of a 42-year-old female who is 39 weeks' pregnant with her third child and is having contractions 1 : 3 (one every three minutes).

Pre-arrival information
The patient is conscious and breathing.

Windscreen report
The house appears is well maintained with a small garden. A male is waiting at the door for you.

Entering the location
You are greeted by a man who appears panicked.

Clinical Cases in Paramedicine, First Edition. Edited by Sam Willis, Ian Peate, and Rod Hill.
© 2021 John Wiley & Sons Ltd. Published 2021 by John Wiley & Sons Ltd.

On arrival with the patient

You are shown to a female who is on her knees in the lounge, leaning forward and breathing heavily through an apparent contraction.

SYSTEMATIC APPROACH

Danger

Nil.

Response

Alert on the AVPU scale.

Airway

Clear.

Breathing

Respiration rate 20 bpm. Effort: normal. Accessory muscle use: no.

Circulation

Heart rate: 90 bpm. Effort: normal. Heart regularity: regular. Capillary refill time: 2 seconds.

Vital signs

RR: 20 bpm

HR: 90 bpm

BP: 120/78 mmHg

SpO_2: 99%

Lead II ECG: normal sinus rhythm

Exposure

The patient is fully clothed, but appears to be bearing down. The room is warm and there is adequate lighting.

TASK

Look through the information provided in this case study and highlight all of the information that might concern you as a paramedic.

What questions regarding the patient's pregnancy and previous birth history do you want to ask?

First, the estimated date of delivery (EDD) needs to be established to ensure the birth is not pre-term. The patient's birth history should include how many times she has given birth and the type of birth (vaginal or caesarean), complications such as shoulder dystocia or postpartum haemorrhage. Her place of booking will give an indication of her risk level; consultant bookings mean a level of complications are noted, whereas a home or midwife booking means no known complications are present.

The onset of the contractions will give an indication as to how long she has been in labour, although this is not a rule as all labour lengths will be different. You also need to know if her membranes are intact and if they are broken, then the colour of the water is important.

What factors would you consider if you were going to transport to hospital?

Birth on the ambulance should be avoided. It is impractical and there is very limited space. There is also a huge restriction on optimum maternal birth position, as well as the inability to control the temperature should the baby be born en route.

CHAPTER 14: OBSTETRIC CASES

The distance to the unit needs to be considered as well as the time of day, since traffic can slow the journey, as can weather such as snow.

Case Progression

SYSTEMATIC APPROACH

Danger
Nil.

Response
Alert on the AVPU scale.

Airway
Clear.

Breathing
Remains the same.

Circulation
Remains the same.

Vital signs
RR: 20 bpm
HR: radial 90 bpm
BP: not repeated due to condition

Exposure
Consent is gained to remove the patient's pyjama trousers and inspect her vulva, where a bulge of intact membrane is noted. As the next contraction builds the presenting part advances and the waters break, revealing clear liquor.

What would your next action be?

The room is already warm, but heat and light should be ensured as well as maintaining dignity. An area should be prepared for newborn resuscitation as well as collecting some extra towels, warmed if possible or placed on a warm radiator.

Encourage pushing as the presenting part advances to the crowning point, at which slow, steady, small breaths or panting should be encouraged. The flat of the hand can be placed over the head to prevent rapid birth of the head and reduce perineal tearing.

Case Progression

The baby's head is born and there is a brief pause of approximately 60 seconds before the next contraction. The rest of the body is born through a process of lateral flexion into your awaiting hands.

What would you do next?

The baby must first be dried thoroughly with a warm, dry towel while you are performing a visual inspection of their condition at birth. The baby should then be placed skin to skin with the mother. At 1 minute of age the APGAR score should be performed and recorded. It is very important that the umbilical cord remains intact while it is still pulsating and is not clamped and cut until it has gone flat, white and opaque. This not only provides the baby with their complete blood volume, but is providing a vital oxygen supply while the pulmonary system is adapting to extrauterine life. There are many other proven benefits of waiting until pulsation ceases, including improved iron stores and neurological development. For more information see BloodtoBaby (2019).

> **Case Progression**
>
> Once the baby is dry and skin to skin, you cover them with a further warm towel and maintain their temperature. You monitor the mother's blood loss and observe for signs of the placental delivery.
>
> The mother experiences a further contraction, there is a gush of approximately 100 mL of blood and the cord is noted to lengthen at the vulva.

What is happening here and how should it be managed?

The third stage is nearing completion here. The lengthening of the cord signifies that the placenta has separated and dropped down into the lower segment of the uterine cavity. This is normally followed by a further urge to push or bear down again, and the mother is able to push the placenta out as she has the baby. The timing of placental delivery can vary, but in a normal physiological third stage (i.e. one that is not medically controlled by drugs, only carried out by a midwife/doctor) the third stage should take no more than 60 minutes. After 60 minutes the placenta is said to be retained. Due to the increased risk of postpartum haemorrhage with a retained placenta, it is recommended that if there is no evidence that the placenta will be born on scene, the clinician should after 30 minutes, consider moving to the nearest maternity facility to ensure a timely placental delivery.

When the placenta is about to be expelled there are several features you may see:

- The cord will lengthen at the vaginal entrance.
- The uterus may rise up on abdominal palpation, making it easier to palpate.
- There will be a gush of blood, which can be 200–300 mL – this is normal as the placenta separates from the wall of the uterus.
- The mother may get an urge to push as the placenta descends into the lower segment of the uterus.
- Assist the mother into an upright position, since gravity will assist with the expulsion. Encourage the mother to empty her bladder if this is possible using a urine collector, as the toilet is not recommended unless you have a bedpan. Do *not* pull on the cord in any way; if the placenta has not separated, the uterus can be unavoidably inverted. Encourage the mother to push with the contraction to assist with the delivery. This stage can be very painful, so appropriate analgesia should be provided. Place the delivered placenta into a suitable bag, ensuring the mother's name is on the bag. Note the time of the delivery and document all findings.

LEVEL 1 CASE STUDIES
Cord prolapse

Information type	Data
Time of origin	15:50
Time of dispatch	16:03
On-scene time	16:18
Day of the week	Monday
Nearest hospital	15 minutes
Nearest backup	15 minutes
Patient details	Name: Catherine Spinks DOB: 08/09/1984

> **CASE**
>
> You are dispatched to attend a 36-year-old female who is reported to be 34 weeks' pregnant with her fourth child and has been advised to call for an ambulance by her midwife. She reports her waters have broken and feels as if there is 'something hanging from her vagina'. She is alone in the house.

Pre-arrival information
The patient is conscious and breathing.

Windscreen report
The property is a small, maisonette-type flat with stair access to the front. No obvious activity outside.

Entering the location
You enter the open door. A woman is shouting 'up here' from upstairs as you announce your arrival.

On arrival with the patient
She is on her hands and knees on the bathroom floor.

SYSTEMATIC APPROACH

Danger
Nil, although you note the bathroom floor is wet.

Response
Alert on the AVPU scale.

Airway
Clear and patent.

Breathing
Respiration rate: 22 bpm. Effort: normal. No accessory muscle use.

Circulation
Heart rate: 100 bpm. Effort: normal. Heart regularity: regular. Capillary refill time: 2 seconds.

Vital signs
RR: 22 bpm
HR: 100 bpm
BP: not taken as yet
SpO$_2$: not taken as yet no peripheral cyanosis
Lead II ECG: not taken as yet

Exposure
When you ask about the presenting complaint, the patient raises her dress, exposing her vulval area. A loop of prolapsed cord approximately 5 cm long is visible at the introitus.

TASK
Look through the information provided in this case study and highlight all of the information that might concern you as a paramedic.

What makes this situation time critical now?

The exposed loop of cord is potentially being compressed by the presenting part of the foetus, as well as being exposed to the external environment, making it vulnerable to vasospasm in the cool external temperature. The greater the duration of the insult onto the cord, the greater the risk is of hypoxic acidosis and mortality of the foetus.

What should your actions be now?

The rapid removal of the patient onto the vehicle should be done without delay. You want to avoid use of the patient transfer chair, as sitting down directly onto the cord will cause further compression. The patient should be assisted to walk out to the vehicle quickly but safely. Once on the vehicle, then one attempt to replace the exposed cord back into the vagina should be attempted. This reduces the risk of further prolapse from walking out to the vehicle as well as being done in a more controlled environment.

Case Progression

SYSTEMATIC APPROACH

Danger
Nil.

Response
Alert on the AVPU scale.

Airway
Clear.

Breathing
Remains the same.

Circulation
Heart rate: 90 bpm. Effort: strong. Heart regularity: regular. Capillary refill time: 1 second.

Vital signs
RR: 22 bpm
HR: 90 bpm
BP: not taken as treating time-critical patient
SpO$_2$: not taken as treating time-critical patient

Exposure
Using a dry pad you replace the small amount of cord into the vagina, leaving the dry pad in place.

What position on the ambulance trolley should the patient be assisted into and why?

The patient should be placed in the right lateral position with her hips raised upwards. The left lateral position can be used, but in most ambulances this position places the woman facing the wall, where no eye contact and reassurance can be given directly. The hips are raised upwards to attempt to release the pressure of the presenting part on the cord and cause less insult on the cord. Using a pillow or several blankets can raise the hips, or if large vacuum splints are available these are ideal, as they do not compress as much as a pillow. The trolley harness should *always* be worn and the woman *never* transferred in the knee chest/all fours position. If there is a midwife or appropriately trained clinician present, then filling of the urinary bladder could be considered, especially if there is a prolonged transfer time. The distention of the bladder causes the presenting part to be lifted upwards, decreasing the pressure on the cord. Equipment required includes a Foley catheter, IV giving set, 500 mL normal saline and a clamp or spigot.

What information should be clearly passed on in the pre-alert/information call?

Situation, Background, Assessment findings and Recommendations (see Table 14.1).

Table 14.1 SBAR

Situation	Visible cord prolapse since 15:50
Background	36 YOF 34/40 pregnant G4P3
	Spontaneous rupture of membranes at 15:50 and cord prolapsed Spoke with midwife who advised 999
Assessment	On inspection 5 cm loop of cord visible, replaced into the vagina at 16:25, then assisted into exaggerated Sims' position
Recommendations	We would like a team to meet us at the ambulance entrance
	Our ETA is 8 minutes

LEVEL 2 CASE STUDY
Postpartum haemorrhage

Information type	Data
Time of origin	05:30
Time of dispatch	06:00
On-scene time	06:20
Day of the week	Wednesday
Nearest hospital	30 minutes
Nearest backup	10 minutes
Patient details	Name: Tara Tompkinson
	DOB: 31/12/1974

CASE
You are dispatched to a 45-year-old female in advance labour. Your update en route informs you that this is the patient's fifth child and she has an urge to push. The next update you get 5 minutes before you make scene, at 06:15, is that the baby has been born and is crying. The emergency operations centre also informs you that the woman has a history of bleeding after giving birth.

Pre-arrival information
The patient is conscious and breathing. The baby is pink and crying.

Windscreen report
The area outside the bungalow appears to be safe. There are a few people gathered around the entrance and children running in the driveway.

Entering the location
Neighbours meet you at the door, offering to carry things and assist. You are led into the bathroom where the patient is sat on a towel on the floor, supported by the bathtub, with evidence of bleeding between her legs. The baby, who looks very large, is skin to skin with a towel over the top and is crying lustily.

On arrival with the patient
She looks pale and overwhelmed.

SYSTEMATIC APPROACH
Danger
Nil.

Response
Alert on the AVPU scale.

Catastrophic haemorrhage
Not present, however blood evident on the floor.

Airway
Clear.

Breathing
The patient is speaking in full sentences, no difficulty in breathing, respiration rate 20 bpm.

Circulation
Radial present, normal rhythm and volume 90 bpm.

Vital signs
RR: 20 bpm
HR: 90 bpm
BP: 110/60 mmHg
SpO$_2$: 99%

Exposure
You gain consent to see if there are signs of active bleeding and any evidence of placental expulsion. The towel is wet with amniotic fluid and blood, making it difficult to estimate the full amount of bleeding. You give an estimated blood loss (EBL) of 400 mL at this point and mark the time as 06:28. You note the cord is still pulsating, there is no sign of placental separation.

TASK
Look through the information provided in this case study and highlight all of the information that might concern you as a paramedic.

What risk factors are present for postpartum haemorrhage (PPH)?

Factors known to be present at time of arrival:

- Previous PPH.
- Advanced maternal age (over 40 years).
- Precipitate labour (this is assumed as the onset time was 30 minutes before the call time).
- Grand multiparity (it is her 5th baby).
- Overdistention of the uterus (multiple pregnancy, polyhydramnios, macrosomic foetus – the baby appears very large).

In the UK 18% of births will experience a PPH and a major PPH complicates 1.3% of births. Other factors that put women at risk of developing a PPH include:

- Previous retained placenta.
- Placenta praevia or accreta.
- Antepartum haemorrhage, especially from placental abruption.
- Pre-eclampsia.
- BMI over 35.
- Existing uterine abnormalities, e.g. fibroids.
- Low maternal haemoglobin level, below 9 g/dL (less able to tolerate haemorrhage).
- Prolonged labour.

- Previous caesarean section.
- Placental abruption.
- Pyrexia in labour.

Placental expulsion has yet to occur. How can the delivery of the placenta be encouraged?

Natural oxytocin should be maximised at this point. Skin-to-skin bonding is encouraged and the natural maternal hormones, particularly oxytocin, are produced. Oxytocin, which is required for uterine contraction in the third stage, often referred to as the hormone of love, is produced during the immediate bonding between a mother and her baby. Placing the baby skin to skin helps to increase the amount of oxytocin produced by putting the baby to the breast and encouraging feeding; even if the baby does not feed, stimulation of the nipple will suffice, there will be further oxytocin produced and this in turn will assist in the contracting of the uterus, helping to reduce bleeding. Skin to skin with a dried baby will also help to regulate the temperature of the newborn. Assisting the mother into an upright or squatting position can also help in expulsion, as gravity helps the placenta move downwards. Do not pull on the cord: this is a technique only to be performed in conjunction with medical third-stage management.

What are the four causes of PPH?

The causes of PPH are known as the 4Ts:

- Tone (uterine atony).
- Tissue.
- Tears (or trauma to the genital tract).
- Thrombin (coagulopathies).

Eliminating each cause will help you to treat and manage the PPH.

Case Progression

SYSTEMATIC APPROACH

Danger
Nil.

Response
Alert on the AVPU scale.

Airway
Clear.

Breathing
Patient is speaking in full sentences, no difficulty in breathing, respiration rate 22 bpm.

Circulation
Radial, normal rhythm and volume 100 bpm.

Vital signs
RR: 22 bpm
HR: 100 bpm
BP: 90/60 mmHg
SpO_2: 97%
Blood sugar: 5.5 mmol/L
Temperature: 36.5 °C
Lead II ECG: sinus rhythm

Exposure
EBL is now 600 mL, placenta was expelled by maternal effort at 06:36. Patient is suffering a postpartum haemorrhage.

What is the first-line treatment for this PPH?

With the placenta expelled, the uterine fundus needs to be massaged in order to help it contract and stop further bleeding. To perform uterine or fundal massage, locate the uterine fundus with the hand facing downwards, cupping the fundus, which should be at the level of the umbilicus. The contracted uterus should feel hard and firm and sit just below the umbilicus. However, if the uterus feels soft and boggy, then fundal massage should be performed. As the fundus of the uterus is massaged in a circular motion, it will encourage contractions and should ultimately stem the blood flow. This can be an uncomfortable procedure, so it is important to remember to inform the patient of what you are about to do and why, gain consent, and ensure appropriate analgesia is utilised. This procedure must only be performed if the placenta has been delivered. While performing uterine massage clots may be expelled from the vagina; this is to be expected, as any tissue retained needs to be expelled. Do not stop if you get clots, carry on – it's working, remember the next T: tissue.

If the uterus has been massaged and contraction achieved, careful monitoring should be observed because if the uterus has lost tone PPH is more likely to happen again. Uterine contraction can be enhanced further by the production of natural oxytocin, as already discussed.

What is your stepwise process for managing this PPH? Include any drugs that can be utilised.

- Follow the ABC approach and use oxygen if hypoxia is present.
- Feel for the uterine fundus and assess.
- Perform uterine massage and observe for clots.
- Check the placenta for completeness.
- Give Syntometrine if available and BP is lower than 140/90 mmHg or misoprostol if BP above 140/90 mmHg.

If both drugs are available and Syntometrine has been given after 15 minutes and bleeding has not settled, give misoprostol.

- Check for perineal trauma and apply pressure if present and there is active bleeding.
- Gain IV (large-bore cannula) access and consider fluids.
- Transport under emergency conditions to nearest obstetric unit.
- Place a pre-alert including estimated blood loss.
- Give tranexamic acid en route; do not delay time on scene to administer this.

LEVEL 2 CASE STUDY
Shoulder dystocia

Information type	Data
Time of origin	01:15
Time of dispatch	01:43
On-scene time	01:50
Day of the week	Wednesday
Nearest hospital	10 minutes
Nearest backup	15 minutes
Patient details	Name: Jasmine Everett DOB: 12/04/1982

> **CASE**
> You are dispatched to a 38-year-old female in advanced labour with an urge to push. Two double-crewed ambulances have been assigned; however, your backup is a considerable distance away. You are informed this is the patient's fourth baby and labour has progressed quickly.

Pre-arrival information

Conscious and breathing.

Windscreen report

The address is a farmhouse up a small lane. No obvious activity outside.

Entering the location

You are greeted by a male who appears distressed.

On arrival with the patient

The patient is sat on the kitchen floor on a towel, her waters have broken, there is evidence of fluid on the floor that looks clear and she is instinctively bearing down with contractions.

SYSTEMATIC APPROACH

Danger

Nil.

Response

Alert on the AVPU scale.

Airway

Clear, pale.

Breathing

20 bpm, regular, no difficulty in breathing.

Circulation

Radial pulse present and regular, 80 bpm.

Vital signs

RR: 20 bpm

HR: 80 bpm

BP: not taken due to obvious second stage of labour

SpO$_2$: not taken

Blood sugar: not taken

Lead II ECG: not taken

Exposure

Due to the spontaneous rupture of membranes and the urge to push, you deduce the patient is in the second stage of labour. When she is not contracting you gain consent to raise her dress and inspect the vulva. On exposure you view the presenting part and as she pushes with the next contraction, the presenting part moves forward rapidly and the head is born. You await restitution of the head and with the next contraction urge the patient to push, but there is no spontaneous birth of the body. This happens again on the second contraction. There is no birth after two contractions with good maternal effort.

TASK

Look through the information provided in this case study and highlight all of the information that might concern you as a paramedic.

What is your diagnosis and why?

Shoulder dystocia. Failure of the birth after two contractions leads to the diagnosis of shoulder dystocia, where the anterior shoulder of the foetus becomes stuck behind the symphysis pubis. In order to facilitate this birth, manoeuvres must be utilised to assist with the birth.

Using a stepwise approach, describe your next steps (do not include manoeuvres at this point).

- Inform your emergency operations centre.
- Request a midwife if available locally as well as backup/status of second crew.
- Prepare for newborn resuscitation.
- Do not pull downwards on the foetal head when performing axial traction, as this can cause a brachial plexus injury.
- Maternal pushing should be discouraged, as this can lead to further impaction.
- *Never* apply fundal pressure, as this can cause foetal complications and uterine rupture.

What is the first manoeuvre you would utilise? How is this performed and why?

McRoberts manoeuvre. The patient is laid flat, with any pillows from under her back removed. One ambulance clinician should, on each leg then lift the legs upwards and abducted them around the woman's abdomen. If there is only one ambulance assistant, then a relative or another person on scene should be utilised to hold the other leg. The patient will not be able to hold the position correctly herself.

McRoberts position changes the diameters within the pelvis, straightening the lumbosacral angle, rotating the maternal pelvis upwards and increasing the anterior–posterior diameter of the pelvis. This is an effective intervention, with reported success rates as high as 90% which is why it must be performed effectively. The procedure is performed for 30 seconds. Maternal pushing is discouraged and axial traction is applied to the foetal head.

Case Progression

SYSTEMATIC APPROACH

Airway
Clear.

Breathing
Respiration rate 20 bpm, regular.

Circulation
Heart rate 100 bpm, regular, strong radial.

Vital signs
RR: 20 bpm
HR: 100 bpm
BP: not taken as birthing
SpO$_2$: not taken

The McRoberts manoeuvre is performed for 30 seconds with axial traction applied to the foetal head. There is no progress on the birth.

What would be your next steps in your management of this situation?

Suprapubic pressure should be utilised next, together with the McRoberts manoeuvre. Applying suprapubic pressure reduces the foetal bisacromial diameter and rotates the anterior foetal shoulder into the wider oblique pelvic diameter. The shoulder is then freed to slip underneath the symphysis pubis with the aid of routine axial traction.

(a) McRoberts manoeuvre   (b) Supra pubic pressure

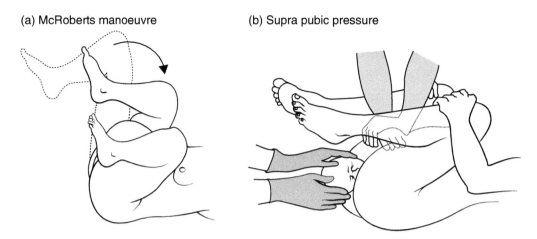

Figure 14.1 McRoberts manoeuvre. Reproduced with permission from Woolcock, M. (ed.) (2018) *Pre-obstetric Emergency Training: A Practical Approach*, 2nd ed. Chichester: Wiley-Blackwell.

Suprapubic pressure is applied by placing the hands in the CPR grip just above the mother's symphysis pubis (see Figure 14.1). The direction of the pressure is very important and must be pushing from the direction of the foetal back, so the attendant should be stood on the side at which the occiput is present. If there is only one ambulance clinician and the person holding the other leg is a layperson, then you must ensure before you commence McRoberts that the ambulance clinician is on the correct side if suprapubic pressure should be required.

The pressure should be performed in a constant downward motion for 30 seconds and then in an intermittent motion for a further 30 seconds, both accompanied by axial traction.

If the foetus fails to birth after the first three manoeuvres, then in the final step you should position the mother over into all fours.

Position the mother on her hands and knees, with her hips well flexed and bottom elevated and her head as low as possible. For the next 30 seconds apply axial traction to the foetal head in order to try to deliver the posterior shoulder from the sacral hollow first. In some studies this has been shown to have a success rate of 83%.

If all the manoeuvres have been unsuccessful, what is the next step for an undelivered foetus?

If after 30 seconds the shoulders still fail to be delivered, undertake a time-critical transfer to the nearest consultant-led obstetric unit. Do not await the arrival of the midwife.

If the mother is upstairs in the house, she cannot sit on a carry chair for extraction, so she should be assisted to walk. The best way to assist this is to get her dressing gown, ask her to put it on and tie the cord over her abdomen. Then get her to pull the tails of the dressing gown through her legs so this forms a sling. She will then need to walk backwards down the stairs, which may help to further move the diameters within the pelvis and may help to dislodge the shoulder. The sling effect of the gown should help to catch the baby if it is born halfway down the stairs – remember that this movement may facilitate and precipitate the birth, so do not move your hands too far away from the foetal head. It also serves to protect the woman's modesty as she is walked out of the house to the awaiting ambulance.

Once in the ambulance, position the patient in a lateral position, ideally right lateral, so that you can maintain eye contact and verbally communicate. Fully strap her in, as her safety is paramount. Place a blanket or pillow between her knees to prevent undue pressure on the foetal head. If contractions continue she may use Entonox, and if she needs to keep pushing do not discourage, but do not actively encourage pushing.

A pre-alert/inform call should be placed to the nearest consultant obstetric unit. Request the team to meet you at the ambulance entrance, as there are internal manoeuvres the obstetric team can perform that are outside the paramedic scope of practice.

LEVEL 3 CASE STUDY
Breech birth

Information type	Data
Time of origin	02:00
Time of dispatch	02:10
On-scene time	02:20
Day of the week	Sunday
Nearest hospital	20 minutes
Nearest backup	15 minutes
Patient details	Name: Betty May DOB: 14/02/1996

CASE
You are dispatched to attend a 24-year-old female who is 38 weeks' pregnant. You are informed that she is alone in the property and has called 999 with an urge to push.

Pre-arrival information
The patient is conscious and breathing.

Windscreen report
The property is on a housing estate and the house and garden around are well maintained.

Entering the location
You are greeted by a female who appears distressed, bending down as she gets a contraction.

SYSTEMATIC APPROACH
Danger
Nil.

Response
Alert on the AVPU scale.

Airway
Clear.

Breathing
Regular, respiration rate 20 bpm, no shortness of breath, breathing normally and talking between contractions.

Circulation
Regular, radial present, 88 bpm.

Vital signs
RR: 20 bpm
HR: 88 bpm
BP: not taken at this time
SpO$_2$: not taken at this time

Exposure

As you are talking to the patient, she is showing signs of the second stage of labour. She is having contractions regularly every 2 minutes lasting at least 60 seconds and is bearing down with each one. She tells you that she feels like 'the baby is coming'. You move her into the lounge area, where she takes her pyjama trousers off and you notice external signs of the second stage of labour: she is contracting every 2 minutes, is bearing down with contractions, there is vulval and anal dilatation and with the next contraction her waters break. As the presenting part becomes visible, you see a string of what looks like black toothpaste emerging out of it.

TASK

Look through the information provided in this case study and highlight all of the information that might concern you as a paramedic.

What is happening and what are your initial reactions?

The baby is in the breech presentation, with the bottom being born first. This occurs in appropriately 3–4% of babies at term, although it is more common in the pre-term birth (RCOG, 2017a). Labour with a baby in the breech position will progress through the stages of labour the same as a head-down or cephalic presentation, but on inspection at the vaginal opening the following may be visible:

- Buttocks.
- Feet or soles of the feet.
- Swollen or bruised genitalia.
- Frank meconium, in a string like black toothpaste.

The optimum position for the woman to birth is the all fours position. This position allows gravity to play a really important role and enables the paramedic to remain hands off as long as the progress is normal. If the mother declines to move into all fours, then position her on the edge of a chair, sofa or bed, to ensure that the baby has sufficient space to be able to hang and allow gravity to perform most of the birth.

Why is gravity so important when dealing with a breech birth?

The baby in the breech presentation has to have enough room to allow gravity to assist with the birth. There needs to be minimal handling of the baby as it is birthing to prevent stimulation of the baby; however, if there is slow or no progress with delivery, do not be afraid to touch the baby to assist in the birth if there is a need. Gravity assists in making sure that the baby's head descends into the pelvis in the correct diameters. If there is pulling on the body this can cause extension of the head, and if there is holding of the body this can prevent the baby's head from descending into the pelvis altogether.

Case Progression

You support the patient to move into an all fours position as she leans over the sofa. As she pushes, more of the presenting part becomes visible and it is evident that the breech is descending. With the next push the bottom and male genitals appear.

Describe the process of the birth up to the point of the arms.

Once the presenting part is visible (the bottom), it will advance and withdraw in a similar way to a head. When the widest part of the bottom is born it is known as the 'rumping', like crowning when the head is born, just the opposite way.

Once the rumping has occurred, the bottom will twist and the legs should now be directly facing you. This is when you need to remember the mantra 'tum to bum'. This will help you to remember the way the baby should be positioned. They should always be in the tum to bum in all fours it is baby's tum to mum's bum.

Once the baby is born up to the umbilicus, then a timer should be started. The Breech Birth network recommend that the baby should be born within 3–5 minutes of the umbilicus becoming visible. These births are a lot quicker than a cephalic birth. Do not touch the baby at this point, and neither should you pull or touch the umbilical cord for any reason. Most definitely do not cut or clamp the umbilical cord until the head is born, even if you think it looks tight in any way. If the baby is in the frank position, then the legs should birth within 30 seconds of each other. Encourage the mother to bear down and push continually not just with contractions and if all is progressing normally do not touch the baby, don't worry if it has its feet on the floor/bed ground.

What characteristics can you look for to inform you of the condition of the baby at this point?

There are several points you can look for that will give you an indication as to the condition of the baby at this point:

- The baby will have good tone.
- The baby will be a good colour, i.e. purple/blue.
- The cord will be full.
- The valley of the cord will be visible (the crease that runs up the chest wall will be like a valley).
- The baby will then do the characteristic 'tummy crunches' movement that is normal to encourage the birth of the arms and head.

Do not interfere with the baby during the crunches. These are the natural movements that the baby will make in order to get them into the position needed to get the arms and head born. Do not worry if the baby does not crunch, but this can lead to a slower birth, and this baby will be more likely to need resuscitation.

Do not pull on the infant's trunk or hold on to them in an attempt to expedite the birth, as this may cause the baby to raise their arms in utero, causing nuchal arms (arms that are raised over the head).

Describe the birth from the arms to the head.

With the mother in the upright position or all fours with effective contractions, the arms should birth spontaneously following the baby performing the abdominal crunches. The arms will normally follow each other in a prayer position with the hands together. Once the arms are free, then again leave the baby and do not interfere with the natural physiology. This is often the most unnerving time and the point at which most clinicians want to take hold and lift the baby upwards, as they fear that the neck will be damaged. This is the worst thing you can do right now. If you hold the baby at this point the head will not engage in the pelvis, and it may stop the baby from being born at all.

Once you see the chin the head is almost there. The head has to contend with the curve of the pelvis the same way as with a cephalic birth, just the opposite way around.

So the first time you touch this baby is when the head emerges and you are there to catch the baby as the head is freed from the birth canal.

If there is a slow descent of the baby, a few key tips are recommended by the Breech Birth Network (2016):

- Encourage movement: get the mother to rock her hips from side to side to shake the baby downwards.
- Get the mother to adopt the 'running start' position like a runner in the blocks of a race with one knee lifted. This will open the outlet of the pelvis.
- When the chin is born a shoulder press can be utilised. This is done by pushing the baby backward towards the mother's abdomen, which will facilitate the birth of the head. This replaces the need for the Mauriceau–Smellie–Veit manoeuvre if the mother was not in an all fours position, as the baby would need lifting upwards to complete the birth through what would be an upward curve of the pelvis.

LEVEL 3 CASE STUDY
Placenta praevia

Information type	Data
Time of origin	13:50
Time of dispatch	14:00
On-scene time	14:15

(Continued)

Information type	Data
Day of the week	Monday
Nearest hospital	10 minutes
Nearest backup	10 minutes
Patient details	Name: Renuka Manuka
	DOB: 28/03/1982

CASE

You are dispatched to a 38-year-old female who is 34 weeks' pregnant with her fourth pregnancy. The information you receive states she is suffering with a per vagina (PV) bleed. No further information is available, as the controller informs you that there is a language barrier.

Pre-arrival information

The patient is conscious and breathing.

Windscreen report

The area outside the house appears to be safe. The house is not well maintained and there are several old, broken-down vehicles on the driveway.

Entering the location

You are greeted by a female who appears pale and distressed, repeatedly saying 'bleeding' and 'danger'. You can see fresh red blood smeared on her knees.

SYSTEMATIC APPROACH

Danger

Nil.

Response

Alert on the AVPU scale.

Airway

The patient is talking to you.

Breathing

Respiration rate 22 bpm, shallow and panicked.

Circulation

Heart rate 102 bpm, radial present, irregular, bounding.

Exposure

When you place your hand on the patient's abdomen it feels soft and she does not wince as if in pain. She shows you a pad with approximately 100 mL of fresh red blood soaked in, but you are not able to gain consent to expose her vulva to see if the bleeding is active.

TASK

Look through the information provided in this case study and highlight all of the information that might concern you as a paramedic.

Your patient is suffering from an antepartum haemorrhage (APH). What is this and how is it classified?

An APH is any frank blood loss from the genital tract, after 24 completed weeks of pregnancy, until the onset of labour. APH occurs in and complicates 3–5% of pregnancies (RCOG, 2014). It is often unpredictable and is a result of the inability of the pregnant patient to compensate for haemorrhage, due to the physiological adaptations of pregnancy. In the pregnant patient deterioration is often rapid and unexpected.

According to the Advanced Life Support Group (2010) there are several factors that lead to an increased risk of suffering from an APH:

- Maternal age over 40 years.
- Presence of complex medical problems, e.g. obesity or diabetes.
- Women who have had more than one previous pregnancy.
- Previous caesarean section.
- Known placenta praevia.
- Use of crack cocaine.
- Coagulation problems.
- Previous history of APH.
- Hypertension.
- Polyhydramnios (an excess of amniotic fluid).

The RCOG Green-top Guideline 63 (2014) uses the following descriptions when describing blood loss from an APH:

- Spotting – staining, streaking or blood spotting noted on underwear or sanitary protection.
- Minor haemorrhage – blood loss of less than 50 mL that has settled.
- Major haemorrhage – blood loss of 50–1000 mL with no signs of clinical shock.
- Massive haemorrhage – blood loss of greater than 1000 mL and/or signs of clinical shock.

The common causes of minor APH include cervical erosion, marginal placental bed bleeding or a blood-stained show. Major APH is mainly due to placental abruption and placenta praevia. The difficulty with estimating blood loss from APH is that the bleeding can be either concealed and not visible externally or revealed and visible, or a combination of both.

List the clinical differences between the two main types of APH.

See Table 14.2.

Table 14.2 Clinical differences between the two main types of antepartum haemorrhage

Clinical sign	Placenta praevia	Placental abruption
Warning haemorrhage	Yes	No
Abdominal pain	No, usually painless	Yes, can be severe
Blood loss colour	Frank fresh red	Dark red/brown
Onset	At rest, postcoital	After trauma/exertion
Degree of shock	Proportional to loss	Disproportional to loss
Consistency of uterus	Soft, non-tender	Tense, hard, 'wooden'

Case Progression

SYSTEMATIC APPROACH

Airway
Clear.

Breathing
Respiration rate 24 bpm.

Circulation
Heart rate 125 bpm. Effort: strong. Heart regularity: regular.

Vital signs
RR: 24 bpm
HR: 125 bpm
BP: 100/60 mmHg
SpO$_2$: 96%

Exposure
You notice that there is a set of pregnancy handheld records on the counter top, and you ask if it is OK to read them, to which the patient agrees. Highlighted at the top of the examination page in large red letters are the words 'Placenta Praevia'.
    There is blood now actively tricking down the patient's legs, you estimate a total amount of 200 mL.

The pregnancy notes state that the woman has placenta praevia. What is this condition?

Placenta praevia is a condition where the placenta is abnormally sited within the uterus. Rather than implanting within the upper portion of the fundus, the placenta imbeds within the lower segment. This is a condition occurring in approximately 1 in 200 pregnancies (AACE, 2017). There are different degrees of placenta praevia depending on how low the placenta is sited within the uterus and how close or how much of the cervix is covered. If there is any portion of placenta on or over the cervix, then the woman is unable to have a vaginal birth due to the risk of bleeding and will be scheduled for a caesarean section.

The condition is diagnosed by ultrasound scan at around 20 weeks (depending on local policy when this is performed). If it is diagnosed then further follow-up scans will be arranged for later on the pregnancy, normally around 36–37 weeks. If you attend a woman who has had no antenatal care and is losing fresh red blood, then you must consider placenta praevia as a potential cause. At term there is over 700 mL of blood per minute provided to the uterus (Open Anesthesia, 2018), so if any portion of the placenta is bleeding from any cause, catastrophic bleeding can ensue.

What are your next actions in this case?

- Rapid assessment of the patient is vital when dealing with a major APH. This is a time-critical, life-threatening emergency and rapid transport to an obstetric facility is vital.
- Monitor O$_2$ saturations. If oxygen saturation falls, remember to ensure oxygen therapy is used in order to prevent any further foetal compromise.
- Assess the amount of bleeding you can see and remember to take any blood-soaked pads with you to the obstetric unit.
- *Do not* administer Syntometrine or misoprostol for an APH, as the foetus is still in situ. Tranexamic acid may be considered, but can only be administered in accordance with your local policies and procedures.
- Do not delay time on scene for cannulation: this should be done en route if bleeding is serious and continuous. Two large-bore cannulae should be inserted early, as maternal shutdown often occurs quickly due to sudden onset of hypovolaemic shock.
- IV fluid therapy should be used in order to maintain a systolic BP above 90 mm/Hg by giving 250 mL bolus doses of sodium chloride. However, it is important to remember that pregnant patients may lose up to 30% of their circulating blood volume without a significant change in their observations, so if you believe the patient is bleeding then do not wait until the BP falls.
- Careful assessment of foetal movements should be made in order to assess foetal viability. It is important to remember to be tactful, as further anxiety and alarm may cause exacerbation of the situation.
- It is important to remember the woman's pain and titrate pain relief accordingly. The use of paracetamol, Entonox and morphine may be considered according to the pain score. It is nevertheless important to

remember that utilisation of morphine should be done with caution, especially if the patient is hypotensive and at risk of respiratory depression.

- Ensure the woman is kept nil by mouth and allow her to adjust her position according to her comfort. The supine position should be avoided and a right lateral tilted position is the preferred option.
- A concise pre-alert to the receiving obstetric facility is important. Including an estimation of blood loss is key, as staff can gather the required assistance needed to deal with specific events. The SBAR handover tool would be suitable for passing on the pre-alert message.

Provide an SBAR handover on this case.

See Table 14.3.

Table 14.3 SBAR handover

Situation	Actively bleeding, known placenta previa
Background	38 YOF 34/40 pregnant G4P3
	Spontaneous APH started approximately 15 minutes ago
Assessment	On inspection of pads fresh red blood seen, approximately 200 mL, but is continually bleeding now, abdomen soft. BP 100/60 mmHg, HR 125 bpm
Recommendations	We would like a team to meet us at the ambulance entrance
	Our ETA is 8 minutes

References and further reading

Advanced Life Support Group (2009) *Pre-Obstetric Emergency Training (POET)*. Cambridge: Wiley-Blackwell.

AAFP (2012) *Advanced Life Support in Obstetrics Provider Manual*. Leawood, KS: American Academy of Family Physicians.

Association of Ambulance Service Chief Executives (AACE) (2017) *JRCALC Supplementary Guidelines*. Bridgewater: Class Professional Publishing.

Association of Ambulance Chief Executives (AACE), Joint Royal Colleges Ambulance Liaison Committee (JRCALC) and Mansfield, A. (2018) *Emergency Birth in the Community*. Bridgewater: Class Professional Publishing.

BloodtoBaby (2019) Optimal cord clamping. https://www.bloodtobaby.com/research (accessed 11 July 2020).

Breech Birth Network (2016) The midwife, the mother and the breech. https://breechbirth.org.uk/2016/06/03/the-birth-of-leliana/ (accessed 1 July 2019).

Cornthwaite, K., Crofts, J., Draycott, T. et al. (2015) *Training for Obstetric Emergencies: PROMPT and Shoulder Dystocia*. London: The Health Foundation. emc (2019) Syntometrine ampoules. https://www.medicines.org.uk/emc/product/865 (accessed 7 February 2019).

FIGO (2012) *Treatment of Postpartum Haemorrhage with Misoprostol*. London: International Federation of Gynecology and Obstetrics.

Joint Royal Colleges Ambulance Liaison Committee (JRCALC) (2017) *JRCALC Clinical Practice Supplementary Guidelines 2017*. Bridgewater: Class Professional Publishing.

MBRRACE-UK (2017) *Saving Lives, Improving Mothers' Care – Lessons Learned to Inform Maternity Care from the UK and Ireland Confidential Enquiries into Maternal Deaths and Morbidity* 2013–15. Oxford: National Perinatal Epidemiology Unit, University of Oxford.

NHS Litigation Authority (2012) *Ten Years of Maternity Claims*. London: NHS Litigation Authority.

NICE (2017) *Intrapartum Care for Healthy Women and Babies (CG190)*. London: National Institute for Health and Care Excellence. Open Anesthesia (2018) Uteroplacental blood flow. https://www.openanesthesia.org/uteroplacental_blood_flow/ (accessed 4 January 2018).

Pilbery, R. (2011) Meningococcal disease. *Standby CPD*, 1(7).

Practical Obstetric Multi-Professional Training (2017) *Course Manual*, 3rd edn. Cambridge: Cambridge University Press.

Reitter, A. & Walker, S. (2019) *Practical insight into upright breech birth from birth videos: A structured analysis*. 4th European Congress on Intrapartum Care, Turin, Italy.

RCOG (2012) *Shoulder Dystocia (Green-top Guideline No. 42)*. London: Royal College of Obstetricians and Gynaecologists.

RCOG (2014) *Antepartum Haemorrhage (Green-top Guideline No. 63)*. London: Royal College of Obstetricians and Gynaecologists. https://www.rcog.org.uk/globalassets/documents/guidelines/gtg_63.pdf (accessed 20 December 2017).

RCOG (2017a) *Management of Breech Presentation (Green-top Guideline No. 20b)*. London: Royal College of Obstetricians and Gynaecologists.

RCOG (2017b) *Umbilical Cord Prolapse (Green-top Guideline No. 50)*. London: Royal College of Obstetricians and Gynaecologists.

Say, L., Chou, D., Gemmill A. et al. (2014) Global causes of maternal death: A WHO systematic analysis. *Lancet Global Health*, 2(6): e323–e333. doi: 10.1016/S2214-109X(14)70227-X

Sayed Ahmed, W.A. & Hamdy, M.A. (2018) Optimal management of umbilical cord prolapse. *International Journal of Women's Health*, 10: 459–465. doi: 10.2147/IJWH.S130879

Smith, L.A., Price, N., Simonite, V. & Burns, E.E. (2013) Incidence of and risk factors for perineal trauma: A prospective observational study. *BMC Pregnancy and Childbirth*, 13(1): 59.

Spillane, E. (2019) Obstetric emergencies in low risk settings. In *Obstetric and Intrapartum Emergencies*, 2nd edn (eds E. Chandraharan & S. Arulkumaran), Cambridge: Cambridge University Press.

Tully, G. (2012) FlipFLOP: Four steps to remember. *Midwifery Today*, 103.

Walker, S., Breslin, E., Scamell, M. & Parker, P. (2017) Effectiveness of vaginal breech birth training strategies: An integrative review of the literature. *Birth*, 44(2): 101–109.

Walker, S., Parker, P. & Scamell, M. (2018) Expertise in physiological breech birth: A mixed methods study. *Birth*, 45(2): 202–209.

Walker, S., Reading, C., Silverwood-Cope, O. & Cochrane, V. (2017) Physiological breech birth: Evaluation of a training programme for birth professionals. *Practising Midwife*, 20(2): 25–28.

Walker, S., Scamell, M. & Parker, P. (2016) Principles of physiological breech birth practice: A Delphi study. *Midwifery*, 43: 1–6.

Walker, S., Scamell, M. & Parker, P. (2018) Deliberate acquisition of competence in physiological breech birth: A grounded theory study. *Women and Birth*, 31(3): e170–e177.

WHO (2017) *WHO Recommendation on Tranexamic Acid for the Treatment of Postpartum Haemorrhage*. Geneva: World Health Organisation.

WHO (2017) *WHO Recommendations on Prevention and Treatment of Postpartum Haemorrhage and the WOMAN Trial*. Geneva: World Health Organisation. https://www.who.int/reproductivehealth/topics/maternal_perinatal/pph-woman-trial/en/ (accessed 19 January 2018).

WOMAN Trial Collaborators (2017) Effect of early tranexamic acid administration on mortality, hysterectomy, and other morbidities in women with post-partum haemorrhage (WOMAN): An international, randomised, double-blind, placebo-controlled trial. *The Lancet*, 389(10084): 2081.

Woollard, M., Hinshaw, K., Simpson, H. & Wieteska, S. (eds) (2009) *Pre-hospital Obstetric Emergency Training*. Oxford: Wiley-Blackwell.

Chapter 15

Remote area cases

Steve Whitfield[1] and Kerryn Wratt[2]

[1] Griffith University School of Medicine, Gold Coast, and Queensland Ambulance Service, Brisbane, QLD, Australia
[2] RescueMED and Australasian Wilderness & Expedition Medicine Society, Omeo, VIC, Australia

LEVEL 1
Hypothermia

Information type	Data
Time of origin	16:45
Time of dispatch	17:15
On-scene time	17:34
Day of the week	Saturday
Nearest hospital	2 hours
Nearest backup	Flight intensive care crew, 45 minutes
Patient details	Name: Roberto Robertson
	DOB: 12/04/1965

CASE

You have been called to a remote alpine area for a 55-year-old male who has been reported slurring his words and 'walking funny' while bush walking on a track.

Pre-arrival information

The area is difficult to access and requires 60 minutes of driving, a 45-minute boat ride and a 1 km walk. You will be met by Parks staff and police to assist with safe access and extrication.

Windscreen report

On arrival you note it is now dark and cold. It has been snowing, with 30 cm or so settled on the ground but none falling now. There is a persistent light breeze. The weather appears to be clearing. You are greeted by Parks staff, who check you are well equipped for the environment and assist you with access to the patient.

Clinical Cases in Paramedicine, First Edition. Edited by Sam Willis, Ian Peate, and Rod Hill.
© 2021 John Wiley & Sons Ltd. Published 2021 by John Wiley & Sons Ltd.

Entering the location

At a bush hut, you find a middle-aged male who appears distressed. He states he become concerned when a walker he passed on the track earlier did not make it to the hut as darkness set in. He states he then walked back up the track and found the patient collapsed and in distress. He returned to the hut and utilised the UHF radio there to contact the ranger, who initiated ambulance and rescue services.

On arrival with the patient

After an approximately 1 km walk you arrive at the male patient. He is wrapped in a silver blanket, lying in snow on a track. His clothing is wet.

Patient assessment triangle

General appearance

The patient is conscious, responding to voice, and looks at you when you talk to him. He is cold to touch and his clothes are wet. He is shivering uncontrollably and slurring his words considerably.

Circulation to the skin

Skin is cool and pale.

Work of breathing

Breathing is slow but adequate.

SYSTEMATIC APPROACH

Danger

There are significant environmental dangers (cold, wet, wind, remoteness). You are well prepared and supported by the ranger and police.

Response

Not alert, but responding to voice on the AVPU scale.

Airway

Clear.

Breathing

Respiration rate: 12 bpm. Effort: normal. Accessory muscle use: no. Auscultation: equal air entry with no abnormal sounds.

Circulation

Heart rate: 56 bpm. Character: weak. Heart regularity: regular. Capillary refill time: >2 seconds.

Vital signs

RR: 12 bpm
HR: 56 bpm
BP: 110/70 mmHg
SpO$_2$: Not reading due to cold
Blood sugar: 5 mmol/L
Temperature: not reading due to cold
Lead II ECG: sinus bradycardia with significant artefact; there is a positive deflection at the J point

Exposure

Skin is cool to touch and wet.

TASK

Look through the information provided in this case study and highlight all of the information that might concern you as a paramedic.

Using what you know about the case at this point, including what you may have seen and how the patient is presenting to you, which vital signs should you undertake first?

It would be important to identify the cause of the patient's altered conscious state and rule out a neurological cause of his slurred speech. Therefore obtaining a temperature and a measure of blood glucose would be useful, as well as a focused neurological exam. It is important to take a full set of vital signs on every patient as part of a structured approach.

Once you have undertaken the essential vital signs, what would your next action be?

Begin to manage the patient's temperature utilising an understanding of the mechanisms of heat transfer (Radiation, Evaporation, Conduction, Convection) and current hypothermia best practice guidelines. The initial aims are to ensure the patient does not become colder or deteriorate into a non-perfusing cardiac rhythm. This would include handling the patient gently and keeping him horizontal, as well as setting up a shelter (tent or bothy bag) and placing the patient in a hypothermia wrap with added heat sources (self-heating blankets or bottles of warm water against the body, but not directly against the skin to avoid burns). Once in the shelter, remove the patient's wet clothes and complete the hypothermia wrap with consideration of toileting needs. An early situation report utilising the IMIST mnemonic would be essential to ensure timely backup and that an appropriate extrication plan is in place given the remote location.

Which of the following non-technical skills do you think are important to be able to safely treat this patient?
a. Effective verbal communication.
b. Effective non-verbal communication.
c. Empathy.
d. Reassurance.
e. Situational awareness.
f. All of the above.

f. All of the above.

Case Progression

The patient is now in a shelter, in a hypothermia wrap with dry clothes on and warmed water bottles placed inside the hypothermia wrap. The bottles are strong and wrapped in clothing to ensure they do not burn the patient.

Patient assessment triangle
General appearance
The patient is now alert, with some shivering.

Circulation to the skin
Still cool and pale.

Work of breathing
Normal, quiet breathing.

SYSTEMATIC APPROACH
Danger
Nil.

Response
Alert on the AVPU scale.

Airway
Clear.

Breathing

Respiration rate: 16 bpm. Effort: normal. Accessory muscle use: no. Auscultation: clear, no added sounds.

Circulation

Heart rate: 60 bpm. Character: weak. Heart regularity: regular. Capillary refill time: >2 seconds.

Vital signs

RR: 16 bpm
HR: 60 bpm
BP: 110/85 mmHg
SpO$_2$: 96%
Blood sugar: 5 mmol/L
Temperature: 33.8 °C
Lead II ECG: sinus rhythm

Exposure

Skin is dry.

What kinds of questions would you ask this patient specifically related to hypothermia as part of the history-taking process?

See Table 15.1.

Table 15.1 History-taking questions

Hypothermia

How long have you been in the environment?
What have you had to eat/drink today? When?
When did you start to feel cold and/or lethargic?

Medication history

Do you take any medications?
If so, which ones and how frequently?
Specifically do you take beta blockers?

F/SH (family and social history)

Any specific family medical history?
Do you drink alcohol? If so, how much and how often?
Who do you live with?
What do you do for work?

Past medical history (PMH)

Do you have any medical conditions?
Specifically any history of stroke, diabetes, hypertension or coronary artery disease?

Differential diagnoses (DDx) – What else could this be?

Stroke
Metabolic disorder
Overdose

Given the patient's improvement as listed in the case progression and his response to treatment, what are your choices now for what to do next?

Continue to protect the patient from any further temperature reduction with full hypothermia wrap and added heat source(s). After ensuring the patient is able to protect his airway, one could provide a warm caloric drink to sip on. After 30 minutes of active temperature management and given the current vital signs, the patient should start to be prepared for transport. Utilise on-scene resources to transport the patient the 1 km back to the hut. At this point a further sitrep and confirmation of the extrication plan should be performed, specifically clarifying the availability of a helicopter assist to provide transport to a definitive treatment facility.

LEVEL ONE CASE STUDY
Heat illness

Information type	Data
Time of origin	12:15
Time of dispatch	12:17
On-scene time	12:34
Day of the week	Saturday
Nearest hospital	3 hours
Nearest backup	Flight intensive care crew, 60 minutes
Patient details	Name: Deano Donaldson DOB: 01/02/2005

CASE
You have been called to a remote beach for a 15-year-old male who has been reported slurring his words and stumbling while walking on a track.

Pre-arrival information
The area is difficult to access by road and requires 4×4 access that exceeds 60 minutes of off-road driving. The patient is part of a school group on a remote field trip and two teachers are on scene administering first aid.

Windscreen report
On arrival you note the outside temperature is 41 °C. The sky is blue, cloudless and there is no breeze and only limited shady cover from shrubs. You are greeted by a teacher who directs you to the patient, 300 m away under a shrub.

On arrival at the patient
You are greeted by a second teacher who appears distressed. She states that the students had been on a planned walk along the beach track after breakfast. The planned route was roughly 6 km, but their departure was delayed for unforeseen reasons. Concerns were raised when the student stumbled and teachers noted he was slurring his words. They sat the patient down in the shade of a shrub, but he did not improve. The patient is supine under a shrub, fully clothed in a long-sleeved shirt and hiking boots. His clothes are wet, but you notice his skin is dry and pale.

Patient assessment triangle
General appearance
The patient is mumbling incoherently. He is hot to touch, has dry skin and his clothes are wet. Compared to other students he presents as slightly obese.

Circulation to the skin
Skin is hot, dry and pale.

Work of breathing
Breathing is fast and shallow.

SYSTEMATIC APPROACH
Danger
The sun is beating down on the scene and, although in the shade, the position is very hot.

Response
Not alert, mumbling incoherently.

Airway
Clear.

Breathing
Respiration rate: 32 bpm. Effort: increased. Accessory muscle use: yes. Auscultation: equal air entry with no abnormal sounds.

Circulation
Heart rate: 166 bpm. Character: weak. Heart regularity: regular. Capillary refill time: >2 seconds.

Vital signs
RR: 32 bpm
HR: 166 bpm
BP: 80/50 mmHg
SpO_2: 90% on air
Blood sugar: 2.1 mmol/L
Temperature: 40.2 °C
Lead II ECG: sinus tachycardia with significant artefact

Exposure
Skin is hot to touch and dry.

TASK
Look through the information provided in this case study and highlight all of the information that might concern you as a paramedic.

What occurs to the human body as a result of continued exposure to extreme heat?

Thermoregulation fails as a result of environmental heat exposure exceeding the body's capacity to maintain homeostasis. The human body cools itself by sweating, but some conditions surpass this ability. Numerous factors affect cooling in hot environments. These can include obesity, cardiovascular disease, drug and alcohol use, and both youth and older age.

How is heat stroke different to heat exhaustion?

Heat stroke is life-threatening and occurs when thermoregulation completely fails (the body is unable to cool down and temperature rises catastrophically). It is often cited as a temperature above 40 °C with significant neurological dysfunction. Heat exhaustion is characterised by only minor changes in mental status, lassitude, headache and ongoing sweating.

Describe the clinical features of heat stroke.

- High core body temperature.
- Red or pale dry skin (no sweating).
- Tachycardia.
- Tachypnoea.
- Altered conscious state.
- Nausea/vomiting.

Based on the case study information, what are some of your clinical priorities?

- The environment is too hot, this patient must be removed from the current scene, ideally carried to the vehicle and placed inside (shade, air-conditioning, medical interventions). Remove clothing and commence active cooling. Immersion in cool water is advised, although it may not be practical here; alternatively, the patient can be sprayed with water and fanned to improve evaporative heat loss.
- Provide airway support (basic or advanced airways).
- Provide oxygenation (high-flow oxygen).
- Provide circulatory support (IV fluid challenge).

Case Progression

The patient is now in the vehicle on the stretcher with an oxygen mask and IV fluids running.

Patient assessment triangle
General appearance
The patient still has altered consciousness.

Circulation to the skin
Warm and pale.

Work of breathing
Fast, accessory muscle use.

SYSTEMATIC APPROACH
Danger
Nil.

Response
Responds to pain on the AVPU scale (grimace).

Airway
Clear – OP tube in situ.

Breathing
Respiration rate: 24 bpm. Effort: increased. Accessory muscle use: yes. Auscultation: clear, no added sounds.

Circulation
Heart rate: 120 bpm. Character: weak. Heart regularity: regular. Capillary refill time: >2 seconds.

Vital signs
RR: 24 bpm
HR: 120 bpm
BP: 100/75 mmHg
SpO$_2$: 93% 15 L non-rebreather
Blood sugar: 4.1 mmHg
Temperature: 38.7 °C
Lead II ECG: sinus tachycardia

Exposure
Skin feels warm to touch.

Describe the specific history you wish to obtain regarding this patient.

- Symptoms: as above.
- Allergies: iodine (anaphylaxis).

- Medications: Otodex.
- Past medical history: myringoplasty (2 years ago), slight obesity.
- Last ate: breakfast at 07:00, drank water (unknown).
- Events leading up to: walking for 3 hours in ambient temperatures exceeding 40 °C.

Based on the patient's marginal improvement as listed in the case progression and the patient's responses, what are your clinical priorities and considerations?

- Protect the patient from negative environmental consequences (heat and hypothermia from cooling).
- Maintain airway patency and oxygenation to achieve perfusion.
- Maintain circulatory support for normal systolic pressures.

LEVEL 2 CASE STUDY
Envenomation – snake bite

Information type	Data
Time of origin	09:15
Time of dispatch	09:16
On-scene time	09:29
Day of the week	Thursday
Nearest hospital	3 hours
Nearest backup	Flight intensive care crew, 60 minutes
Patient details	Name: Dora Edwards DOB: 14/02/1965

CASE

You have been called to a remote camp site for a 55-year-old female bitten by a seen snake while walking on a remote bush track.

Pre-arrival information

The area is difficult to access by road and requires 4×4 access that exceeds 45 minutes of off-road driving. The patient is a foreign tourist who has been camping, felt a sting on her left thigh and saw a 'long black snake' moving away.

Windscreen report

On arrival you see the patient walking towards the ambulance with a dressing on her thigh. She appears well perfused and alert.

Entering the location

The patient's partner greets you while telling the patient to sit back down on a camp chair. He states that they were walking approximately 500 m away when he heard her squeal. They both observed a black-looking snake slither away. He describes a 1 in bite on her left thigh. They decided to walk back and call an ambulance.

On arrival with the patient

The patient is sitting in a camp chair with her leg elevated on another chair. She states that she has a slight headache and some non-specific abdominal pain.

Patient assessment triangle
General appearance

She is fit and healthy, GCS 15/15 (Eyes 4, Speech 5, Motor 6). She is speaking in full sentences and able to maintain posture.

Circulation to the skin
Skin appears well perfused.

Work of breathing
Breathing is normal.

SYSTEMATIC APPROACH

Danger
Currently no obvious dangers.

Response
Alert on the AVPU scale.

Airway
Clear.

Breathing:
Respiration rate: 22 bpm. Effort: normal. Accessory muscle use: no. Auscultation: equal air entry with no abnormal sounds.

Circulation
Heart rate: 105 bpm. Character: normal. Heart regularity: regular. Capillary refill time: <2 seconds.

Vital signs
RR: 22 bpm
HR: 105 bpm
BP: 120/70 mmHg
SpO_2: 96% on air
Blood sugar: 4.1 mmol/L
Temperature: 37.1 °C
Lead II ECG: sinus tachycardia

Exposure
Her skin is well perfused and a quick observation behind the dressing reveals twin puncture marks approximately 2.5 cm in width on the left thigh.

TASK
Look through the information provided in this case study and highlight all the information that might concern you as a paramedic.

Based on the case study information, and being aware that the potential for paralysis exists with some envenomations, describe your clinical priorities.

Given that the patient saw the snake immediately following the bite, determining the cause of this case is not difficult. However, preempting the likely development and attempting to prevent deterioration are paramount in managing this patient. Snake venom mostly moves through the lymphatic system and can significantly alter central nervous system function. It is therefore imperative to slow the movement of the venom. The application of a pressure immobilisation bandage and splinting the affected limb greatly reduce lymphatic drainage. Potential airway and respiratory muscle paralysis may require airway management and ventilation, limiting movement and urgent transport to hospital.

Describe in detail the method of applying a pressure immobilisation bandage and explain the mechanism for this intervention – how it slows the venom.

Most bites occur in tissue and muscle. The venom proteins are often too large to travel through capillary walls, meaning the method of transport is predominantly via lymphatic drainage. Although lacking high-level evidence, the current practice of applying pressure immobilisation bandaging is widely accepted as best practice in the setting of Elapidae bite. A pressure bandage (10–15 cm wide) is placed directly over the bite and wound, down the limb to the most distal portion and back up to the most proximal area. Multiple bandages may be used.

Using the information provided and some relevant external sources, list and describe at least four non-specific envenomation symptoms that can be present.

- Nausea.
- Vomiting.
- Headache.
- Abdominal pain.
- Diarrhoea.
- Diaphoresis.

Case Progression

You have applied two pressure immobilisation bandages and splinted the legs together to limit movement. The patient is located in the ambulance on the stretcher.

Patient assessment triangle
General appearance
The patient is pale, claims to have a numb tongue and lips and is slurring her speech.

Circulation to the skin
Warm and pale.

Work of breathing
Fast, shallow.

SYSTEMATIC APPROACH
Danger
Nil.

Response
Responds to voice on the AVPU scale.

Airway
You notice when the patient speaks that she is accumulating saliva and some blood around her gums.

Breathing
Respiration rate: 28 bpm. Effort: increased. Accessory muscle use: no. Auscultation: clear, no added sounds.

Circulation
Heart rate: 130 bpm. Effort: weak radial pulse. Heart regularity: regular. Capillary refill time: >2 seconds.

Vital signs
RR: 28 bpm
HR: 130 bpm
BP: 90/60 mmHg
SpO$_2$: 92% on air
Blood sugar: 4.6 mmol/L
Temperature: 37.3 °C
Lead II ECG: sinus tachycardia

Exposure
Skin feels warm to touch.

Describe the specific history you would want to obtain regarding this patient.

- Symptoms: as above + time of bite, distance moved post-bite, onset time of first symptoms.
- Allergies: nil.
- Medications: Nordette.
- Past medical history: none.
- Last ate: breakfast at 07:00, drank alcohol last night (unsure of amount).
- Events leading up to: walking down a beach track when bitten.

Without immediate access to antivenom, and based on the patient's deterioration as described in the case progression, what are your clinical priorities and considerations?

- This is a time-critical patient requiring urgent emergency transport without delay.
- Maintain airway patency and ventilation to achieve oxygenation.
- Maintain circulatory support, aiming for normal systolic pressure.
- Keep limb splinted and bandaged.

LEVEL 2 CASE STUDY
Animal attack

Information type	Data
Time of origin	13:06
Time of dispatch	13:10
On-scene time	16:20
Day of the week	Sunday
Nearest hospital	42 minutes by road
Nearest backup	20 minutes by helicopter
Patient details	Name: Peter Sandringham DOB: 01/06/1948

CASE
You are responding to a 72-year-old male who is reported to have been bitten by a goanna at a remote beach location.

Pre-arrival information
The report is of a goanna attacking a dog and subsequently biting the dog's owner. The male patient is reported to have a large laceration on the lower leg that is bleeding heavily. The patient is located at a remote beach location. Helicopter assistance is not immediately available.

Windscreen report
You arrive after driving a significant distance along a beach. You note a male patient seated in a four-wheel drive vehicle with a blood-soaked bandage on his leg and a number of bystanders assisting. There appears to be a large amount of blood on the vehicle seat and sand around the patient.

On arrival with the patient
The patient is conscious, but appears pale and sweaty with a large laceration on his lower leg that is still actively bleeding.

Patient assessment triangle
General appearance
The patient is conscious and alert.

Circulation to the skin
Skin is pale and sweaty.

Work of breathing
Normal breathing.

SYSTEMATIC APPROACH

Danger
You are in a remote coastal location. Be aware of environmental dangers (sun, wind, animals).

Response
Alert on the AFPU scale and orientated to time, place, person, event.

Airway
Clear.

Breathing
Respiration rate: 18 bpm. Effort: normal. Accessory muscle use: no. Auscultation: equal air entry with no abnormal sounds.

Circulation
Heart rate: 130 bpm. Character: weak. Heart regularity: regular. Capillary refill time: >2 seconds. Patient is still actively bleeding, with blood visible on the car seat and in the sand.

Vital signs
RR: 18 bpm
HR: 130 bpm
BP: 100/60 mmHg
SpO_2: Not reading
Blood sugar: 5 mmol/L
Temperature: 35.2 °C
Lead II ECG: sinus tachycardia

Exposure
Skin is cool to touch. Chest wall movement is normal.

TASK
Look through the information provided in this case study and highlight all of the information that might concern you as a paramedic.

Using what you currently know about the case at this point, including what you may have seen and how the patient is presenting to you, what is your immediate clinical priority?

The patient appears to be suffering a significant uncontrolled haemorrhage. As this is potentially life-threatening, the haemorrhage needs to be immediately arrested utilising direct pressure and if necessary a tourniquet. Once the bleeding has stopped, it would be important to confirm the patient's perfusion status including conscious state, heart rate, blood pressure and capillary return.

Once the haemorrhage has been arrested, what is your ongoing plan of action?

The patient appears to have lost a significant amount of blood. After confirming that *all* haemorrhage has been controlled, position the patient supine, with preference for this being on the ambulance stretcher or alternatively reclining the vehicle seat back as far as possible. It would also be important to ensure the patient's temperature is maintained in a normal range to avoid the deleterious effects of hypothermia in a trauma patient. Provide pain relief, with options including methoxyflurane via a Penthrox inhaler and/or intranasal fentanyl. Insert a large-bore cannula (18 or 16 gauge) into a large vein, ensure this is patent and set up fluid at a TKVO rate. Preference would be to deliver blood or similar products if these were available and the patient was actively bleeding. Once IV access is established, manage the patient's pain with IV medications, with a preference for fentanyl.

Which of the following non-technical skills do you think are important to be able to safely treat this patient?
a. Effective verbal communication.
b. Effective non-verbal communication.
c. Empathy.
d. Reassurance.
e. Situational awareness.
f. All of the above.

f. All of the above.

Case Progression

The patient's haemorrhage has stopped and the pain is under control.

Patient assessment triangle
General appearance
The patient remains alert and orientated.

Circulation to the skin
Skin is pale but dry.

Work of breathing
Normal breathing.

SYSTEMATIC APPROACH

Danger
Nil.

Response
Alert.

Airway
Clear.

Breathing
Respiration rate: 18 bpm. Effort: normal. Accessory muscle use: no. Auscultation: clear, no added sounds.

Circulation
Heart rate: 104 bpm. Character: strong. Heart regularity: regular. Capillary refill time: 2 seconds.

Vital signs
RR: 18 bpm
HR: 104 bpm
BP: 110/85 mmHg
SpO$_2$: 90%
Blood sugar: 5 mmol/L
Temperature: 36.2 °C
Lead II ECG: sinus rhythm

Exposure
No accessory muscle use.

What kinds of questions would you ask this patient specifically related to his encounter with the lizard as part of the history-taking process?

See Table 15.2.

Table 15.2 History-taking questions

Animal attack
What happened? Where does it hurt? Do you know where you have been bitten?
When did this occur?
Are there any abnormal sensations distal to (at the furthest point away from) the injury site?
Can you describe the animal that bit you?

Medication history
Are you on any blood-thinning agents (aspirin, warfarin, apixaban, dabigatran, clexane, clopidogrel)?
Have you had tetanus vaccinations + 10-year boosters?
Do you take any other medications?
If so, which ones and how frequently?

F/SH (family and social history)
Any specific family medical history?

Past medical history (PMH)
Do you suffer from any bleeding disorders?
Do you have any other medical conditions?

Given the patient's improvement as listed in the case progression, and your current location, what are your choices now for what to do next?

It is important that the patient's condition is monitored closely. Particular attention should be given to the patient's wounds and the possibility of rebleeding occurring. The extrication plan needs to be put in motion with a particular decision regarding the best method of patient transport from the scene to definitive care. This decision will depend on the availability of transport resources. Options may include aircraft, watercraft or land-based transport. Fixed-wing aircraft will require a landing area appropriate for the aircraft's capabilities. Rotary-wing aircraft, if available, have the advantage of landing in a smaller area. Watercraft viability will depend on sea state and prevailing weather conditions. Land transport can be utilised if other options are not appropriate, ensuring regular re-evaluation of the patient's condition in order to quickly identify likely or actual deterioration.

LEVEL 3 CASE STUDY
Diving injury

Information type	Data
Time of origin	10:15
Time of dispatch	10:16
On-scene time	11:34
Day of the week	Saturday
Nearest hospital	3 hours
Nearest backup	Flight intensive care crew, 60 minutes
Patient details	Name: David Ligton
	DOB: 30/06/1985

CASE
You have been called to a diving vessel on a reef where a 35-year-old male has surfaced in respiratory distress during a scuba dive.

Pre-arrival information
The local marine rescue unit has been tasked to aid in your response and transport you and your equipment to the vessel. The area is in open water and the vessel has limited working space. The patient is located on the lower aft deck. Eight other scuba divers are on the vessel, none with medical training.

Windscreen report
On arrival the weather is warm and sunny, water conditions are 0.5 m SE. The vessels are moored together by the respective skippers and you make your way across to the dive boat.

Entering the scene
You are directed to the lower aft deck, where a patient in a wetsuit is positioned against the bulkhead left lateral in the sun. Diving equipment is lying close, by with two divers examining the patient's dive computer, gauges, oxygen tank and buoyancy control device (BCD). As you approach, they clear you a path to the patient and remove the equipment from the immediate area.

On arrival with the patient
He is alert, anxious, coughing and speaking in broken sentences. You notice he is shivering. Stuttering, he says that he has completed two dives this morning with what he describes as a standard diving profile with safety stops. He states that on surfacing to the boat he lost consciousness initially and has no recollection of how he got on the boat. His dive partner states that he was assisted onto the boat by the members of the team.

Patient assessment triangle
General appearance
The patient is in a wetsuit and shaking.

Circulation to the skin
Skin on his hands (the only visible part) is cool and pale.

Work of breathing
Breathing is fast and shallow.

SYSTEMATIC APPROACH
Danger
The vessel is bobbing gently in the swell and this makes it difficult to stand.

Response
Alert and orientated.

Airway
Clear, coughing.

Breathing
Respiration rate: 20 bpm. Effort: increased. Accessory muscle use: yes. Auscultation: equal air entry with full-field fine crackles.

Circulation
Heart rate: 110 bpm. Effort: weak radial. Heart regularity: regular. Capillary refill time: >2 seconds.

Vital signs
RR: 20 bpm
HR: 110 bpm
BP: 145/80 mmHg
SpO_2: 90% on air
Blood sugar: 5.1 mmol/L
Temperature: 36.2 °C
Lead II ECG: sinus tachycardia

> **TASK**
> Look through the information provided in this case study and highlight all of the information that might concern you as a paramedic.

Describe the fundamental differences between decompression sickness (DCS) and arterial gas embolism (AGE), and describe some of the suspected clinical features.

DCS is a result of bubbles of nitrogen and other dissolved gases expanding in the tissue as pressure decreases, causing local damage. AGE is caused by a rapid and uncontrolled over-inflation of the lungs (usually from a decrease in ambient pressure), which causes subsequent alveolar rupture. This allows the noxious passage of air into arterial circulation via the pulmonary vein. The symptoms of DCS include:

- Fatigue.
- Joint and muscle aches or pain.
- Clouded thinking.
- Numbness.
- Weakness.
- Paralysis.
- Rash.
- Poor coordination or balance.

Based on the case information, clinical features and initial history, list your clinical priorities to best manage this patient.

- Expose the patient and remove the wetsuit – provide warming to prevent hypothermia.
- Maintain airway patency – consider high-flow oxygen if available.
- Auscultate the patient.
- Head-to-toe assessment identifying any rashes, haemorrhages or fluid loss.
- Respiratory examination for signs of pneumothorax.
- Consider oral hydration or IV isotonic fluids (you must avoid fluid overload, which can worsen potential pulmonary oedema).
- Urgently consider need for hyperbaric opinion and medical recompression.

Considering the mechanism already described in the case details, list several complications (potential or suspected) that may arise from the pressure change.

- Barotrauma – damage to the tissue from gas-filled tissue expanding.
- Ear barotrauma – damage to the tympanic membrane affecting balance and hearing, causing dizziness or headache.
- Pulmonary barotrauma – rupture of the alveoli affecting breathing, perfusion, consciousness.

> **Case Progression**
>
> You have removed the wetsuit from the patient with shears and have covered him in a dry blanket. He is now located on a scoop with a pillow, but he wishes to maintain a left lateral position. You have administered high-flow oxygen at 15 Lpm as well as gained IV access for a small fluid challenge.
>
> **Patient assessment triangle**
> *General appearance*
> The patient is pale, with a notable red rash covering his midsection and back. He states he feels dizzy, has pins and needles in his hands and feet, and seems anxiously short of breath.

Circulation to the skin
Warm and pale.

Work of breathing
Laboured.

SYSTEMATIC APPROACH

Danger
The movement of the vessel continues.

Response
Responds to voice on the AVPU scale.

Airway
Clear, speaking in broken sentences.

Breathing
Respiration rate: 24 bpm. Effort: laboured. Accessory muscle use: no. Auscultation: equal air entry, full-field fine crackles.

Circulation
Heart rate: 120 bpm. Character: normal radial. Heart regularity: regular. Capillary refill time: >2 seconds.

Vital signs
RR: 24 bpm
HR: 120 bpm
BP: 130/75 mmHg
SpO_2: 93% 15 L non-rebreather
Blood sugar: 4.1 mmol/L
Temperature: 36.7 °C
Lead II ECG: sinus tachycardia

Exposure
Skin feels warm – obvious rash.

Given that DCS has a wide and sometimes varying range of presentations, outside of a standard history, what are some of the other details or considerations you should be bearing in mind regarding this patient?

- What was the maximum depth of the dive?
- What was the planned duration of the dive?
- What was the actual duration of the dive?
- What was the gas mixture used?
- Is it a diving site that is known to the team?
- What was the visibility like underwater?
- Has the patient been unwell/drinking?
- Did anyone notice any difficulty while diving?
- Was there a rapid ascent?
- What equipment was used (dive computer with dive profile)? If the diver has a dive computer and is referred to the hyperbaric facility, send the computer with them.
- Was there any bounce diving during this dive?
- What were the planned decompression stop time and depth?
- What was the actual decompression stop?

- How many dives have been logged in the past 24 hours?
- What was the surface interval between dives ?
- Has the patient flown prior to this dive?
- Any past history of DCS?
- Past medical history and medication.

Based on the patient's marginal improvement as listed in the case progression, and the patient's responses, what are your clinical priorities and considerations?

- Protect the patient from negative environmental consequences (heat and cold).
- Maintain airway patency and oxygenation to achieve perfusion.
- Maintain circulatory support, aiming for normal systolic pressure.
- Consider attempting contact with the hyperbaric chamber and, if possible, transmit imagery of the rash to them as well as patient details.
- If there is any chest pain, breathing difficulties, unconsciousness or declining neurologically, then this patient should be transported to the closest emergency department for assessment.

LEVEL 3 CASE STUDY
Acute altitude illness

Information type	Data
Time of origin	11:10
Time of dispatch	11:30
On-scene time	11:50
Day of the week	Wednesday
Nearest hospital	5 hours trekking
Nearest backup	20 minutes in non-medical helicopter (if available)
Patient details	Name: Sara Jane Waters DOB: 12/05/1988

CASE
You are the identified medic on a multiday trek. It is day 12 and today you will climb to the highest point of the trek at 5,643 m. You are walking at the rear of the group of 12 trekkers while ascending. At approximately 5,200 m you note that one of your team, a 32-year-old female, has drifted to the back, is stumbling and when questioned appears disorientated.

Pre-arrival information
Having reviewed each participant's medical history prior to the trek, you know that this patient has a history of mild asthma. You treated her for headache and nausea while at base camp the day before. When you checked in on her this morning she indicated she felt OK, with some very mild nausea and a headache. She hadn't slept well and didn't feel like breakfast.

Windscreen report
You are on a well-used track with many trekkers and porters passing by. There is heavy cloud cover at your current elevation, but this appears to dissipate at lower levels. It is cold with a light, intermittent breeze.

On arrival with the patient
You initially note that the patient is having trouble walking, is stumbling and lacks coordination. You help her to sit down and on questioning note that she is very confused.

Patient assessment triangle
General appearance
The patient is conscious and alert, but in no way orientated.

Circulation to the skin
Skin is warm and pink.

Work of breathing
Increased.

SYSTEMATIC APPROACH

Danger
There are significant environmental dangers (altitude, cold, wind, remoteness). You are well prepared for this and have the support of a substantial team of porters.

Response
Alert but significantly disorientated on the AVPU scale. The patient cannot recall where she is or why, the date or day of the week, or even her own name.

Airway
Clear.

Breathing
Respiration rate: 26 bpm. Effort: increased. Accessory muscle use: mild. Auscultation: equal air entry with no abnormal sounds.

Circulation
Heart rate: 110 bpm. Character: strong. Heart regularity: regular. Capillary refill time: 2 seconds.

Vital signs
RR: 26 bpm
HR: 110 bpm
BP: 150/95 mmHg
SpO_2: Not reading due to cold
Blood sugar: 5 mmol/L
Temp: not reading due to cold
Lead II ECG: sinus tachycardia

Exposure
Skin is warm to touch. Chest wall movement is slightly increased. You note that that the neurological deficits are bilateral and affect upper and lower limbs.

TASK
Look through the information provided in this case study and highlight all of the information that might concern you as a paramedic.

Using what you currently know about the case at this point, including what you may have seen and how the patient is presenting to you, which vital signs should you undertake first?

The patient appears to be neurologically affected, so you would want to identify potential causes. These would include hypoxia, hypercarbia, hypotension, hypothermia and hypoglycaemia. Identify her SpO_2 level, as well as blood pressure, temperature, blood glucose level and CO_2 level if able. Also undertake a focused neurological assessment to understand her complete neurological deficits and identify if this could be an acute event such as a stroke.

Once you have undertaken the essential vital signs, what would your next action be?

The patient is clearly disorientated with significant neurological deficit. Utilise your UHF radio to ask the team leader to stop the group and provide immediate shelter to undertake further assessment in a sheltered environment. Ask for assistance to warm the pulse oximeter, thermometer and glucometer to ensure they are functional. This presentation (acute onset of ataxia and disorientation at altitude) is likely to be associated with high altitude cerebral oedema (HACE). The immediate treatment for this is descent until the symptoms resolve, normally 300–1000 m. While preparing for descent, administer oxygen that the porters are carrying for this circumstance and closely monitor the patient's SpO_2, targeting 90%. This would be quickly followed by 8 mg dexamethasone (IM, IV or oral).

Which of the following non-technical skills do you think are important to be able to safely treat this patient?
a. Effective verbal communication.
b. Effective non-verbal communication.
c. Empathy.
d. Reassurance.
e. Situational awareness.
f. All of the above.

f. All of the above.

Case Progression

The patient is now in a shelter with oxygen running and 8 mg dexamethasone administered while you are organising the descent.

Patient assessment triangle
General appearance
The patient is alert but remains disorientated, although her level of understanding appears to be improving.

Circulation to the skin
Warm and pink.

Work of breathing
Normal breathing.

SYSTEMATIC APPROACH
Danger
Nil.

Response
Alert but disorientated on the AVPU scale.

Airway
Clear.

Breathing
Respiration rate: 18 bpm. Effort: normal. Accessory muscle use: no. Auscultation: clear, no added sounds.

Circulation
Heart rate: 96 bpm. Character: strong. Heart regularity: regular. Capillary refill time: 2 seconds.

Vital signs
RR: 18 bpm
HR: 96 bpm
BP: 130/85 mmHg
SpO_2: 90%
Blood sugar: 5 mmol/L
Temperature: 36.2 °C
Lead II ECG: sinus rhythm

Exposure
No accessory muscle use.

What kinds of questions would you ask this patient specifically related to altitude illness as part of the history-taking process?

See Table 15.3.

Table 15.3 History-taking questions

Altitude illness
What symptoms have you felt today? Headache? Nausea? Lethargy?
What have you had to eat/drink today? When?
What has your ascent profile been on this trip? How many days above 2500 m?
At what altitudes have you been sleeping?
Have you had any altitude illness previously? AMS? HACE? HAPE?
If so, when? Where? How high? How did you recover?
What altitudes have you been exposed to previously?

Medication history
Have you been taking altitude illness prophylaxis medication? Which (acetazolamide or dexamethasone)?
Do you take any other medications?
If so, which ones and how frequently?

F/SH (family and social history)
Any specific family medical history?
Do you drink alcohol? If so, how much and how often?
Who do you live with?
What do you do for work?

Past medical history (PMH)
Do you have any medical conditions apart from asthma?

Differential diagnoses (DDx) – What else could this be?
Hypoxia
Hypothermia
Stroke
Metabolic disorder
Overdose

Given the patient's improvement as listed in the case progression, and the patient's responses, what are your choices now about what to do next?

- Descend towards the closest medical help. If the patient is unable to walk despite the initial treatment, consider utilising a yak or donkey, or carrying her utilising the group and/or porters.

- Continue oxygen therapy as long as oxygen is available or until symptoms resolve.
- Continue dexamethasone 4 mg every 6 hours.
- Communicate with helicopter operators to assess availability of helicopter extrication should the patient not improve or if she deteriorates.

References and further reading

Department of Environment and Science (2019) Snakes of Central Queensland. https://environment.des.qld.gov.au/wildlife/animals/living-with/snakes/near-you/central-qld (accessed 18 October 2019).

Dow, J., Giesbrecht, G., Danzl, D.F. et al. (2019) Wilderness Medical Society clinical practice guidelines for the out-of-hospital evaluation and treatment of accidental hypothermia: 2019 update. *Wilderness & Environmental Medicine*, 30(Suppl 4): S47–S69. doi: 10.1016/j.wem.2019.10.002

Giesbrecht, G.G. (2018) 'Cold card' to guide responders in the assessment and care of cold-exposed patients. *Wilderness & Environmental Medicine*, 29(4): 499–503. doi: 10.1016/j.wem.2018.07.001

Johnson, M., Boyd, L., Grantham, H. & Eastwood, K. (2014) *Paramedic Principles and Practice ANZ*. St Peters: Harcourt.

Laskowski-Jones. L. & Jones, L.J. (2018) Management of cold injuries. In *Wilderness EMS* (ed. S. Hawkins), Philadelphia, PA: Wolters Kluwer, pp. 241–254.

Lipman, G., Gaudio, F., Eifling, K. et al. (2019) Wilderness Medical Society practice guidelines for the prevention and treatment of heat illness: 2019 update. *Wilderness & Environmental Medicine*, 30(Suppl 4): S33–S46. doi: 10.1016/j.wem.2018.10.004

Luks, A.M., Auerbach, P.S., Freer, L. et al. (2019) Wilderness Medical Society practice guidelines for the prevention and treatment of acute altitude illness: 2019 update. *Wilderness & Environmental Medicine*, 30(Suppl 4): S3–S18. doi: 10.1016/j.wem.2019.04.006

Quinn, R.H., Wedmore, I., Johnson, E. et al. (2014) Wilderness Medical Society practice guidelines for basic wound management in the austere environment. *Wilderness & Environmental Medicine*, 25(3): 295–310. doi: 10.1016/j.wem.2014.04.005

Smith, B., Bledsoe, B.E. & Nicolazzo, P. (2018) General management of trauma in the wilderness. In *Wilderness EMS* (ed. S. Hawkins), Philadelphia, PA: Wolters Kluwer, pp. 371–392.

Thalmann, E.D. (2004) Decompression illness: What is it and what is the treatment? DAN: Divers Alert Network. https://www.diversalertnetwork.org/medical/articles/Decompression_Illness_What_Is_It_and_What_Is_The_Treatment (accessed 18 October 2019).

Zafren, K. (2018) Management of altitude illness. In *Wilderness EMS* (ed. S. Hawkins), Philadelphia, PA: Wolters Kluwer, pp. 271–288.

Zafren, K., Giesbrecht, G.. Danzl, D.F. et al. (2014) Wilderness Medical Society practice guidelines for the out-of-hospital evaluation and treatment of accidental hypothermia: 2014 update. *Wilderness & Environmental Medicine*, 25(Suppl 4), S66–S85. doi: 10.1016/j.wem.2014.10.010

Chapter 16 Mining emergencies

Paul Grant[1] and Curtis Northcott[2]

[1] Registered Paramedic, Mines Emergency Rescue and Response (MERR), QLD, Australia
[2] RMA Medical Rescue and Registered Paramedic, Mount Isa, QLD, Australia

---

CHAPTER CONTENTS

Level 1:	Febrile seizure
Level 1:	Monoarticular trauma (ankle dislocation)
Level 2:	Unstable angina
Level 2:	Heat stroke
Level 3:	Chemical burns
Level 3:	Hyperglycaemic hyperosmolar non-ketotic syndrome

LEVEL 1 CASE STUDY
Febrile seizure

Information type	Data
Time of origin	11:06
Time of dispatch	11:10
On-scene time	11:15
Day of the week	Sunday
Nearest hospital	5 hours
Nearest backup	Intensive care paramedic on duty, immediate Royal Flying Doctor Service, 6 hours
Patient details	Name: Regina Rodriguez DOB: 05/05/2015

CASE

The Emergency Response Team have been called to a 5-year-old-female who has collapsed to the ground in a local park. The nearest mine site has established a medical response protocol as part of a collaborative emergency services agreement with the local Indigenous community.

Pre-arrival information
A sitrep confirms the young female is actively seizing. The caller is unsure if the patient is breathing or has a pulse. The call centre encourages the responder to monitor the patient until medical assistance arrives.

Windscreen report
The area outside the local park appears safe. A group of people are trying to assist the patient.

Entering the location
You are greeted by a distressed parent, who tells you that their daughter has a history of seizures and has been shaking on the ground for the past 5 minutes.

Clinical Cases in Paramedicine, First Edition. Edited by Sam Willis, Ian Peate, and Rod Hill.
© 2021 John Wiley & Sons Ltd. Published 2021 by John Wiley & Sons Ltd.

On arrival with the patient

The patient is actively seizing on the grass in the park. Her mother is screaming and distraught, her father is in a state of distress but is actively talking to you. You also note vomit coming out of the patient's mouth.

Paediatric assessment triangle
General appearance
The patient is unconscious and actively seizing.

Circulation to the skin
Central cyanosis and mildly pale.

Work of breathing
Abnormal position.

SYSTEMATIC APPROACH
Danger
Nil.

Response
Nil – the patient is seizing.

Airway
Unable to assess as the patient is seizing. The airway in compromised due to the presence of trismus and vomit.

Breathing
Unknown as the patient is seizing.

Circulation
Unknown as the patient is seizing.

Vital signs
Unknown as the patient is seizing.

Exposure
The 5-year-old patient is placed on the stretcher in the ambulance at the end of the seizure and her clothes removed to allow a thorough head-to-toe examination is performed.

TASK

Look through the information provided in this case study and highlight all the information that might concern you as a paramedic.

List several causes of seizures.

- Hypoglycaemia (Halawa et al., 2015; Brennan & Whitehouse, 2012).
- Meningococcal septicaemia (Larsen et al., 2019).
- Septic shock (Reznik et al., 2017).
- Febrile convulsions (Leung et al., 2018).
- Idiopathic seizure disorder (Dragoumi et al., 2013).
- Cardiac disorders, e.g. dysrhythmias, long QT syndrome, hypertrophic obstructive cardiomyopathy (Sabu et al., 2016; Scalais et al., 2013).
- Epilepsy.

What pharmacological agents are available to stop this seizure? What are the routes of administration and what dosages would be appropriate for this case?

- Pharmacology agent: midazolam. Presentation 5 mg/1 mL. Route of administration: IM, IV, rectal, buccal, nasal.
- Common drug calculation formulas:
  - Weight (kg) = (Age*3) + 7
  - Dose (mg) = Weight*(mg/kg)
  - $Volume\,(mL) = \dfrac{Required\,Strength}{Stock\,Strength} * Stock\,Volume$
  - $Midazolam\,quick\,method\,(mg) = \dfrac{\left(\left(Age*3\right)+7\right)*2}{10}$
  - $Midazolam\,quick\,method\,(mL) = \dfrac{\left(\left(Age*3\right)+7\right)*2*2}{100}$
- Dosage calculation – IM
  - Weight (kg) = (5*3) + 7 = 22 kg
  - Dose (mg) = Weight*(mg/kg) = 0.2*22 = 4.4 mg
  - $Quick\,method\,(mg) = Weight\,(kg) = \dfrac{22*2}{10} = 4.4\,mg$
- Volume dosage – IM
  - Weight (kg) = (5*3) + 7 = 22 kg
  - $Volume\,(mL) = \left(\dfrac{4.4\,mg}{5\,mg}\right)*1 = 0.88\,mL$
  - $Quick\,method\,(mL) = \dfrac{88}{100} = 0.88\,mL$
  - Total dosage = 4.4 mg/0.88 mL
- Dosage calculation – nasal
  - Weight (kg) = (5*3) + 7 = 22 kg
  - Dose (mg) = Weight*(mg/kg) = 0.2*22 = 4.4 mg
  - $Quick\,method\,(mg) = Weight\,(kg) = \dfrac{22*2}{10} = 4.4\,mg$
- Volume Dosage – nasal
  - Weight (kg) = (5*3) + 7 = 22 kg
  - Remember to add 0.1 mL for dead space
  - $Volume\,(mL) = \left(\left(\dfrac{4.4\,mg}{5\,mg}\right)*1\right)+0.1\,mL = 0.98\,mL$
  - $Quick\,method\,(mL) = \dfrac{88}{100}+0.1 = 0.98\,mL$
  - Total dosage = 4.4 mg/0.98 mL for nasal midazolam

Case Progression

4.4 mg/0.88 mL of IM midazolam has been administered and high-flow oxygen has been applied to the patient. Approximately 5 minutes have now passed since the midazolam was administered and oxygen placed onto the patient's face.

  The parents tell you that their daughter has a history of seizures, but they have been able to manage them in the past.

Patient assessment triangle
General appearance
The patient is in a lethargic state.

Circulation to the skin
The patient is extremely pale.

Work of breathing
Increased effort and rate of breathing.

SYSTEMATIC APPROACH
Danger
Nil.

Response
Verbal on the AVPU scale.

Airway
Clear.

Breathing
Accessory muscle use: no. Auscultation: clear, no added sounds. Effort: normal.

Circulation
Capillary refill time: >2 seconds. Effort: strong. Pulse regularity: regular.

Vital signs
RR: 35 bpm
HR: 170 bpm
BP: Systolic 60 palp
SpO$_2$: 89%
Blood sugar: 6.2 mmol/L
Temperature: 39.8 °C
Lead II ECG: sinus tachycardia

Exposure
A mottled purpuric rash, non-blanching, has been found on the patient's torso.

TASK
Look through the information provided in this case study and highlight all the information that might concern you as a paramedic.

How do you differentiate a blanching rash from a non-blanching rash?

A non-blanching rash does not fade when pressed down for a short period of time (Thomas et al., 2016; Szima et al., 2017). You can even pull the skin tight and the colour will not fade.

What is your diagnosis of this patient? Using your clinical judgement, what is the management of this child going to be?

The patient has a mottled purpuric rash, non-blanching, found on her torso, tachypnoea and has had a seizure. The differential diagnosis is meningococcal septicaemia.

With this, you should arrange rapid critical care paramedic backup and early notification to the Royal Flying Doctor Service. The patient should receive ceftriaxone and IV fluids. The dosage that this patient requires is as follows:

- 50 mg/kg (maximum dosage 1 g)
- Weight (kg) = (5*3) + 7 = 22 kg
- 22 kg*50 mg = 1100 mg
- Total maximum dose 1 g
- Thus, the patient requires a dosage of 1 g

How do you prepare ceftriaxone for IM, IV and IO routes of administration?

- IM preparation: Reconstitute 1 g ceftriaxone with 3.6 mL water for injection in a 10 mL syringe to achieve a final concentration of 1 g/4 mL (250 mg/mL).
- IV preparation: Reconstitute 1 g ceftriaxone with 9.6 mL water for injection in a 10 mL syringe to achieve a final concentration of 1 g/10 mL (100 mg/mL). This should be provided as a slow push over 3–5 minutes.
- IO preparation: Reconstitute 1 g ceftriaxone with 9.6 mL water for injection in a 10 mL syringe to achieve a final concentration of 1 g/10 mL (100 mg/mL). This should be provided as a slow push over 3–5 minutes. An IO should only be undertaken if it is within your scope of practice in paramedicine.

Why do ambulance services allow paramedics to administer a broad-spectrum antibiotic in this type of clinical case?

The initiation of antibiotics in the out-of-hospital setting varies by service and country.

When patients receive antibiotics, in the first hour they have a survival rate of 79.9%; the mortality rate for each hour's delay in administration increased by 7.6% and resulted in a decrease in survival over the following 6 hours (Martin & Weiss, 2015; Rhodes et al., 2017; Gaieski et al., 2010; Sterling et al., 2016; Joo et al., 2014). Thus, broad-spectrum antibiotics should be given within 1 hour of diagnosis (Daniels et al., 2011; Johnston et al., 2017; Robson et al., 2009), antibiotic administration reflects on patient outcomes and maximisers the chances of survival. More importantly, the time of administration of antibiotics and source of infection are independently associated with mortality (Qian et al., 2018).

A study by Alam et al. (2018) compared early antibiotic administration in the hospital versus earlier antibiotic administration in the ambulance. A randomised trial (n=2672) compared patients who received antibiotics in the ambulance (n=1535) to patients who were recognised to be septic, but received no pre-hospital antibiotics (n=1137). The study found that the treatment group received antibiotics a median of 96 minutes earlier than usual care, decreasing to 70 minutes during the study. There was no difference either between groups in the primary outcome of 28-day mortality, with treatment group mortality 7.8% and usual care mortality 8.2%, or in the secondary outcomes of 90-day mortality, ICU admission rate, and ICU and hospital lengths of stay. However, patients who received usual care had a higher hospital readmission rate (10.5% vs 6.6%).

Why is the patient being provided with additional IV fluids and what is the fluid resuscitation rate going to be?

When administering fluids, the aim is to correct hypovolemic states, augment cardiac output and restore organ perfusion in patients who have sepsis-induced hypoperfusion (Rhodes et al., 2017; Semler & Rice, 2016; NICE, 2016; Robson et al., 2009).

Jozwiak et al. (2018) discuss the dynamics of variables in fluid resuscitation regarding fluid responsiveness and individualisation in regard to initial fluid infusion. During the first 3 hours of resuscitation a fixed volume at 30 mL/kg is recommended (Jozwiak et al., 2018). Nevertheless, caution is required in patients who have sepsis-induced hypoperfusion, since there is the risk of pulmonary or systemic oedema for patients who are receiving aggressive fluid administration (Byrne, 2017; Semler & Rice, 2016).

The overall aim when treating patients with sepsis-induced hypoperfusion is a mean arterial pressure of >85 mmHg or systolic BP >100 mmHg (Rhodes et al., 2017; Jozwiak et al., 2018; Byrne, 2017; Leone et al., 2015; Singer et al., 2016; NICE, 2016; Robson et al., 2009).

Evidence shows (Kelm et al., 2015) that reduced hospital mortality has been shown in patients who receive adequate initial fluid resuscitation compared to those who receive delayed fluid resuscitation (18.3% vs 56.6%, p<0.001).

What is more, the odds of hospital mortality are lower among severe sepsis patients treated with pre-hospital IV fluids alone (p<0.01). The evidence supporting this claim shows a strong correlation of a positive fluid balance with an increased risk of fluid overload and subsequent mortality (Seymour et al., 2014).

The paediatric population may require 60 mL/kg of 0.9% isotonic normal saline within 15 minutes of identification of sepsis (Brierley et al., 2009).

LEVEL 1 CASE STUDY
Monoarticular trauma (ankle dislocation)

Information type	Data
Time of origin	13:00
Time of dispatch	13:02
On-scene time	13:20
Day of the week	Wednesday
Nearest hospital	4 hours (Royal Flying Doctor Service depending on priority)
Nearest backup	Onsite assistance and telehealth with medical officer
Patient details	Name: Steven Magill
	DOB: not recorded

CASE
An emergency call is made via radio describing an underground coal mine worker injuring his ankle and being in extreme pain. The worker was walking in a pool of water holding two heavy equipment bags when he stumbled and fell. The responders assisted the worker to a safe place and described his ankle as at a 90° angle.

Pre-arrival information
Immediately a differential diagnosis of a dislocated ankle was made, the first responders were advised to keep the worker warm and reassure him that help was on the way, and not to attempt any manipulation on his ankle.

Windscreen report
The underground mining operational area is a pool of water and the ground conditions are extremely hazardous. The workers were setting up the blasting area when the accident occurred.

Entering the location
The area was saturated with water, which had created pools.

On arrival with the patient
The worker was sitting up, leaning forward, and he was showing signs of extreme pain and stated that the pain was excruciating.

Patient assessment triangle
General appearance
The worker is in obvious pain, he is covered in mud and is cold and wet. His ankle is being supported by a work colleague and it is externally rotated laterally at 90°.

Circulation to the skin
He has cold hands, it is difficult to see if his face is pale as he is covered in mud. There is noted pallor in the affected limb.

Work of breathing
There is equal rise and fall of the chest with effective ventilation. No added sounds are heard. The rate is increased.

SYSTEMATIC APPROACH

Danger

The area is hazardous and caution is needed with simple tasks.

Response

Alert on the AVPU scale.

Airway

Patent.

Breathing

Accessory muscle use: no. Auscultation: clear, no added sounds. Effort: normal.

Circulation

Unknown at this stage.

Vital signs

RR: 24 bpm

HR: 120 bpm

BP: 135/100 mmHg

Blood sugar: 5.9 mmol/L

SpO_2: 97%

Temperature: 36.2 °C

GCS: 15/15 (E4, V5, M6)

Patient's weight: 130 kg

Exposure

The patient is wet, cold and shivering.

TASK

Look through the information provided in this case study and highlight all the information that might concern you as a paramedic.

Based on the information given in this case, what is your differential diagnosis?

The patient has a dislocated ankle and/or fracture.

A dislocated ankle often occurs in conjunction with a fracture or complete rupture of the ankle ligaments. It is rare, as all the ligaments on one side of the ankle must rupture. The force that is required to dislocate an ankle joint is considerable. The patient weighs approximately 130 kg and he was carrying two large equipment bags when he stood on a submerged object and rolled his ankle laterally. The patient was also wearing safety boots that support the ankle, which indicates that the ankle was placed under an enormous amount of force when it dislocated. This mechanism of injury would suggest a fracture due to the excessive forces the ankle was placed under.

What are your main considerations and your immediate actions in this case?

The patient is in danger of hypothermia and you must address this immediately while assessing the injury. Complete a primary survey, stabilise the patient and administer pain relief. Once the patient has been stabilised, the boot should be cut off without moving the ankle, which would be a challenge in this environment.

The emergency service officers who are assisting you should prepare a vacuum splint and assist in its application with extreme care. The ankle should be placed in the vacuum splint and supported in the current position with a pillow. The distal neurovascular function should be monitored regularly for sensory and motor response.

Case Progression

The team has stabilised the worker's leg and placed it in a vacuum splint, thus immobilising his leg. A pillow has been placed under his injured ankle for support. His wet clothes have been removed and several thermal blankets placed around his body. The patient's ankle is kept in the lateral position even though neurovascular sensory and motor function is compromised. The patient's external capillary refill time is >5 seconds, which is concerning, but the paramedic does not attempt a midline alteration of the patient's ankle in the current environment. The case is time critical, and there is an obvious danger of ischaemia or, worse, muscular necrosis.

Patient assessment triangle
General appearance
Warm and stable. Prominent protrusion of the talus bone and the ankle is laterally rotated at 90°.

Circulation to the skin
Injury area cold, pallor, capillary refill time >5 seconds.

Work of breathing
Faster than usual, but otherwise good quality.

SYSTEMATIC APPROACH
Danger
The patient is placed in the ambulance carefully and there is no obvious danger.

Response
Precautions due to analgesia administration.

Airway
Patent.

Breathing
Accessory muscle use: no. Auscultation: clear, no added sounds. Effort: normal.

Circulation
Injured area poor circulation. Patient is warm and stable.

Vital signs
RR: 18 bpm
HR: 85 bpm
BP: 115/85 mmHg
SpO_2: 98%
Blood sugar: 6.2 mmol/L
Temperature: 36.9 °C
Lead II ECG: sinus rhythm
Weight: 130 kg

What analgesia would be appropriate in this case?

- After consent has been given and the appropriate contraindications have been discussed (Borobia et al., 2019), immediately administer 3 mL methoxyflurane to subdue the pain.
- Once the paramedic has gained peripheral venous access (Ahmadi et al., 2016):
  - IV: 2–4 mL morphine over 1–5 minutes as a slow push.
  - IM: An option would be to administer 5 mL morphine IM initial dose if the environment is too hazardous to place an IV line.

- Or:
  - Nasal: 25–50 µg fentanyl equally divided and administered in each nostril, to a maximum of 200 µg.
  - IV: 25 µg fentanyl, to a maximum of 100 µg.
- Caution must be taken when administering narcotic analgesia as it could cause CNS depression and as such a reversal agent should always be available (Ahmadi et al., 2016).

Should the joint should be realigned if neurovascular compromise is identified (remember you are in a remote setting), for example revealing a cold, discoloured and pulseless foot?

Yes, under the directions of a medical officer.

Case Progression

The patient is taken to the medical centre, where the paramedic escalates the emergency to the Royal Flying Doctor Service, who indicate that it will be at least a 5 hour delay due to the current workload.

There are several telehealth discussions between the paramedic and the emergency medical officer, and the decision is made to realign the ankle due to the extended time it would take to get to definitive care and given the patient's condition. The medical centre is set up for the paramedic to conduct the procedure under the direction of the emergency medical officer via telehealth consultation. This is accomplished by in-line traction with counter-traction.

What pharmacological agents could be used for undertaking anaesthesia in a remote environment?

Induction for anaesthesia (Sinner & Graf, 2008; Kurdi et al., 2014; Newton & Fitton, 2008; Rosenbaum & Palacios, 2019):

- Agent: ketamine hydrochloride
- Route: IV
- Dose: 0.25–2 mg/kg single dose
- Weight 130 kg
- 2 mg*130 kg = 260 mg
- Total maximum dose: 150 mg
- Syringe preparation
  - Mix 200 mg (2 mL) ketamine with 18 mL water for injection in a 20 mL syringe to achieve a final concentration of 10 mg/mL.
  - *All syringes must be labelled appropriately.*
  - Total maximum dose: 150 mg
  - $Volume = \dfrac{Drug\ Dose * Drug\ volume}{Stock\ Strength}$
  - $Volume = \dfrac{150\ mg * 20\ mL}{200\ mg} = 15\ mL$
  - Required dosage 150 mg in 15 mL

Relaxant (FDA, 2008):

- Agent: rocuronium
- Route: IV
- Dose: 0.6–1.2 mg/kg
  - Weight 130 kg
  - 2 mg*130 kg = 260 mg.
  - Total maximum dose: 150 mg

LEVEL 2 CASE STUDY
Unstable angina

Information type	Data
Time of origin	22:45
Time of dispatch	23:00
On-scene time	23:15
Day of the week	Tuesday
Nearest hospital	5 hours
Nearest backup	Intensive care crew, 3 hours
	Royal Flying Doctor Service, 4 hours
Patient details	Name: Ben Dilkin
	DOB: 01/08/1964

CASE

You have been called to a 56-year-old male with a sudden onset of chest pain while driving mobile plant.

Pre-arrival information

The patient is conscious, breathing and being attended by the emergency services officer (ESO).

Windscreen report

The patient is lying supine next to the mobile plant on the go line.

Entering the location

Site access is clear and safe.

On arrival with the patient

The patient is supine on the ground, clutching his chest, with the Emergency Services Officers assisting him. As you arrive at the patient, the ESO tells you that the patient has a history of hypertension.

Patient assessment triangle

General appearance

The patient is alert and looks to have visible chest discomfort (Levine's sign), is diaphoretic and has vomited.

Circulation to the skin

Mild pallor.

Work of breathing

Pursed lips, tachypnoea.

SYSTEMATIC APPROACH

Danger

Nil.

Response
Alert on the AVPU scale.

Airway
Clear, patent.

Breathing
Accessory muscle use: no. Auscultation: clear air entry, no added sounds. Effort: mildly increased.

Circulation
Capillary refill time: 2 seconds. Heart regularity: regular. Mild pallor to the peripheries. Radial pulse effort: weak.

Vital signs
RR: 20 bpm
HR: 105 bpm
BP: 140/90 mmHg
SpO_2: 94%
Blood sugar: 5.0 mmol/L
Temperature: 36.5 °C
GCS: 15/15 (E4, M5, V6)
Lead II ECG: sinus tachycardia with ST elevation in I and aVL; ST depression III and aVF;
ST elevation in V3–6

Exposure
No obvious abnormalities found on the exposure of the chest.

History (OPQRST)
Onset (what they were doing) – driving a dump truck.
Provocation (what makes the pain better or worse) – nothing, it is continuous discomfort.
Quality (how it is described) – tight, griping.
Radiation (whether it moves anywhere) – into the upper abdomen.
Severity (1–10) – 7
Timing (how long they have had it) – 1 hour 15 minutes

TASK
Look through the information provided in this case study and highlight all the information that might concern you as a paramedic.

What should you consider in terms of the location of this patient and resource management?

Extrication, Emergency Escalation Process (EEP) and additional resources such as intensive care paramedics, Helicopter Emergency Medical Service (HEMS), Royal Flying Doctor Service (RFDS).

What should the paramedic assess first? What are the treatment priorities?

The first assessment is the primary survey: DRABCDE. Treatment priorities are as follows:

- Rest and reassurance (reassurance assists the patient to stay calm).
- Thorough history taking – SAMPLE, OPQRST.
- Aspirin 300 mg (Wee et al., 2015; Dai & Ge, 2012).
- Glyceryl trinitrate (GTN) 400 µg initially, thereafter as required (Boden et al., 2015; Wee et al., 2015).
- Ondansetron 8 mg IV.

- Fentanyl 50 µg IV (Weldon et al., 2016).
- 12 Lead ECG (Wee et al., 2015).
- Oxygen, but only in the presence of hypoxia or low oxygen saturations (Andell et al., 2019).

What is the pre-flight clinical intervention regarding peripheral access that must be adhered to on a patient who is being emergency evacuated by the RFDS?

Most patients undergoing air transport require at least one site of IV access. More seriously ill patients and those requiring ongoing fluids, blood or drug infusions need two peripheral IV lines, to ensure backup access if one line fails (as commonly occurs). It is key to remember always to work distally and an attempt always is made in a peripheral vein, unless otherwise indicated for a major resuscitation.

According to Thoracic Society of Australia and New Zealand guidelines, should the patient be provided with supplemental oxygen given his current SpO2 status?

No – TSANZ recommends that SpO_2 is maintained between 92 and 96%. If oxygen falls below this range, titration of oxygen administration should occur (Beasley et al., 2015).

Case Progression

The diagnosis based on the ECG is sinus rhythm with an anterolateral STEMI (Burns, 2019). The following medications have now been administered: 300 mg aspirin, 400 µg GTN, an initial dose of analgesia provided via the IM route due to the environment. The patient is then transported back to the mine site medical centre, where IV access is obtained in the right dorsal venous arch following an unsuccessful attempt in the right antecubital fossa (ACF) vein.

Patient assessment triangle
General appearance
The patient is unresponsive.

Circulation to the skin
Central cyanosis.

Work of breathing
Cheyne–Stokes respirations.

SYSTEMATIC APPROACH
Danger
Nil.

Response
Unconscious on the AVPU scale.

Airway
Clear.

Breathing
Effort: increased. Accessory muscle use: yes. Auscultation: clear, no added sounds.

Circulation
Capillary refill time: not recorded. Effort: weak. Heart regularity: regular.

Vital signs
RR: 35 bpm
HR: 155 bpm
BP: 175/115 mmHg
Blood sugar: 6.8 mmol/L
SpO_2: 96%
Temperature: 36.5 °C
12 Lead ECG: global STEMI
Approximately 3 minutes after these vital signs are taken, the patient collapses and becomes unresponsive.

> **TASK**
> Look through the information provided in this case study and highlight all the information that might concern you as a paramedic.

Now the patient has collapsed, what are the immediate actions that should be taken?

- Follow the chain of survival: early recognition, early CPR, early defibrillation, early hospital care (Hasselqvist-Ax et al., 2015; Wissenberg et al., 2013).
- Follow your providers' life support guidelines (Basic Life Support or Advanced Life Support); remember it is key that BLS or ALS is provided in the first 6 minutes (Kurza et al., 2018).
- Notification to RFDS/HEMS for immediate evacuation to definitive care.

What further options would a critical care paramedic have in this situation given the remote setting?

- Critical care paramedics might have the option for dual-antiplatelet therapy (DAPT), including clopidogrel 300 mg loading dose if thrombolysis is planned, 600 mg if percutaneous coronary intervention (PCI) is planned (Khan et al., 2016; Yudi et al., 2016).
- Ticagrelor 180 mg loading dose, 90 mg BD for moderate- to high-risk non-ST elevation acute coronary syndrome (NSTEACS) treated conservatively or invasively, and STEMI planned for primary PCI (Yudi et al., 2016).
- Prasugrel 60 mg may be used in place of clopidogrel in patients with STEMI of less than 12 hours where PCI is planned, or NSTEACS after angiography and before PCI (Yudi et al., 2016).

LEVEL 2 CASE STUDY
Heat stroke

Information type	Data
Time of origin	13:00
Time of dispatch	13:05
On-scene time	13:10
Day of the week	Saturday
Nearest hospital	3 hours
Nearest backup	3 hours
Patient details	Name: Mark Hibson DOB: 12/09/1985

> **CASE**
> You are called to a 35-year-old male in a delirious state at a mining site. You deploy to the emergency with two emergency service officers (ESOs).
>
> **Pre-arrival information**
> Situational reports are sent every few minutes to the response team while you travel. First responders have been instructed to secure the scene and commence basic life support protocols, and have stripped the patient down to his underwear. Medical assistance ETA 5 minutes. You note that this is the third day of an extreme heatwave and the workers have been working in the area during this time.
>
> **Windscreen report**
> The temperature is stifling, rising above 50 °C in the immediate area.
>
> **On arrival with the patient**
> The patient is lying on a bed in the medical facility in only his underwear. A fan has been placed next to him and one of the first responders is spraying a fine mist of cold water over his body (Evaporative cooling).

Patient assessment triangle
General appearance
The patient appears fatigued.

Circulation to the skin
A first responder says the worker was not sweating when they placed him in the medical centre and was not himself, stating he was saying things that didn't make sense.

Work of breathing
Tachypnoea.

SYSTEMATIC APPROACH
Danger
The patient has been removed from the hazardous environment.

Response
Pain on the AVPU scale.

Airway
Clear and patent.

Breathing
Accessory muscle use: no. Auscultation: clear. Effort: labored.

Circulation
Radial pulses palpated, weak, fast.

Vital signs
RR: 32 bpm
HR: 120 bpm
BP: 116/52 mmHg
SpO_2: 94% on room air
Blood sugar: 5.2 mmol/L
Temperature: 40.0 °C
GCS 10/15 (E4, V2, M4)
ECG Lead II: sinus tachycardia

Exposure
Active cooling in progress.

TASK
Look through the information provided in this case study and highlight all the information that might concern you as a paramedic.

What are the two types of heatstroke? Name and describe them.

- Classic: The classic type affects individuals with an underlying chronic medical condition, most often older patients (Székely et al., 2015).
- Exertional: The exertional type generally occurs in younger, otherwise healthy individuals undergoing prolonged heavy exercise or heavy work tasks under high ambient temperature and humidity (Székely et al., 2015).

What are the potential locations where icepacks can be placed to assist in the cooling of this patient?

Icepacks should be placed on the groin, axillae and back of the neck. Excess clothing should also be removed to assist with rapid cooling (Bouchama et al., 2007). Ice sheet cooling is also another method that can be used, through wrapping the patient in bedsheets that have been soaked in ice water to reduce the patient's body temperature (Butts et al., 2017).

Case Progression

The patient is in the mine site medical centre where active cooling has begun, by placing ice packs on the groin, axillae and back of the neck. The medical centre air conditioner is at 16 °C. IV access has been obtained in the left antecubital fossa (ACF) following an unsuccessful attempt in the right ACF vein.

SYSTEMATIC APPROACH

Danger
Nil.

Response
Alert on the AVPU scale.

Airway
Clear.

Breathing
Accessory muscle use: yes. Auscultation: clear, no added sounds. Effort: increased.

Circulation
Capillary refill time: not recorded. Effort: moderate. Heart regularity: regular.

Vital signs
RR: 32 bpm
HR: 112 bpm
BP: 115/80
Blood sugar: 5.2 mmol/L
SpO$_2$: 85%
Temperature: 36.5 °C
12-Lead ECG: sinus tachycardia

Exposure
As stated for cooling. No injuries identified.

What treatment should be provided to this patient?

- IV access bilateral 16 gauge cannula administration of cold saline.
- Aggressively treat hypovolemia and hypotension, commence fluid challenge.
- Continuous monitoring is paramount.
- Ice packs wrapped in towels placed in specific locations.
- Spray fine mist from a bottle of cold water onto the patient.
- Fan directed at specific areas.
- Patient's vital signs must be monitored closely during the cooling process.
- If the patient's body temperature drops below normal (36 °C), he will be at risk of hypothermia.

Why is it important to monitor the skin during the cooling process?

The integumentary system, particularly for patients who have prolonged icepacks placed on skin that is not covered appropriately, is susceptible to damage (Butts et al., 2017; Tan et al., 2017). Covering ice packs with a towel or sheet and regularly adjusting the site of application will mitigate this risk (Tan et al., 2017).

LEVEL 3 CASE STUDY
Chemical burns

Information type	Data
Time of origin	13:55
Time of dispatch	14:00
On-scene time	14:05
Day of the week	Sunday
Nearest hospital	7 hours
Nearest backup	Intensive care support, 3 hours Royal Flying Doctor Service, 5 hours
Patient details	Name: Janine Scleen DOB: 16/06/1975

CASE
You have been called to a 45-year-old woman who is suffering alkaline burns. An emergency activation has been initiated, indicating the location of the emergency is in the processing plant on a mine site.

Pre-arrival information
A sitrep confirms the patient is unconscious and is displaying agonal breathing.

Windscreen report
The area outside the processing plant appears to be safe.

Entering the location
First on the scene is the Emergency Services Officer (ESO), who has not approached the patient due to the danger of the hazardous environment. However, the ESO is instructing the emergency response team (ERT) to don the appropriate PPE and undertake an emergency extrication.

On arrival with the patient
The ERT has removed the patient from the hazards.

Patient assessment triangle
General appearance
The patient was found unconscious and lying prone in hazardous chemicals prior to your arrival. The ERT has removed the patient and she is now lying supine on a stretcher and displaying signs of agonal respiration.

Circulation to the skin
Mild peripheral pallor and central cyanosis.

Work of breathing
Tachypnoea.

SYSTEMATIC APPROACH
Danger
The patient was lying prone in chemicals and has now been extricated from the hazard.

Response
Unconscious on the AVPU scale.

Airway
Possible compromised airway due to chemical burns, pulmonary aspirations and vomitus matter partially occluding the airway.

Breathing

Accessory muscle use: yes. Auscultation: coarse crackles. Effort: increased.

Circulation

Capillary refill time: 4 seconds. Effort: weak. Heart regularity: regular.

Vital signs

RR: 35 bpm

HR: 250 bpm

BP: 130/90 mmHg

Blood sugar: 5.0 mmol/L

SpO_2: 80%

Temperature: 36.6 °C

Lead II ECG: supraventricular tachycardia (SVT)

Exposure

Signs of alkaline burns on the face and front of the patient's body.

TASK

Look through the information provided in this case study and highlight all the information that might concern you as a paramedic.

What are the clinical risks to this patient?

The initial risk for this patient is pulmonary aspiration and, as the patient was lying prone in a pool of hazardous chemical, continual burns from the chemical (Gorguner & Akgun, 2010).

Consider the scene and baseline vital signs. What should you address immediately?

The patient is presenting as acutely unwell and has the potential to deteriorate rapidly. The immediate priority for the onsite paramedic is removing the patient from the area (which has been done) and immediately neutralising the chemical reaction that is occurring with Diphoterine, following up with irrigation for 20 minutes, with copious amounts of water to cease the burning process (Friedstat et al., 2015). The initial treatment that needs to be started is the removal of the active chemical, suction of the airway and further airway management (Khan et al., 2011). This can be achieved with a second generation supraglottic device, an i-gel. Early intubation is key if there is suspected airway burn (Dhimar et al., 2017).

What type of shock state(s) is associated with a burn victim? Explain your answer.

Shock in a burns patient is a combination of *distributive* and *hypovolemic* shock. The recognition of these shock states is noted by intravascular volume depletion, low pulmonary artery occlusion pressure (PAOP), increased systemic vascular resistance and depressed cardiac output (Lee et al., 2014; Wurzer et al., 2018).

What type of information should be sought during history taking from a patient who has suffered from any type of burns?

- Exact mechanism:
  - Type of burn agent.
  - How did it encounter the patient?
  - What first aid was performed?
  - What treatment has been started?

- ○ Is there a risk of concomitant injuries (such as fall from a height, road traffic crash, explosion)?
- ○ Is there a risk of inhalational injuries (did the burn occur in an enclosed space)?
- Exact timing:
  - ○ When did the burn occur?
  - ○ How long was first aid applied for?
  - ○ How long was the patient exposed to the chemical?
- Exact injury:
  - ○ Scald – What was the liquid? Was it boiling or recently boiled? Was there a solute in the liquid?
  - ○ Electrocution injury – What was the voltage? Was it a domestic or industrial situation? Was there any flashing or arcing? What was the contact time?
  - ○ Chemical – What was the chemical? (Hettiaratchy & Papini, 2004)

Case Progression

The patient has been removed from the danger, neutralisation of the chemical has occurred and irrigation of the patient is complete. An i-gel has been inserted, O_2 @ 15 liters, and intermittent positive-pressure ventilation (IPPV) is currently occurring at a rate of 17 breaths per minute along with maintaining normothermia. Continuous monitoring of the patient is occurring as a priority.

Patient assessment triangle
General appearance
The patient is lying supine on a stretcher in the onsite medical centre.

Circulation to the skin
Pallor.

Work of breathing
Decreased from the initial baseline.

SYSTEMATIC APPROACH
Danger
Nil.

Response
Unconscious on the AVPU scale.

Airway
Secured with the insertion of an i-gel.

Breathing
Accessory muscle use: yes. Auscultation: clear, no added sounds. Effort: decreased.

Circulation
Capillary refill time: 3 seconds. Effort: strong. Heart regularity: regular.

Vital signs
RR: 17 BPM
HR: 105 bpm
BP: 125/85 mmHg
SpO_2: 96%
Blood sugar: 5.0 mmol/L
TBSA: 25%
Temperature: 35.2 °C
IV access: Via the external jugular vein
Lead II ECG: sinus tachycardia
Weight: approximately 85 kg

How much fluid would you administer to a burn victim? What fluid would you administer in this case and why? What does fluid do for the burn victim?

- The fluid administration required for this patient is calculated using the Parklands formula = 4 mL × TBSA% × Victim weight (kg) (Endorf & Dries, 2011). Since the patient is 85 kg and has 25% TBSA, then she is going to require:

$$\text{Parklands formula} = 4 \text{ mL} \times 25\% \times 85 \text{ kg} = 8500 \text{ mL}$$

- The fluid the patient should be receiving is Ringer's lactate solution (Vivóa et al., 2016; Haberal et al., 2010; Todd et al., 2007).
- Not only are you providing the patient with a source of fluid replacement, you are also assisting with the loss of intravascular fluid that has occurred to the burned area and the formation of oedema in areas that are not burned. As a result of this, you are preventing shock and organ failure occurring, since you are providing the patient with organ perfusion.

PRACTICAL TIP

IV access facilitates a route for fluid replacement and further IV medications. Fluid replacement is critical in the first 24 hours after a burns incident to ensure the patient remains hemodynamically stable. An isotonic crystalloid solution as given to this patient promoting tissue perfusion.

Severe burns are often very painful, therefore paramedics will administer analgesia to assist patients in coping with the pain and anxiety. This patient was found unconscious, therefore negating the need for analgesia. While pre-hospital care is being administered, the patient's vitals and volume of IV fluid administered are regularly noted on the Patient Care Record (PCR) form.

LEVEL 3 CASE STUDY
Hyperglycaemic hyperosmolar non-ketotic syndrome

Information type	Data
Time of origin	Medical centre visit while on duty
Time of dispatch	12:30
Day of the week	Monday
Nearest hospital	90 minutes
Nearest major hospital	180 minutes
Patient details	Name: James Sherry
	DOB: 1962

CASE

A 58-year-old male attends the onsite medical centre at a mine site showing signs of distress and fatigue.

On arrival with the patient

His clinical presentation reveals xerostomia, polydipsia, polyuria, weakness and fatigue. There is an increase in his work of breathing and his respiratory rate is 23 BPM. The patient is sitting on a chair while the physical exam is carried out. A quick history assessment reveals the patient has type II diabetes and hypertension, which he controls with medications.

Patient assessment triangle
General appearance

The patient is of African descent. You have difficulty understanding his strong accent. He appears to be extremely fatigued and shows signs of confusion.

Circulation to the skin
Warm, dry skin peripherally.

Work of breathing
Increased.

SYSTEMATIC APPROACH

Danger
Nil.

Response
Voice on the AVPU scale.

Airway
Open and patent.

Breathing
Rate is increased and fruity odour is detected.

Circulation
Capillary refill time: 2–3 seconds. Pulse: regular–regular.

Vital signs
RR: 23 BMP
HR: 120 bpm
BP: 105/70 mmHg
SpO$_2$: 94% (mild hypoxia)
Blood sugar: a reading of HI is display and no numerical value shown on the monitor
Temperature: 38.2 °C
GCS: 13/15 (E2, V5, M6)
Lead II ECG: sinus tachycardia

Exposure
The patient is sitting in a cool environment.

TASK
Look through the information provided in this case study and highlight all the information that might concern you as a paramedic.

What differential diagnoses can be made from this patient presentation?

- Hyperglycaemic crisis.
- Hyperglycaemic hyperosmolar non-ketotic syndrome (HHNS) – predominantly found in people living with type II diabetes.
- Diabetic ketoacidosis (DKA) – predominantly found in people living with type I diabetes.

What are the main differences between the differential diagnoses?

See Table 16.1.

Table 16.1 DKA and HHNS differentiation

Diabetic Ketoacidosis (DKA)	Hyperglycaemic Hyperosmolar Non-Ketotic Syndrome (HHNS)
Absolute (or near-absolute) insulin deficiency, resulting in • Severe hyperglycaemia	Severe insulin deficiency, resulting in • Profound hypoglycaemia and hyperosmolality (from urinary free water losses)
• Ketone body production • Systemic acidosis	• No significant ketone production or acidosis
Develops over hours to 1–2 days	Develops over days to weeks
Most common in type I diabetes, but increasingly seen in type II diabetes	Typically presents in type II or previously unrecognised diabetes Higher mortality rates

Sources: Maletkovic & Drexler (2013); Fayfman et al. (2017); Levine & Sanson (2012).

What treatment options can be initiated immediately in a remote setting?

It depends on the scope of practice:

- IV fluids (Fayfman et al., 2017; Waldhäusl et al., 1979).
- Oxygen if indicated, clinical judgement required.
- Insulin, under medical officer directive and permissible under the scope of practice (Fayfman et al., 2017).
- Electrolyte replacement, under medical officer directive and permissible under the scope of practice (Fayfman et al., 2017).

What are the three main symptoms of diabetes?

Polyphagia (excessive hunger), polydipsia (increased thirst) and polyuria (frequent, excessive urination) (Clark et al., 2007; Ramachandran, 2014).

What do the HI and LO symbols indicate on a blood sugar level (BSL) monitor?

HI and LO are symbols that indicate when scan results are beyond the reportable range of a BSL monitor. HI will be displayed when the result is above 27.8 mmol/L. LO will be displayed when the result is below 2.2 mmol/L. These ranges may vary between different manufacturers.

People with low or high blood sugar readings need to make quick treatment decisions. 'RR LO' is an abbreviation for 'reportable range, low limit', which means the blood sugar is dangerously below normal.

Case Progression

Signs and symptoms
- Increased thirst.
- Fatigue.
- Frequent urination.
- Increased hunger.

Allergies
Nil known.

Medications
- Captopril (ACE inhibitor, hypertension) – non-compliant.
- Metformin (diabetes) – non-compliant.

Pertinent past history
- Chronic hypertension and type II diabetes.
- Later investigations revealed chronic hepatic and renal diseases.

Last oral intake
Fluids all day consisting of copious amounts of fruit juice and water.

Events leading up to the illness
The past 3 days the patient has felt extremely fatigued. He has not taken any medication for the last week as he has left it at home.

Out-of-hospital treatment
- Fluid replacement: IV fluid challenge, reassess hypotension and titrate (Levine & Sanson, 2012).
- Mild hypotension: administer 0.9% sodium chloride (10 mL/kg/h) for the initial hour, followed by a maintenance programme to stabilise the patient (Maletkovic & Drexler, 2013; Levine & Sanson, 2012).
- Electrolyte replacement: in-hospital treatment (Maletkovic & Drexler, 2013).
- Insulin therapy – not on the scope from the medical officer.

What are the four principles of biomedical ethics?

Autonomy, beneficence, non-maleficence and justice (Gillon, 1994; Jotterand, 2005).

Explain the ethic principle of autonomy.

Autonomy is Latin for 'self-rule'. Paramedics have an obligation to respect the autonomy of other people, which means respecting the decisions made by others concerning their own lives. The patient has autonomy of thought, intention and action when making decisions regarding healthcare procedures. Therefore, the decision-making process must be free of coercion or coaxing. For a patient to make a fully informed decision, they must understand all the risks and benefits of the procedure and the likelihood of success.

References and further reading

Ahmadi, A., Bazargan-Hejazi, S., Heidari Zadie, Z. et al. (2016) Pain management in trauma: A review study. *Journal of Injury and Violence Research*, 8(2): 89–98. doi: 10.5249/jivr.v8i2.707

Alam, N., Oskam, E., Stassen, P.M. et al. (2018) Prehospital antibiotics in the ambulance for sepsis: A multicentre, open label, randomised trial. *Lancet Respiratory Medicine*, 6(1): 40–50. doi: 10.1016/S2213-2600(17)30469-1

Andell, P., James, S., Östlund, O. et al. (2019) Oxygen therapy in suspected acute myocardial infarction and concurrent normoxemic chronic obstructive pulmonary disease: A prespecified subgroup analysis from the DETO2X-AMI trial. *European Journal of Acute Cardiovascular Care*, Article ID 2048872619848978. doi: 10.1177/2048872619848978

Beasley, R., Chien, J., Douglas, J. et al. (2015) Thoracic Society of Australia and New Zealand oxygen guidelines for acute oxygen use in adults: 'Swimming between the flags'. *Respirology*, 20(8): 1182–1191. doi: 10.1111/resp.12620

Boden, W.E., Padala, S.K., Cabral, K.P. et al. (2015) Role of short-acting nitroglycerin in the management of ischemic heart disease. *Drug Design, Development and Therapy*, 9: 4793–4805. doi: 10.2147/DDDT.S79116

Borobia, A.M., Collado, S.G., Cardona, C.C. et al. (2019) Inhaled methoxyflurane provides greater analgesia and faster onset of action versus standard analgesia in patients with trauma pain: InMEDIATE: A randomized controlled trial in emergency departments. *Annals of Emergency Medicine*, 75(3): 315–328. doi: 10.1016/j.annemergmed.2019.07.028

Bouchama, A., Dehbi, M. & Chaves-Carballo, E. (2007) Cooling and hemodynamic management in heatstroke: Practical recommendations. *Critical Care*, 11: R54. doi: 10.1186/cc5910

Brennan, M.R. & Whitehouse, F.W. (2012) Case study: Seizures and hypoglycemia. *American Diabetes Association Diabetes Care*, 30(1): 23–24. doi: 10.2337/diaclin.30.1.23

Brierley, J., Carcillo, J.A., Choong, K. et al. (2009) Clinical practice parameters for hemodynamic support of pediatric and neonatal septic shock: 2007 update from the American College of Critical Care Medicine. *Critical Care Medicine*, 37(2): 666–688. doi: 10.1097/CCM.0b013e31819323c6

Burns, E. (2019) Anterior myocardial infarction. *Life in the Fast Lane*, 4 June. https://litfl.com/anterior-myocardial-infarction-ecg-library/ (accessed 12 July 2020).

Butts, C.L., Spisla, D.L., Adams, J.D. et al. (2017) Effectiveness of ice-sheet cooling following exertional hyperthermia. *Military Medicine*, 182(9): e1951–e1957. doi: 10.7205/MILMED-D-17-00057

Byrne, L. & Van Haren, F. (2017) Fluid resuscitation in human sepsis: Time to rewrite history? *Annals of Intensive Care*, 7: 4. doi: 10.1186/s13613-016-0231-8

Clark, N.G., Fox, K.M. & Grandy, S. (2007) Symptoms of diabetes and their association with the risk and presence of diabetes. Findings from the Study to Help Improve Early evaluation and management of risk factors Leading to Diabetes (SHIELD). *American Diabetes Association Diabetes Care*, 30(11): 2868–2873. doi: 10.2337/dc07-0816

Dai, Y. & Ge, J. (2012) Clinical use of aspirin in treatment and prevention of cardiovascular disease. *Thrombosis*, 21(8): 1155–1167. doi: 10.1155/2012/245037

Daniels, R., Nutbeam, T., McNamara, G., & Galvin, C. (2011) The sepsis six and the severe sepsis resuscitation bundle: A prospective observational cohort study. *Emergency Medicine Journal*, 28(6): 507–512. doi: 10.1136/emj.2010.095067

Dhimar, A.A., Sangada, B.R., Upadhyay, M.R. & Patel, S.H. (2017) I-Gel versus laryngeal mask airway (LMA) classic as a conduit for tracheal intubation using ventilating bougie. *Journal of Anaesthesiology Clinical Pharmacology*, 33(4): 467–472. doi: 10.4103/joacp.JOACP_113_16

Dragoumi, P., Tzetzi, O., Vargiami, E. et al. (2013) Clinical course and seizure outcome of idiopathic childhood epilepsy: Determinants of early and long-term prognosis. *BMC Neurology*, 13: 206.

Endorf, F.W. & Dries, D.J. (2011) Burn resuscitation. *Scandinavian Journal of Trauma, Resuscitation and Emergency Medicine*, 19: 69. doi: 10.1186/1757-7241-19-69

Fayfman, M., Pasquel, F.J. & Umpierrez, G.E. (2017) Management of hyperglycemic crises: Diabetic ketoacidosis and hyperglycemic hyperosmolar state. *Medical Clinics of North America*, 101(3): 587–606. doi: 10.1016/j.mcna.2016.12.011

FDA (2008) Rocuronium bromide injection. Food and Drug Administration. https://www.accessdata.fda.gov/drugsatfda_docs/label/2008/078717s000lbl.pdf (accessed 12 July 2020).

Friedstat, J., Brown, D.A. & Levi, B. (2017) Chemical, electrical, and radiation injuries. *Clinics in Plastic Surgery*, 44(3): 657–669. doi: 10.1016/j.cps.2017.02.021

Gaieski, D.F., Mikkelsen, M.E., Band, R.A. et al. (2010) Impact of time to antibiotics on survival in patients with severe sepsis or septic shock in whom early goal-directed therapy was initiated in the emergency department. *Critical Care Medicine*, 38(4): 1045–1053. doi: 10.1097/CCM.0b013e3181cc4824

Gillon, R. (1994) Medical ethics: Four principles plus attention to scope. *BMJ*, 309(6948): 184. doi: 10.1136/bmj.309.6948.184

Gorguner, M. & Akgun, M. (2010) Acute inhalation injury. *Eurasian Journal of Medicine*, 42(1): 28–35. doi: 10.5152/eajm.2010.09

Haberal, M., Ebru Sakallioglu Abali, A. & Karakayali, H. (2010) Fluid management in major burn injuries. *Indian Journal of Plastic Surgery*, 43: S29–S36. doi: 10.4103/0970-0358.70715

Halawa, I., Zelano, J. & Kumlien, E. (2015) Hypoglycemia and risk of seizures: A retrospective cross-sectional study. *Seizure*, 25: 147–149. doi: 10.1016/j.seizure.2014.10.005

Hasselqvist-Ax, I., Riva, G., Herlitz, J. et al. (2015) Early cardiopulmonary resuscitation in out-of-hospital cardiac arrest. *New England Journal of Medicine*, 372: 2307–2315. doi: 10.1056/NEJMoa1405796

Hettiaratchy, S. & Papini, R. (2004) Initial management of a major burn: I—overview. *BMJ*, 328(7455): 1555–1557. doi: 10.1136/bmj.328.7455.1555

Johnston, A.N.B., Park, J., Doi, S.A. et al. (2017) Effect of immediate administration of antibiotics in patients with sepsis in tertiary care: A systematic review and meta-analysis. *Clinical Therapeutics*, 39(1): 190–202. doi: 10.1016/j.clinthera.2016.12.003

Joo, Y.M., Chae, M.K., Hwang, S.Y. et al. (2014) Impact of timely antibiotic administration on outcomes in patients with severe sepsis and septic shock in the emergency department. *Clinical and Experimental Emergency Medicine*, 1(1): 35–40. doi: 10.15441/ceem.14.012

Jotterand, F. (2005) The Hippocratic oath and contemporary medicine: Dialectic between past ideals and present reality? *Journal of Medicine and Philosophy*, 30(1): 107–128. doi: 10.1080/03605310590907084

Jozwiak, M., Hamzaoui, O., Monnet, X. & Teboul, J.L. (2018) Fluid resuscitation during early sepsis: A need for individualization. *Minerva Anestesiologica*, 84(8): 987–992. doi: 10.23736/S0375-9393.18.12422-9

Kelm, D.J., Perrin, J.T., Cartin-Ceba, R. et al. (2015) Fluid overload in patients with severe sepsis and septic shock treated with early-goal directed therapy is associated with increased acute need for fluid-related medical interventions and hospital death. *Shock*, 43(1): 68–73. doi: 10.1097/SHK.0000000000000268

Khan, A.A., Williams, T., Savage, L. et al. (2016) Pre-hospital thrombolysis in ST-segment elevation myocardial infarction: A regional Australian experience. *Medical Journal of Australia*, 205(3): 121–125. doi: 10.5694/mja15.01336

Khan, R.M., Sharma, P.K. & Kaul, N. (2011) Airway management in trauma. *Indian Journal of Anaesthesia*, 55(4): 463–469. doi: 10.4103/0019-5049.89870

Kurdi, M.S., Theerth, K.A. & Deva, R.S. (2014) Ketamine: Current applications in anesthesia, pain, and critical care. *Anesthesia Essays and Researches*, 8(3): 283–290. doi: 10.4103/0259-1162.143110

Kurza, M.C., Schmicker, R.H., Leroux, B. et al. (2018) Advanced vs. basic life support in the treatment of out-of-hospital cardiopulmonary arrest in the resuscitation outcomes consortium. *Resuscitation*, 128: 132–137. doi: 10.1016/j.resuscitation.2018.04.031

Larsen, F.T.B.D., Brandt, C.T., Larsen, L. et al. (2019) Risk factors and prognosis of seizures in adults with community-acquired bacterial meningitis in Denmark: Observational cohort studies. *BMJ Open*, 9(7): e030263. doi: 10.1136/bmjopen-2019-030263

Lee, K.C., Joory, K. & Moiemen, N.S. (2014) History of burns: The past, present and the future. *Burns & Trauma*, 2(4): 169–180. doi: 10.4103/2321-3868.143620

Leone, M., Asfar, P., Radermacher, P. et al. (2015) Optimizing mean arterial pressure in septic shock: A critical reappraisal of the literature. *Critical Care*, 19(1): 101. doi: 10.1186/s13054-015-0794-z

Leung, A.K.C., Hon, K.L. & Leung, T.N.H. (2018). Febrile seizures: An overview. *Drugs in Context*, 7: 1–12. doi: 10.7573/dic.212536

Levine, S.N. & Sanson, T.H. (2012) Treatment of hyperglycaemic hyperosmolar non-ketotic syndrome. *Drugs*, 38(3): 462–472. doi: 10.2165/00003495-198938030-00007

Maletkovic, J. & Drexler, A. (2013) Diabetic ketoacidosis and hyperglycemic hyperosmolar state. *Endocrinology and Metabolism Clinics of North America*, 42(4): 677–695. doi: 10.1016/j.ecl.2013.07.001

Martin, K. & Weiss, S.L. (2015) Initial resuscitation and management of pediatric septic shock. *Minerva Pediatrica*, 67(2): 141–158.

Newton, A. & Fitton, L. (2008) Intravenous ketamine for adult procedural sedation in the emergency department: A prospective cohort study. *Emergency Medicine Journal*, 25(8): 498–501. doi: 10.1136/emj.2007.053421

NICE (2016) *Sepsis: Recognition, Diagnosis and Early Management (NG51)*. London: National Institute for Health and Care Excellence. https://www.nice.org.uk/guidance/ng51 (accessed 12 July 2020).

Qian, E., McKown, A.C., Ware, L.B. & Rice, T.W. (2018). *Association between timing of appropriate antibiotics and mortality in sepsis is not influenced by source of infection. American Thoracic Society* 2018 International Conference, San Diego Convention Center, CA.

Ramachandran, A. (2014) Know the signs and symptoms of diabetes. *Indian Journal of Medical Research*, 140(5): 579–581.

Reznik, M.E., Merkler, A.E., Mahta, A. et al. (2017) Long-term risk of seizures in adult survivors of sepsis. *Neurology*, 89(14): 1476–1482. doi:1 0.1212/WNL.0000000000004538

Rhodes, A., Evans, L.E., Alhazzani, W. et al. (2017) Surviving sepsis campaign: International guidelines for management of sepsis and septic shock: 2016. *Intensive Care Medicine*, 43(3): 304–377. doi: 10.1007/s00134-017-4683-6

Robson, W., Nutbeam, T., & Daniels, R. (2009) Sepsis: A need for prehospital intervention? *Emergency Medicine Journal*, 26(7): 535–538. doi: 10.1136/emj.2008.064469

Rosenbaum, S.B. & Palacios, J.L. (2019) *Ketamine*. Treasure Island, FL: StatPearls.

Sabu, J., Regeti, K., Mallappallil, M. et al. (2016) Convulsive syncope induced by ventricular arrhythmia masquerading as epileptic seizures: Case report and literature review. *Journal of Clinical Medicine Research*, 8(8): 610–615. doi: 10.14740/jocmr2583w

Scalais, E., Chafai, R., Van Coster, R. et al. (2013) Early myoclonic epilepsy, hypertrophic cardiomyopathy and subsequently a nephrotic syndrome in a patient with CoQ10 deficiency caused by mutations in para-hydroxybenzoate-polyprenyl transferase (COQ2). *European Journal of Paediatric Neurology*, 17(6): 625–630. doi: 10.1016/j.ejpn.2013.05.013

Semler, M.W. & Rice, T.W. (2016). Sepsis resuscitation: Fluid choice and dose. *Clinical Chest Medicine*, 27(2): 241–250. doi: 10.1016/j.ccm.2016.01.007

Seymour, C.W., Cooke, C.R., Heckbert, S.R. et al. (2014) Prehospital intravenous access and fluid resuscitation in severe sepsis: An observational cohort study. *Critical Care*, 18(5): 533. doi: 10.1186/s13054-014-0533-x

Singer, M., Deutschman, C.S., Seymour, C.W. et al. (2016) The third international consensus definitions for sepsis and septic shock (Sepsis-3). *JAMA Network*, 315(8): 801–810. doi: 10.1001/jama.2016.0287

Sinner, B. & Graf, B.M. (2008) Ketamine. In *Modern Anesthetics: Handbook of Experimental Pharmacology*, vol. 182 (eds J. Schüttler & H. Schwilden), Berlin: Springer. doi: 10.1007/978-3-540-74806-9_15

Sterling, S.A., Miller, W.R., Pryor, J. et al. (2016) The impact of timing of antibiotics on outcomes in severe sepsis and septic shock: A systematic review and meta-analysis. *Critical Care Medicine*, 43(9): 1907–1915. doi: 10.1097/CCM.0000000000001142

Székely, M., Carletto, L. & Garami, A. (2015) The pathophysiology of heat exposure. *Temperature*, 5(4): 452. doi: 10.1080/23328940.2015.1051207

Szima, S., Balazs, G., Elek, N. & Dahlem, P. (2017) Pediatric sepsis: Clinical markers. *Journal of Child Science*, 7(1): e42–e53. doi: 10.1055/s-0037-1603894

Tan, P.M., Teo, E.Y., Ali, N.B. et al. (2017) Evaluation of various cooling systems after exercise-induced hyperthermia. *Journal of Athletic Training*, 52(5): 108–116. doi: 10.4085/1062-6050-52.1.11

Thomas, A.E., Baird, S.F. & Anderson, J. (2016) Purpuric and petechial rashes in adults and children: Initial assessment. *BMJ*, 352: 1285. doi: 10.1136/bmj.i1285

Todd, S.R., Malinoski, D., Muller, P.J. & Schreiber, M,A. (2007) Lactated Ringer's is superior to normal saline in the resuscitation of uncontrolled hemorrhagic shock. *Journal of Trauma*, 62(3): 636–639. doi: 10.1097/TA.0b013e31802ee521

Vivóa, C., Galeiras, R. & del Caz, M.D.P. (2016) Initial evaluation and management of the critical burn patient. *Medicina Intensiva*, 40(1): 49–59. doi: 10.1016/j.medine.2016.01.002

Waldhäusl, W., Kleinberger, G., Korn, A. et al. (1979) Severe hyperglycemia: Effects of rehydration on endocrine derangements and blood glucose concentration. *American Diabetes Association Diabetes Care*, 28(6): 577–584. doi: 10.2337/diab.28.6.577

Wee, Y., Burns, K. & Bett, N. (2015) Medical management of chronic stable angina. *Australian Prescriber*, 38(4): 131–136. doi: 10.18773/austprescr.2015.042

Weldon, E.R., Ariano, R.E. & Grierson, R.A. (2016) Comparison of fentanyl and morphine in the prehospital treatment of ischemic type chest pain. *Prehospital Emergency Care*, 20(1): 45–51. doi: 10.3109/10903127.2015.1056893

Wissenberg, M., Lippert, F.K., Folke, F. et al. (2013) Association of national initiatives to improve cardiac arrest management with rates of bystander intervention and patient survival after out-of-hospital cardiac arrest. *JAMA*, 310(13): 1377–1384. doi: 10.1001/jama.2013.278483

Wurzer, P., Culnan, D., Cancio, L.C. & Kramer, G.C. (2018) Pathophysiology of burn shock and burn edema. In *Total Burn Care*, 5th edn (eds D.N. Herndon & J.H. Jones), Edinburgh: Elsevier, pp. 66–76.

Yudi, M.B., Clark, D.J., Farouque, O. et al. (2016) Clopidogrel, prasugrel or ticagrelor in patients with acute coronary syndromes undergoing percutaneous coronary intervention. *International Medicine Journal*, 46(5): 559–565. doi: 10.1111/imj.13041

Zack-Williams, S.D., Ahmad, Z. & Moiemen, N.S. (2015) The clinical efficacy of Diphoterine® in the management of cutaneous chemical burns: A 2-year evaluation study. *Journal of the Euro-Mediterranean Council for Burns and Fire Disasters*, 28(1): 9–12.

Index

Page locators in **bold** indicate tables. Page locators in *italics* indicate figures. This index uses letter-by-letter alphabetization.

Clinical Cases in Paramedicine, First Edition. Edited by Sam Willis, Ian Peate, and Rod Hill.
© 2021 John Wiley & Sons Ltd. Published 2021 by John Wiley & Sons Ltd.